Difference and Disease

Before the nineteenth century, travellers who left Britain for the Americas, West Africa, India, and elsewhere encountered a medical conundrum: why did they fall ill when they arrived, and why – if they recovered – did they never become so ill again? The widely accepted answer was that the newcomers needed to become 'seasoned to the climate'. Suman Seth explores forms of eighteenth-century medical knowledge, including conceptions of seasoning, showing how geographical location was essential to this knowledge and helped to define relationships between Britain and her far-flung colonies. In this period, debates raged between medical practitioners over whether diseases changed in different climes. Different diseases were deemed characteristic of different races and genders, and medical practitioners were thus deeply involved in contestations over race and the legitimacy of the abolitionist cause. In this innovative and engaging history, Seth offers dramatically new ways to understand the mutual shaping of medicine, race, and empire.

SUMAN SETH is an associate professor in the Department of Science and Technology Studies at Cornell University. His previous publications include *Crafting the Quantum: Arnold Sommerfeld and the Practice of Theory, 1890–1926*. He is the co-editor of the journal *Osiris* and the guest editor of a special issue of *Postcolonial Studies* on 'Science, Colonialism, Postcolonialism' (2009).

Global Health Histories

Series editor:

Sanjoy Bhattacharya, University of York

Global Health Histories aims to publish outstanding and innovative scholarship on the history of public health, medicine and science worldwide. By studying the many ways in which the impact of ideas of health and well-being on society were measured and described in different global, international, regional, national and local contexts, books in the series reconceptualise the nature of empire, the nation state, extra-state actors and different forms of globalization. The series showcases new approaches to writing about the connected histories of health and medicine, humanitarianism, and global economic and social development.

Difference and Disease

Medicine, Race, and the Eighteenth-Century British Empire

Suman Seth

Cornell University, New York

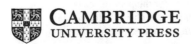

CAMBRIDGE
UNIVERSITY PRESS

University Printing House, Cambridge CB2 8BS, United Kingdom

One Liberty Plaza, 20th Floor, New York, NY 10006, USA

477 Williamstown Road, Port Melbourne, VIC 3207, Australia

314-321, 3rd Floor, Plot 3, Splendor Forum, Jasola District Centre, New Delhi - 110025, India

79 Anson Road, #06-04/06, Singapore 079906

Cambridge University Press is part of the University of Cambridge.

It furthers the University's mission by disseminating knowledge in the pursuit of education, learning and research at the highest international levels of excellence.

www.cambridge.org
Information on this title: www.cambridge.org/9781108407007
DOI: 10.1017/9781108289726

First published 2018
First paperback edition 2020

A catalogue record for this publication is available from the British Library

Library of Congress Cataloging in Publication data
Names: Seth, Suman, 1974– author.
Title: Difference and disease : medicine, race, and the eighteenth-century
British empire / Suman Seth.
Description: Cambridge, United Kingdom; New York, NY:
Cambridge University Press, 2018. | Includes bibliographical references.
Identifiers: LCCN 2018002424 | ISBN 9781108418300 (hardback)
Subjects: | MESH: Geography, Medical – history | Travel-Related Illness |
Climate | Colonialism – history | Racism – history | History, 18th Century |
West Indies | United Kingdom
Classification: LCC RA651 | NLM WZ 70 FA1 | DDC 614.4/2–dc23
LC record available at https://lccn.loc.gov/2018002424

ISBN 978-1-108-41830-0 Hardback
ISBN 978-1-108-40700-7 Paperback

"… bad intentions alone do not invalidate knowledge. For that to happen it takes bad epistemology …"

Johannes Fabian, *Time and the Other*

For Ashima

Contents

Acknowledgements

I did not imagine, when I finished my first book, that I would write this one, which has required that I learn the histories of a new discipline, period, and place. Whatever insight I've managed has come through the support and guidance of many friends and colleagues. Robert Travers has taught me much about the eighteenth-century British Empire; Chris Hamlin was unstinting in his generosity in helping me come to some mastery of the history of eighteenth-century medicine, while Steve Stowe and John Waller introduced me to the historiography of medicine during a sabbatical year at Michigan State University; James Delbourgo offered critical and enormously helpful suggestions for ways to engage with social histories of slavery in the Atlantic World; and both Michael Gordin and Mary Fissell turned critical eyes to my introduction and helped make it both more precise and more reflective of the fields with which it engages. The Science and Technology Studies (STS) department at Cornell has provided a mostly supportive and congenial environment in which to teach and research. My colleagues – including Peter Dear, Steve Hilgartner, Ron Kline, Bruce Lewenstein, Mike Lynch, Trevor Pinch, Sara Pritchard, Jessica Ratcliff, Margaret Rossiter, Phoebe Sengers, Rebecca Slayton, and Malte Ziewitz – can be counted on to engage seriously and deeply. Special thanks to Rachel Prentice and to Ann Johnson, who I miss terribly. Much love to my broader Cornell and Ithaca family: Cynthia Brock, Shelley Feldman, Deb van Galder, Trina Garrison, Durba Ghosh, Sara Hatfield, Deirdre and George Hay, Geo Kloppel, Patricia Lia, Hope Mandeville, Vlad Micic, Lucinda Ramberg, Mark and Evan Stevens, Stacey Stone, and Marne, Larry, Maya, and Casey Honigbaum. Ray Craib and Jenny Mann remind me regularly of the kind of scholar and person I'd like to be. Holly Case, Nicole Giannella, Murad Idris, and Theresa Krüggeler left Ithaca a while ago, but they are – and always will be – family.

Various chapters of this book were presented at The Institute for Comparative Modernities and the STS Colloquium Series, Cornell University; the Vanderbilt History Seminar, Vanderbilt University; Universidad Autonoma de Yucatan; Louisiana State University; the Porter Fortune Symposium, University of Mississippi; Halle University; the Science, Technology, and Society Colloquium at the University of Michigan;

the University of California, Los Angeles; History of Science and Technology Colloquium, Johns Hopkins University; the History and Philosophy of Science Colloquium, University of Sydney; the Science and Society Speaker Series, Drexel University; the History Colloquium, Princeton University; the Gallatin School of Individualized Study, New York University; the University of Pennsylvania; and the Politics Department at the University of Virginia. A special thanks to those, like Suzanne Marchand and Nonny de La Peña, who opened their homes to me on my travels. Matt and Janelle Stanley were generous in every possible way. They are, both metaphorically and literally, the people I'd want in my corner in a fight. For invitations, questions, and comments, thanks to Sanjoy Bhattacharya, Richard Blackett, Tom Broman, Debbie Coen, Steffan Igor Ayora Diaz, Tony Grafton, Rana Hogarth, Sarah Igo, Myles Jackson, Bill Jordan, Stephen Kenny, Fabio Lanza, Theresa Leavitt, Natalie Melas, Lisa Messeri, Emmie Miller, Ole Molvig, Sarah Naramore, Deirdre Cooper Owens, Susan Scott Parrish, Kapil Raj, Ruth Rogaski, Richard Rottenburg, Simon Schaffer, Londa Schiebinger, Alistair Sponsel, Helen Tilley, Gabriela Vargas-Cetina, Keith Wailoo, Aaron Windel, and Anya Zilberstein. In terms of the final product, I could not have asked for a more professional, engaged, or fun editor than Lucy Rhymer. The team at Cambridge, including Daniel Brown, Sue Barnes, and Nicola Howcroft, were exceptional. Readers will join me in thanking Janelle Bourgeois for her work on the index.

New projects need the support of old friends. Laura Stark is the epitome of thoughtful, open, and engaged humanistic research and thinking. She is also dear to me beyond measure. Any day in which I see Heidi Voskuhl – H-Dog – is a great one. Mary Terrall, Helen Tilley, and Elaine and Norton Wise remain both mentors and role models. Angela Creager is, quite simply, the best. Seeing and learning from Warwick Anderson, Ofer Gal, Daniela Helbig, and Hans Pols continues to be one of my favourite things about returning to Sydney University. Thanks to Arlan and Carol Smith for many years of love and care. Sharrona Pearl's ideas about my arguments and writing have made this book immeasurably better, just as I am a better person for knowing her. I don't know how her unflagging generosity is possible. I would be lost without friends like Lisa Bailey, Scott Bruce, Johanna Crane, James Cunningham, Katy Hansen, Kevin Lambert, Anne Lester, Dan Magaziner, Valeri Kiesig, Erika Milam, Tania Munz, Anjali Singh, Richard Staley, and Chuck Wooldridge, who comfort the heart and inspire the mind. Patrick McCray is the God of Thunder.

Amber Lia-Kloppel has been tireless in helping me find images for my front cover. She has been equally tireless in making me feel joyful and cared for and grounded. I look forward to repaying favours and incurring new debts to her and Isabella in the years to come. My father has never once doubted in my success, even when my own confidence would break. My siblings, Sanjay and Vanita, are my best and quickest readers, to be counted on to tell me what works and what is dull or unnecessary. Vastly more importantly, they – and Kelly, Raju and Nishad – are to be counted on for love and laughter, food and foolishness.

Mindy Smith has been my best friend and strongest support for the years this work has taken and for many more besides. She has been reader, sounding-board, advisor, and critic. Thanking her for her part in this project would do little justice to all the debts she's owed. Books are written while lives are forged and it's the lives that matter most. Together, we've raised a daughter who is the best thing I will ever produce. It's to our daughter – who has never known a time when I was not working on this project – that this book is dedicated.

Introduction: Difference and Disease

One morning in late December, 1750, two physicians in Kingston, Jamaica fought a duel to the death. After an ever-more contentious debate, in print, over the preceding several months, the two confronted one another in person. Intemperate language led to blows, then to the offer and acceptance of a challenge. Very early on the 29th, Parker Bennet arrived at John Williams' house, armed with sword and pistols, and called his adversary out. Williams, according to a later report, loaded his pistols with 'Goose or Swan shot', affixed his sword to his wrist with a ribband, and opened his door enough to present his pistol, shooting Bennet in the chest. Bennet, by this version of events at least, was considerably more chivalrous and having delivered his own arms to his servant, reeled backwards under the force of the shot to get them. Pursuing him, Williams fired a second time, catching Bennet in the knee. By this point, Bennet had reached his sword, which he now found to be stuck so firmly in its scabbard that he could not draw it. Williams, drawing his own weapon, struck Bennet under the right arm and ran him through, before turning to make his exit from the scene. Bennet, somehow still alive, caught his opponent before he could make his escape. Having finally worked his own sword free, his thrust pierced Williams beneath his right clavicle, severed the jugular vein, and broke off in the body. Williams died almost instantly, while Bennet survived him by roughly four hours (one assumes just long enough to offer a story that reflects considerably better on his honour than his adversary's).[1]

Although the two had known one another for several years and had possibly harboured grudges for some time, the immediate cause of their dispute was a book Williams had published earlier in 1750, *An Essay on the Bilious,*

---

[1] John Williams and Parker Bennet, *Essays on the Bilious Fever: Containing the Different Opinions of Those Eminent Physicians John Williams and Parker Bennet, of Jamaica: Which Was the Cause of a Duel, and Terminated in the Death of Both* (Jamaica and London: T. Waller, 1752). The duel is discussed briefly in Richard B. Sheridan, *Doctors and Slaves: A Medical and Demographic History of Slavery in the British West Indies, 1680–1834* (Cambridge: Cambridge University Press, 1985), 68; and G. M. Findlay, 'John Williams and the Early History of Yellow Fever', *The British Medical Journal* 2, no. 4574 (1948).

or Yellow Fever of Jamaica.[2] On reading, the *Essay* seems insufficient to have produced such an effect, for it is a reasonably innocuous medical work, no more critical of other authors and physicians than most others of its time. What seems to have incensed Bennet, however, was a relatively brief passage in Williams' Preface, which drew a distinction between practitioners who had been in the West Indies for some time – and who hence possessed adequate local knowledge and experience – and those who had arrived more recently, having possibly been trained at an elite medical institution in one of Europe's metropolitan centres. 'It appears to me', wrote Williams, 'that no man, let his genius or stack of learning be what it will, can be a judge of the disorders of this country without faithful observation and experience; yet the passion for novelty is so great amongst us that some persons sacrifice life itself to it'. Williams appended a Latin tag from Virgil's 'Aenied' (*quae tanta insania cives?* 'Oh what great insanity is this, citizens?') before continuing:

A new comer, whose head is filled with theory and darling hypotheses, by some will be trusted before a man who ... hath made himself acquainted with the diseases of the country, and prudently follows the vestigial of nature; never sacrificing his patient to any favourite hypothesis.[3]

Bennet was precisely such a 'new comer', having obtained his medical degree in Edinburgh in 1745.[4] And his gloss on Williams remarks, published in *An Enquiry into the Late Essay on the Bilious Fever*, provides an idea of how quickly the discussion would devolve:

The second paragraph in the 4th page is a very extraordinary one, and requires a small paraphrase ... *Oh ye men of* Jamaica! *Are ye not a parcel of blockheads? To trust your lives in the hands of a NEW COMER! Of a man who has been at the University! Who has attended the nasty lectures of* Morgagni, Albinus, *or* Monroe, *whose head is filled with the whimsical notions of* Boerhaave! *And who knows no more of diseases than what he has learned by seeing the trifling practice of* European *hospitals! – Come to me! I am your faithful* Hippocrates *of* Jamaica![5]

If he was young and new to Jamaica, Bennet nonetheless also claimed relevant experience: 'some of us have been in *Africa*, on board *Guineamen*, and in other islands of the *West-Indies*, as well as he; consequently are equally entitled to write upon and cure the *yellow fever*'.[6] Yet Bennet would draw on relatively little of that experience in making a mockery of Williams' probity, competence, Latin, erudition, and – with repeated references to his opponent

[2] John Williams, *[an] Essay on the Bilious, or Yellow Fever of Jamaica* (Kingston, Jamaica: William Daniell, 1750).

[3] Williams and Bennet, iv.

[4] Brief biographical material on each man is offered in Findlay.

[5] Williams and Bennet, 60 1.

[6] Ibid., 61.

as *Mr.* John Williams – his lack of a degree.[7] Williams replied in print with a poem, describing '*Bennet*, whose trifling writings no point hit:/That fop in learning, and that fool in wit'.[8] Bennet in turn responded with an attack on Williams' 'bad poetry, false measure, and vile logic', referring to the poem as the 'idle nonsense of a conceited dunce' and its author as 'a forward cringing fop'.[9] Why Williams thought it would be helpful to reply at this point is not clear. Perhaps he saw that the alternative to words was a violence the end of which could not be predicted. In any case, reply he did, defending himself against charges that he had prescribed a deadly quantity of opium to some of his unfortunate patients by appending supportive letters from the apothecaries who had filled his prescriptions. He also responded to the central point of Bennet's original indignation.

But you were pleased to take offence at the Preface, I hear; where I say, 'a new comer must be liable to more errors in his practice, than a person who hath had a great share of observation and experience', or words to that purpose. Pray, Sir, is not this Truth? Would doctor Mead deny this? And would not that great man be at a loss himself on his first arrival in a southern climate?[10]

The final document in Williams' *Letter to Doctor Bennet* was dated 27 November 1750. Both men would be dead a little over a month later.

The story of Bennet and Williams is a bizarre one. But it is also revealing, opening a door towards a more general set of questions that this book seeks to examine: what determined the social status of medical practitioners in the metropole and far-flung colonies? Which of several competing epistemologies and ontologies were correct? Was there something that bound the diseases of the tropics together and marked them as distinct to those of more temperate regions of the earth? How might one become habituated to a climate and a range of distempers radically different from that in which one was born? Let me elaborate on these questions before I turn, in the next section, to my historical and historiographical stakes.

At the heart of Bennet and Williams' deadly disagreement, we can see, were concerns over who had the appropriate training, social standing, and experience to speak to medical matters in the colonies. That socio-political question could not be resolved, of course, without simultaneously considering a second set of questions: to what extent were the diseases of the Indies really different to those of Northern Europe? If they were essentially the same, surely one might prefer the ministrations of a physician who had received a degree from

---

[7] E.g. ibid., 75.
[8] Ibid., 33–4.
[9] Ibid., 36, 39.
[10] Ibid., 48.

one of the leading universities in Europe, and who could claim – as Bennet did, practice in European hospitals? If the disease environments were radically different, on the other hand, one might well call in a doctor whose knowledge went beyond the ailments afflicting the inhabitants of London or Edinburgh.

The question sounds strange to our modern ears, for we are familiar with tropical medicine as a particular speciality. As a child in Australia, born to Indian parents, I remember well the trepidation that accompanied excitement at the thought of visits to relatives in Delhi. Foul-tasting quinine tablets and painful shots always diluted my enthusiasm for the journey, as did almost ritualised discussions between adults about the relative likelihood of us contracting cholera, typhoid, or malaria. But tropical medicine was born at the end of the nineteenth century, and in 1750 Bennet and Williams were on the cusp of a new understanding of illness between the tropics.

When, then, and why did Anglophone physicians begin to see the diseases of warm climates as different in kind, not merely degree, from those of cooler locations to the north? Relatedly, when and why did medically significant differences *within* northern Europe – which had been an object of considerable interest for some time – begin to pale in significance relative to a larger difference between Europe and the tropics? A sizeable part of the answers to these questions came in analyses of the disease that was the subject of Williams' first essay: yellow fever. It was an irony utterly lost on the two rancorous combatants that the fever in question gained much of its intellectual interest from the fact that it, like Williams, seemed to distinguish sharply between those who were habituated to the climate of the West Indies, and those who were new to it. The fever was particularly fatal, Williams noted, 'to strangers, *Europeans*, and *North Americans*'. If one survived the first attack, however, one was unlikely to be afflicted again. At the very least, a second bout of the fever would be considerably less violent. Today, when we point to the transmission of the yellow fever virus through the bite of mosquitoes, we invoke the body's production of antibodies to explain our acquired immunity. For eighteenth-century physicians, almost no part of this reasoning would have made sense.

According to Williams, newcomers from the North were particularly vulnerable to the disease because they possessed tense fibres and were 'plethoric', having a comparative surfeit of blood, which was also heated upon arrival in the Indies. The warmth caused the blood to expand and become 'rarefied', pressing upon the rigid vessels that contained it. The rarefied blood travelled more quickly through the body, increasing all secretions 'recrementitious and excrementitious' except those by urine and stool. Yet these last two were the body's means of removing excess bile. '[A] redundance of bile', Williams declared, 'together with that stiffness of the fibres, and richness of the blood, are obvious and sufficient causes of their proneness to this fever'. For Williams, then, the best treatment was to bleed strangers on their arrival, reducing their excess blood, a process to be continued until their bodily fibres relaxed, and their 'juices assimilated to the air of the country'.[11] At that point, in common parlance, they could be said to be 'seasoned' to the climate.

Associated, then, with questions concerning socio-political status, conceptual foundations, and geographical taxonomies, another strand that runs through this book is the history of the idea of seasoning. The term dates back to at least the fifteenth century, when one finds the verb *to season* used in a sense very similar to the most common modern understanding: 'to render (a dish) more palatable by the addition of some savoury ingredient'. The word derives from the Old French *saisonner*, meaning 'to ripen, to render (fruit) palatable by the influence of the seasons'. A second, somewhat different and later English term flows from this original French usage, for one also speaks of seasoned timber, or seasoned metal. In this case, a particular treatment, usually related to the way in which the material will later be used, brings it to a kind of maturity or ripeness. The analogous use of the term for people – to be inured to rough conditions by training and experience – appears already in the early seventeenth century.[12] It seems commonplace to speak of seasoned soldiers, in particular, by the 1680s.

The idea of a 'seasoning sickness', however, meaning an illness that habituates the body to a particular environment or climate – and which, crucially, is only experienced once – seems to be a product of the late seventeenth century.[13] Certainly, eighteenth-century travellers, doctors, soldiers, and sailors all paid a great deal of attention to an illness that seemed to be a disease of *place*. Seasoning affected neither 'natives' nor those who had spent a good deal of time in a specific locale. Only those habituated to one location who ventured to another in which they were strangers fell ill. If they survived their affliction, their bodies were then inured to the novelties of the environments in which they now found themselves. And increasingly through the eighteenth century, yellow fever was seen by many as the seasoning sickness *par excellence*.

Bennet and Williams' dispute, then, turned on a number of the differences alluded to in my title. Both men, however, were silent – perhaps because it was beyond dispute? – on what may have been the most important distinction for social life in the West Indies: that between populations enslaved and free. For much of the eighteenth century, that social and legal distinction mattered more for physicians interested in the diseases of the Islands than did questions of race. Doctors treated black slaves, and noted that they often suffered disproportionately from the same diseases that afflicted whites, and sometimes from

---

[11] Ibid., 30.
[12] *Oxford English Dictionary*, 'season, *v*'. Meanings 1a. 4a. 4c.
[13] The *Oxford English Dictionary* cites Daniel Denton's *A Brief Description of New York* (1670) as the first usage of the word 'seasoning' with this meaning.

diseases that seemed distinctive to them. Yet most put those differences down to factors derived from their patients' position as slaves – poor diet, inadequate clothing and housing – or else to different beliefs about the causes and cures of their afflictions. White and black bodies – neither of which were deemed 'native' to the Indies – responded in similar ways to the climate. Matters would begin to change, however, beginning in the 1760s. In later chapters, then, *Difference and Disease* explores the relationship between the theories of what has become known as 'race-science' – and has been examined, particularly for the eighteenth century, almost exclusively within the European metropole – and the theories of medicine and science within a colonial, racially mixed population. The history of medicine, I hope to show, provides an ideal way of exploring the history of an empire defined as much by its structuring differences as by its putative unity, while the history of empire allows us to tease out the locatedness of medical discourse about specific locations.

Difference and the Postcolonial History of Colonial Medicine

For some time, imperial historians have contested the idea that a sense of being British was first created at home and then diffused to the colonies. As scholars including Linda Colley, Christopher Bayly, and others have argued, the colonies and other far-flung places in which Britons found themselves were among the sites in which Britishness was born.[14] It was, at least in part, in the periphery that the centre as we know it was brought into being. In recent years, historians of eighteenth-century medicine have similarly turned away from a near exclusive attention to the metropole and towards a broader analysis of what might be termed 'medicine in a global context'. Among historians of imperial medicine, Mark Harrison's work has been pre-eminent and my own book draws upon and seeks to complement arguments made in his *Medicine in an Age of Commerce and Empire* (2010).[15] Harrison's study aims to provide a history of medicine within the British Empire as a whole, not merely in select colonies, and to describe the circulations of people, knowledge, and practices within and between the centre and peripheries. The book rightly works to diminish differences long critiqued

---

[14] Linda Colley, *Britons: Forging the Nation, 1707–1837* (New Haven and London: Yale University Press, 2009); C. A. Bayly, *Imperial Meridian: The British Empire and the World, 1780–1830* (London and New York: Routledge, 1989). Catherine Hall, *Civilising Subjects: Colony and Metropole in the English Imagination, 1830–1867* (Chicago: University of Chicago Press, 2002). Kathleen Wilson, *The Island Race: Englishness, Empire and Gender in the Eighteenth Century* (London: Routledge, 2003); (ed.) *A New Imperial History: Culture, Identity, and Modernity in Britain and the Empire, 1660–1840* (Cambridge: Cambridge University Press, 2004). See also Kapil Raj, *Relocating Modern Science: Circulation and the Construction of Knowledge in South Asia and Europe, 1650–1900* (Basingstoke: Palgrave Macmillan, 2007).

[15] Mark Harrison, *Medicine in an Age of Commerce and Empire: Britain and its Tropical Colonies, 1660–1830* (Oxford: Oxford University Press, 2010).

within the secondary literature on the history of colonial science. Medical men in the colonies were not derivative drones following the lead of their colleagues in the metropole, but rather proponents of creative 'dissent' – that word used by Harrison to denote not merely a religious position common to many of the leading physicians in the colonies, but also a willingness to work against long-held traditions. Practitioners working in hospitals in the Indies 'rejected the genteel, text-based medicine of the physician elite for an avowedly empirical form of medicine supported by the twin pillars of bedside observation and post-mortem dissection'. Similar changes were occurring in Britain, but they proceeded at a more rapid pace overseas, where colonial practitioners could take 'advantage of unparalleled opportunities for dissection and the correlation of morbid signs with symptoms in living patients'.[16] Physicians in the 'peripheries', then, were *ahead* of those at the so-called centre. As a result, the rational medicine that emerged at the end of the eighteenth century should be understood as being 'as much a product of the colonies as of the infirmaries of revolutionary Paris; or, for that matter, of the hospitals and anatomy schools of Britain'.[17] The difference between metropole and colony is thus at the heart of Harrison's work, as it was for earlier studies, but the advantage is now given to the latter.[18]

I have considerable sympathy for this inversion, and where Harrison and I overlap topically, I have gratefully made use of his many insights and turned my attention towards those differences – in theories, for example, or social status – that are less relevant to the eventual emergence of so-called 'Paris medicine'. But the dominance of the distinction between practitioners in Europe and those in the colonies tends to lead to the diminution of other forms of difference that I try to stress.[19] The role of eighteenth-century medicine in the construction of race, for example, receives a much fuller treatment here than in any previous work.[20] The book's geographic scope is broad, tracking

---

16 Ibid., 27.

17 Ibid., 9.

18 Pratik Chakrabarti, *Materials and Medicine: Trade, Conquest and Therapeutics in the Eighteenth Century* (Manchester: Manchester University Press, 2011).

19 In paying so much attention to difference, I am drawing from recent work in the 'new imperial history'. For a discussion, see Kathleen Wilson, 'Introduction: Histories, Empires, Modernities', in *A New Imperial History: Culture, Identity, and Modernity in Britain and the Empire, 1660–1840*, ed. Kathleen Wilson (Cambridge: Cambridge University Press, 2004). See also Linda Colley, 'Britishness and Otherness: An Argument', *Journal of British Studies* 31 (1992). Hall. Wilson, *The Island Race: Englishness, Empire and Gender in the Eighteenth Century*.

20 In Harrison's book, the discussion of race is largely limited to the period after 1790, in spite of the book spanning the years from 1660 to 1830. An earlier essay is more concerned with the period after 1780 and especially with the early nineteenth century. It is in the 1820s, it is argued there, that 'biological explanations … began to appear in medical texts'. As one reason for this, Harrison points to the abolition of the slave trade in 1807, which 'may have served to focus medical attention more closely on questions of racial difference'. Mark Harrison, '"The Tender Frame of Man": Disease, Climate and Racial Difference in India and the West Indies,

materials derived not only from Britain's 'tropical colonies' – largely the East and West Indies – but also from areas maintained by British representatives of the African slave trade as well as North America. I have also chosen to focus on a long-term, diachronic study of Britain's imperial holdings, rather than a shorter-term synchronic account of exchanges between and across empires in a given location, such as the Caribbean.

Perhaps as a result of its wide geographical scope, which includes but goes beyond the 'Atlantic world', relationships between medicine, slavery, and abolitionism are key elements of this study. I have tried, too, to be attentive to the differences between all of these locations. Among the implications of this attention is the fact that I cannot quite agree with those who have argued that military medical texts are the most important sources for understanding medicine outside of the British Isles in the eighteenth century.[21] The claim might be accurate for India, but it does not seem applicable to the West Indies for much of the century. While tracts on the diseases of soldiers and sailors focused on British bodies in locations described broadly as those 'nearer, or under the line' as William Cockburn phrased it in 1696, or in 'hotter Countries' as he put it in *Sea Diseases* a decade later, 'location-specific' works tended to stress the particularity of their location, radically distinguishing between lands located between the tropics. An over-emphasis on military rather than civilian works can thus also over-emphasise the similarities assumed between locations. In addition, medical men treating soldiers and sailors, as J. D. Alsop has noted, had a rather restricted group of patients under their care: for the most part, they ministered to younger, European men.[22] John Hunter was interested in the question of 'race', writing a dissertation on the varieties of human kind in 1775 before being appointed physician to the army and, from 1781 to 1783, superintendent of the military hospitals in Jamaica. However, in the text that he wrote based on his experiences, *Observations on the Diseases of the Army in Jamaica* (1788), he noted that '[t]he diseases of Negroes fell seldom under my

---

1760–1860', *Bulletin of the History of Medicine* 70, no. 1 (1996): 82, 83. Curtin, similarly, emphasises the period after 1780: Philip D. Curtin, '"The White Man's Grave": Image and Reality, 1780–1850', *Journal of British Studies* 1 (1961); 'Epidemiology and the Slave Trade', *Political Science Quarterly* 83, no. 2 (1968); *The Image of Africa: British Ideas and Action, 1780–1850* (Madison: University of Wisconsin Press, 1964). On relationships between medicine and slavery, I am indebted to the works of Richard B. Sheridan: 'Africa and the Caribbean in the Atlantic Slave Trade', *The American Historical Review* 77, no. 1 (1972); 'The Guinea Surgeons on the Middle Passage: The Provision of Medical Services in the British Slave Trade', *The International Journal of African Historical Studies* 14, no. 4 (1981); *Doctors and Slaves: A Medical and Demographic History of Slavery in the British West Indies, 1680–1834*.

[21] J. D. Alsop, 'Warfare and the Creation of British Imperial Medicine, 1600–1800', in *British Military and Naval Medicine, 1600–1830*, ed. Geoffrey L. Hudson (Amsterdam: Rodopi, 2007), 23. Harrison, *Medicine in an Age of Commerce and Empire: Britain and its Tropical Colonies, 1660–1830*, 14.

[22] Alsop, 37.

observation'.[23] This is to be contrasted to the testimony concerning the slave trade of Dr John Quier and others the same year, in which all three (civilian) physicians noted that they had under their care three to four *thousand* slaves a year as part of their practice.[24] Civilian surgeons and physicians also – unsurprisingly – paid much more attention to the afflictions of women than their military counterparts. One might note, finally, that attention to the many different kinds of patients outside of the metropole makes one rather less sanguine about the 'opportunities' for dissections and other more novel medical practices, for dissections and experimentation were often carried out on the bodies of those – soldiers, perhaps, and often slaves – who could not always easily resist.[25]

At its core, this book is about the mutual shaping of medicine and the eighteenth-century British Empire.[26] As such, I put it forward as an example of the *postcolonial history of colonial medicine*.[27] Such histories were once fairly common,[28] but today historians of science, medicine and colonialism seem loath to engage with postcolonial approaches. Indeed, two recent essays by prominent historians of science and colonialism have been markedly critical of postcolonial methods and their potential utility.[29] Where the issue is antipathy rather than apathy, however, such critiques seem rooted in misunderstandings of the state of postcolonial science studies as it is today. For, in the last few decades, histories of science and colonialism have followed many of the same paths as postcolonial studies. Historians of the colonial past, like postcolonial

---

[23] John Hunter, *Observations on the Diseases of the Army in Jamaica; and on the Best Means of Preserving the Health of Europeans, in That Climate* (London: G. Nicol, 1788), 305.

[24] Assembly. Jamaica., *Two Reports (One Presented the 16th of October, the Other on the 12th of November, 1788) from the Committee of the Honourable House of Assembly of Jamaica, Appointed to Examine into ... The Slave-Trade ... Published, by Order of the House of Assembly, by Stephen Fuller ... Agent for Jamaica.* (London: B. White and Son; J. Sewell; R. Faulder; and J. Stockdale, 1789).

[25] Londa Schiebinger, 'Human Experimentation in the Eighteenth Century: Natural Boundaries and Valid Testing', in *The Moral Authority of Nature*, ed. Lorraine Daston and Fernando Vidal (Chicago: University of Chicago Press, 2004); *Secret Cures of Slaves: People, Plants, and Medicine in the Eighteenth-Century Atlantic World* (Stanford: Stanford University Press, 2017).

[26] For a somewhat similar project, from a different perspective, see Alan Bewell, *Romanticism and Colonial Disease* (Baltimore: Johns Hopkins University Press, 1999).

[27] For a fuller discussion of the relationship between postcolonial science studies and the history of science and colonialism, see Suman Seth, 'Colonial History and Postcolonial Science Studies', *Radical History Review* 127 (2017).

[28] See, for example, Megan Vaughan, *Curing Their Ills: Colonial Power and African Illness* (Stanford: Stanford University Press, 1991); David Arnold, *Colonizing the Body: State Medicine and Epidemic Disease in Nineteenth-Century India* (Berkeley: University of California Press, 1993); Gyan Prakash, *Another Reason: Science and the Imagination of Modern India* (Princeton: Princeton University Press, 1999).

[29] Kapil Raj, 'Beyond Postcolonialism ... And Postpositivism: Circulation and the Global History of Science', *Isis* 104 (2013); James McClellan III, 'Science & Empire Studies and Postcolonial Studies: A Report from the Contact Zone', in *Entangled Knowledge: Scientific Discourses and Cultural Difference*, eds. Klaus Hock and Gesa Mackenthun (Münster: Waxmann, 2012).

theorists today, are sceptical of the telos and boundaries of the nation state; have called into question the dichotomies and divisions of the colonial age as analytic, rather than actors' categories; have stressed the global setting as a way to understand the flows and movement of sciences and technologies; and are fascinated by hybridity and heterogeneity.

In particular, much of the literature in postcolonial science studies has been concerned with the troubling of binaries and boundaries. 'We have to be sensitive', Warwick Anderson and Vincanne Adams have written in a particularly important formulation, 'to dislocation, transformation, and resistance; to the proliferation of partially purified and hybrid forms and identities; to the contestation and negotiation of boundaries; and to recognizing that practices of science are always multi-sited'.[30] A similar move is common in the history of colonialism and science. Indeed, for scholars like Kapil Raj, this is one of the appeals of a circulatory model of knowledge exchange, since such a model does not reify the categories of knowledge into those of coloniser and colonised.[31] Sujit Sivasundaram has made a similar claim, arguing that a focus on the global may allow us to think beyond such binaries and 'fragment traditions of knowledge on all sides'.[32] An excellent recent collection accepts 'it may make sense to conceptualise encounters between Europeans and other peoples as dualistic and antagonistic', but that there is no reason to assume '*essentially* confrontational relations'.[33] Instead, one may look at the go-betweens in exchanges, those who allowed boundaries to be blurred and exchanges to occur, even as they sometimes maintained and objectified the boundaries they transgressed. The volume is thus concerned with people whose tasks involve the *intra* and the *trans:* 'those tricky and often elusive characters who seemed newly important in networks linking cultures and, as often, confusing their boundaries'.[34] There is a good argument to be made that histories of science, medicine, and colonialism are remarkably methodologically close to being postcolonial studies of medicine and technoscience done in the past, and vice versa. And in that situation, there seems little reason for each field not to borrow from and engage with one another more.

---

[30] Vincenne Adams and Warwick Anderson, 'Pramoedya's Chickens: Postcolonial Studies of Technoscience', in *The Handbook of Science and Technology Studies*, ed. Edward J. Hackett et al. (Cambridge, MA: MIT Press, 2007), 183–4.

[31] Raj, *Relocating Modern Science: Circulation and the Construction of Knowledge in South Asia and Europe, 1650–1900*.

[32] Sujit Sivasundaram, 'Sciences and the Global: On Methods, Questions, and Theory', *Isis* 101 (2010): 154. At times, however, Sivasundaram seems to fall into the trap of seeing globalisation as a force of history in its own right, arguing, for example, that '[g]lobalization enabled the precolonial, the colonial, and the postcolonial to fit together', ibid., 156.

[33] Simon Schaffer et al., eds., *The Brokered World: Go-Betweens and Global Intelligence, 1770–1820* (Sagamore Beach: Science History Publications, 2009), xv.

[34] Ibid., xvii.

There is an alternative, however, to the blurring of extant boundaries and it is a valuable one. It is here, in fact, that the value of historical work that engages with postcolonial writings becomes particularly clear. For there is a danger in so much attention being paid to the (important) fact that conceptualised ways of dividing the world did not always hold in practice. We should not understand the critique of an absolute (such as Said's totalising model of the power of colonial epistemologies over the colonised) as a negation.[35] After all, not everyone was able to slip between and over boundaries. That boundaries could be blurred by those sufficiently fortunate or skilled did not mean that many were not bound, limited, and governed within such boundaries. In our valuable attention to the manoeuvrings of those who were, in the omnipresent metaphor of much of this literature, involved in forms of trade and exchange, we should not lose track of those who, usually against their will, were exchanged and traded. We need, then, to pay attention to the functioning of categorical divisions, without reifying them or regarding them as absolutes. One means of doing so is to investigate not the blurring of extant boundaries, but the socially imbricated, tentative, and complex coming-into-being of the categories and binaries in the first place.

Such a task has been integral to postcolonial studies, from Said's germinal *Orientalism* through more recent studies of time and history by Johannes Fabian and Dipesh Chakrabarty.[36] These works inform the analysis here. This book is built around an exploration of the role played by science and medicine in the emergence of three categories fundamental to colonialism: race, particularly in the form of racialised pathologies; the division of the world into 'tropical' and 'temperate' disease zones; and the medical mapping of empire and, in particular, of zones of familiarity and strangeness according to whether newcomers to a location had to undergo a 'seasoning sickness'. Historians of colonialism and imperialism have come to be very wary of an analytic distinction between centres and peripheries. 'The point', insists a recent overview of work in the history of Atlantic science, 'is to distribute knowledge production, to insist on its contingency, and to break away from the geographies of center and periphery as a framework for classifying both people and knowledge'.[37] The point might, as I have suggested, be taken too far, since boundaries and

---

[35] See, for example, Edward W. Said, *Orientalism* (New York: Vintage, 2003).

[36] Johannes Fabian, *Time and the Other: How Anthropology Makes Its Object* (New York: Columbia University Press, 1983). Dipesh Chakrabarty, *Provincializing Europe: Postcolonial Thought and Historical Difference* (Princeton: Princeton University Press, 2000). For related works within the history of science (sometimes without the postcolonial label) see Helen Tilley, 'Global Histories, Vernacular Science, and African Genealogies: Or, Is the History of Science Ready for the World?', *Isis* 101 (2010). For further discussion, see Seth.

[37] Marcelo Aranda et al., 'The History of Atlantic Science: Collective Reflections from the 2009 Harvard Seminar on Atlantic History', *Atlantic Studies* 7 (2010): 499.

divisions, however porous, serve to limit movements.[38] But beyond this, one should ask how such boundaries were conceived of in the first place? How was the ideational distinction between (imperial) centre and periphery, between the place where 'Britons' were home and where they were 'strangers', produced and maintained? How, more particularly, did science and medicine play a role in this production and maintenance and how did this far-from-monolithic or static division change over time?

Such are at least some of the historiographical questions driving my analysis. Structurally, the material below is divided into three parts, within which chapters are arranged roughly chronologically. Part I, 'Locality' is comprised of Chapters 1 and 2; Chapters 3 and 4 make up Part II, 'Empire'; Part III, spanning Chapters 5 to 7, explores the relationships between 'race-medicine and race-science'. The three themes are fairly distinct, but there is considerable overlap, both temporal and substantial, between each part. The conclusion then seeks to bring all into a common conversation. In the next section, I offer a more detailed summary of the argument of each chapter, while simultaneously aiming to provide some sense of the literatures to which I hope to make contributions.

Before embarking upon such detail, and after having supplied some sense of what this book is (or hopes to be), it would be well to be clear about what it is not. I have already noted that my geographical focus is the British Empire: comparative accounts or inter-imperial exchanges are not at the centre of analysis. Such exchanges almost certainly occurred, although perhaps more often at the level of quotidian practice than in the somewhat more formal published documents that make up the bulk of my sources. British texts about the diseases of warm climates tended to be rather parochial in the figures and works outside European metropoles that they cited and by mid-century, British writings were extensive enough that they could provide a seemingly complete set of references on their own.[39] One sees this via patterns of internal citation, but the most striking evidence might be that from a source outside the British Empire. In a prize-winning essay published in English in 1762, Solomon de Monchy, city physician at Rotterdam, proclaimed the pre-eminence of English writers on the diseases of the West Indies. Somewhat idiosyncratically, given the long history of Dutch colonialism and writings on medicine, de Monchy

---

[38] Breaking down the centre/periphery divide has been an essential element of studies that have taken the Atlantic world as their geographical focus. See, e.g. James Delbourgo, *A Most Amazing Scene of Wonders: Electricity and Enlightenment in Early America* (Cambridge, MA: Harvard University Press, 2006); Susan Scott Parrish, *American Curiosity: Cultures of Natural History in the Colonial British Atlantic World* (Chapel Hill: University of North Carolina Press, 2006).

[39] Schiebinger alludes to a similar phenomenon, suggesting that the 'invisible boundaries of empire' may have 'limit[ed] interisland exchange'. Schiebinger, *Secret Cures of Slaves: People, Plants, and Medicine in the Eighteenth-Century Atlantic World*, 181.

suggested of his compatriots that, if they were not 'totally strangers to navigation', they were 'yet little acquainted with the many changes and effects, which
living at sea, and sailing into different climates, very generally produce in the
human constitution'. As a result, he relied, for his own understanding, on 'the
many observations of the English physicians and Surgeons, who, at present, to
the great benefit of that commercial nation, make the Sea-distempers a considerable object of their study, and have written on them from their own experience'.[40] For British medical authors in the colonies, a significant expansion
in their engagement with texts written by their non-Anglophonic counterparts
appears to have begun only towards the end of the eighteenth century.[41]

I draw gratefully throughout the subsequent pages from work in the last few
decades on the social histories of medicine, colonialism and slavery – particularly within the Caribbean and North America. Mine, however, is fundamentally a work of intellectual history, although I mean to signify by this term not
a context-free history of ideas, but rather a profoundly context-laden *history
of arguments*. And, although I rely on printed sources, which suggests that the
subjects of my analysis were members of a fairly elite class in cultural terms,
it would be wrong to imagine that most were even to be numbered among the
economically secure, let alone the wealthy. Some medical writers in the colonies (for example William Hillary, the principal subject of Chapter 2) made
comfortable livings, were regularly cited throughout the empire, and had books
that underwent multiple editions. But the majority of those outside European
metropolitan centres (and often even within them) were far more obscure figures, struggling – like Bennet and Williams – in a difficult medical marketplace. This is intellectual history, then, with a capacious understanding of what
an 'intellectual' might be, and with an aim to recover not simply the best and
boldest ideas of an age, but the thought-worlds and ideational stakes of medical
practitioners of many kinds.

If my sources encompass a fair diversity in terms of economic status or edu-
cational training, it must be acknowledged that they lack in diversity in other
ways. I am attentive to gender as a category of analysis throughout, with a
sustained focus on relationships between gender, sexuality, race, and medicine
in Chapters 5 and 7 in particular. But women enter most of the stories recounted
here as patients rather than practitioners. The voices of non-European medical
practitioners are similarly muted.[42] Some British authors were happy to bolster

---

[40] Solomon de Monchy, *An Essay on the Causes and Cure of the Usual Diseases in Voyages to
the West Indies* (London: T. Becket and P. A. De Hondt, 1762), ii, lv.
[41] See, e.g. Benjamin Moseley, *A Treatise on Tropical Diseases; And on the Climate of the West-
Indies* (London: T. Cadell, 1787).
[42] The vast majority of those providing medical treatment for the enslaved were themselves slaves.
For classic accounts, see for the West Indies, Sheridan, *Doctors and Slaves: A Medical and
Demographic History of Slavery in the British West Indies, 1680–1834*, and for the antebellum

their own claims to the possession of local knowledge by citing more or less reliable 'native' informants, so that one can, at times, get a sense of competing forms of knowledge within the pages of Anglophonic texts. Yet even such mentions tend to be limited. I should be clear, too, on the fact that the absence of non-European voices is also the result of my own authorial choices. I am less interested here, for example, in the specifics of treatments and therapeutics – where indigenous or slave knowledge might more often be cited – than I am in medical theories, where British men of medicine tended to emphasise their own 'rationalist' expertise and to downplay or ignore the contributions or claims of their non-European counterparts.[43]

Locality

Chapter 1 explores the role of Hippocratic ideas about the relationship between health and location – laid out most clearly in the Hippocratic text *Airs, Waters, and Places* – prior to 1700. Our understanding of this material has been

United States, Todd L. Savitt, *Medicine and Slavery: The Diseases and Health Care of Blacks in Antebellum Virginia* (Champaign: University of Illinois Press, 1978); Ronald Numbers and Todd L. Savitt, eds., *Science and Medicine in the Old South* (Baton Rouge: Louisiana State University Press, 1999); Sharla M. Fett, *Working Cures: Healing, Health, and Power on Southern Slave Plantations* (Chapel Hill and London: University of North Carolina Press, 2002). For superb recent accounts of Afro-Caribbean medical knowledge in the Atlantic world, see Karol Weaver, *Medical Revolutionaries: The Enslaved Healers of Eighteenth-Century Saint Domingue* (Urbana and Chicago: University of Illinois Press, 2006); James H. Sweet, *Domingo Álvares, African Healing, and the Intellectual History of the Atlantic World* (Chapel Hill: University of North Carolina Press, 2011); Pablo F. Gómez, 'Incommensurable Epistemologies?: The Atlantic Geography of Healing in the Early Modern Caribbean', *Small Axe* 18 (2014); *The Experiential Caribbean: Creating Knowledge and Healing in the Early Modern Atlantic* (Chapel Hill: University of North Carolina Press, 2017); 'The Circulation of Bodily Knowledge in the Seventeenth-Century Black Spanish Caribbean', *Social History of Medicine* 26 (2013); Schiebinger, *Secret Cures of Slaves: People, Plants, and Medicine in the Eighteenth-Century Atlantic World*.

43 As Karol Weaver notes: 'Although eighteenth-century physicians, plantation surgeons, and white planters used slave remedies, they downplayed the role of the slave healer by placing the remedy within the traditional European therapeutic framework or by making reference to the healing traditions of esteemed nations', Weaver, 74. Willingness to explicitly cite local informants also appears to have changed across time and space. Londa Schiebinger offers the revealing example of differences in the way that Thomson reported his results and sources in a text intended largely for a West Indian audience (*Treatise on the Diseases of Negroes*, 1820) and the way he presented similar materials to a metropolitan audience in the *Edinburgh Medical and Surgical Journal*. 'In his Jamaican *Treatise*', Schiebinger notes, 'Thomson valued "Negro" knowledge; in his European version, this knowledge often fell from view', Schiebinger, *Secret Cures of Slaves: People, Plants, and Medicine in the Eighteenth-Century Atlantic World*, 179. In writing about botanical knowledge, Miles Ogborn observes that British authors in the early eighteenth century were willing to admit that non-Europeans might know about or experiment with nature. By the 1780s, however, such admissions were becoming much rarer: Ogborn, 'Talking Plants: Botany and Speech in Eighteenth-Century Jamaica'. *History of Science* 51 (2013): 275–6. See also Jorge Cañizares-Esguerra, *How to Write the History of the New World: Histories, Epistemologies, and Identities in the Eighteenth Century Atlantic World* (Stanford: Stanford University Press, 2001), 60–129.

shaped, to a sizeable extent, by a comment made in 1707 by Hans Sloane, later to become President of the Royal Society. Sloane declared that he had been informed, before travelling to the West Indies, that 'the Diseases of this place were all different from what they are Europe, and to be treated in a differing Method'.[44] Historians, taking Sloane at his word, have thus often characterised the period before the beginning of the eighteenth century as one in which the orthodox position held that substantially different climates produced radically different diseases. I show, to the contrary, that medical men tended to work with similitudes more than differences, most often analogising warmer climates overseas to warmer seasons at home. Insofar as differences existed – and they obviously did – it was because one found more cases of diseases commonly suffered in English summers in Jamaica all year round. *Contra* Sloane, I have found very few examples of any authors arguing that the diseases of warmer countries were utterly unknown in Europe. Yet one does find several examples of medical men advocating for novel *treatments* in different locations and in this claim we locate, I would contend, the stakes of Sloane's statement. Arguing, in Jamaica, with local practitioners who insisted that their local knowledge might trump that of a metropolitan physician, Sloane rejected any claim that his expertise might not be transferable to his new location. In examining the relationship between differences of places and distempers, then, one is forced simultaneously to an analysis of differences in social standing and the locatedness of claims to expertise.

Chapter 2 continues the analysis of Hippocratic thought by focusing on the author of the most influential text on the diseases of the West Indies for the mid-eighteenth century, William Hillary. Hillary serves as guide through a thicket of interrelating ideas relevant to medicine in warm climates from the 1720s to the 1760s, including the roles of the mechanical philosophy and medical meteorology, and debates between those who favoured contagionist rather than climatic theories of disease causation. Focus on the author of *Observations on the Changes of the Air, and the Concomitant Epidemical Diseases in the Island of Barbadoes* also allows the elaboration of two related arguments. The first involves what has become known as the Hippocratic revival in early eighteenth-century British medicine and points to the ways that a study of the colonies can inform our understanding of the history of medicine within the British Isles. As Chapter 1 shows, *Airs, Waters, and Places* had already, prior to 1700, become a model for understanding the illnesses deemed characteristic

---

[44] Hans Sloane, *A Voyage to the Islands Madera, Barbados, Nieves, S. Christophers and Jamaica, with the Natural History of the Herbs and Trees, Four-Footed Beasts, Fishes, Birds, Insects, Reptiles, &C. Of the Last of Those Islands; to Which Is Prefix'd an Introduction, Wherein is an Account of the Inhabitants, Air, Waters, Diseases, Trade, &C. of That Place, with Some Relations Concerning the Neighbouring Continent, and Islands of America.*, 2 vols. (London: printed by B. M. for the author, 1707 & 1725), 1707, xc.

of a given location. The turn to Hippocratism in the metropole thus happened later than that in the colonies. More significantly, it also had a different object. Authors within Britain tended to emphasise epidemic, rather than endemic illnesses, taking as their touchstone the Hippocratic works, *Epidemics I* and *III*. Contrasting the forms of Hippocratic thought in Britain and its imperial holdings, then – and speaking not of Hippocratism but geographically specific *Hippocratisms* – one can come to a more nuanced and specific understanding of precisely what neo-Hippocratism meant and the different kinds of work it might do. And in Hillary's work – as befits a physician who practiced in both the West Indies and Britain – one can also see how different forms of Hippocratism might be fused. The chapter's second argument takes up a question posed by the material in Chapter 1. If one does not find arguments for the distinctiveness of the diseases of tropical countries before 1700, when do such arguments first emerge? In Hillary, we find part of an answer, one that would bring the issue of slavery and the slave trade to the fore. For Hillary, a putative similarity between the warmth of climates in the West Indies and the Guinea Coast was not sufficient to produce a common disease environment: after all, differences abounded. Where one found diseases common to both locations and unfamiliar within Europe, then, one looked to other causes, such as the movement of human cargo. At mid-century, then, one could not so much speak of the diseases of the Tropics as of the diseases of lands connected by the triangular trade in slaves and goods.

Empire

The first two chapters of this book share a common geographical focus, using close readings of texts (mostly) written in and about the West Indies as a means of unpacking assumptions about the relationships between sickness and place more generally. Chapters 3 and 4 aim to widen the scope of analysis, embracing and elaborating upon the notion of an 'imperial medicine'. It seems obvious to note that the metaphorical health of the British Empire rested on the literal health of its subjects, both military and civilian. Yet in many ways, historians of eighteenth-century British imperialism have tended to take the history of medicine for granted. Almost incredible death rates from disease, of course, form the backdrop for any narrative of imperial expansion. And death rates could, at times, reach such levels that they were marshalled by those agitating for political change, or for alterations in the organisation and structure of the armed forces. For many imperial historians, however, *theories* of disease – their causation and treatment – function as an effectively irrelevant superstructure in relation to vastly more significant basal facts of morbidity and mortality. Ideas that appear laughably antiquated to modern eyes merely help explain why tropical service was deadly and to be avoided when possible.

Medical history, when invoked, functions in a supportive role for a more fundamental political, social, or intellectual history of empire and imperialism.

And yet, as I show in Chapter 3, theories of disease and their relationships to place can be used as profoundly illuminating sources for understanding a basic issue: How did Britons conceive of their empire? How did they conceptualise the relationship between centres and peripheries? How did relations of similitude and difference shape reactions to places deemed utterly foreign or suitably home-like? Answers, of course, changed over time. Dividing the century into rough thirds, Linda Colley has argued that the period up to the end of the Seven Years War was one in which the empire could be regarded as largely homogenous.[45] The spectacular expansion in imperial territories after the victories of the war, however, led to a sense that the Empire was suddenly unfamiliar, a feeling that began to dissipate after the loss of the American colonies. Medical discourse allows one to paint a somewhat different narrative, although the turning points remain roughly the same. As is made clear by insistences on 'seasoning' new arrivals to different climes, homogeneity was never a medical assumption about far-flung lands. The Seven Years War marks a turning point in imperial conceptions of self, but this is because before mid-century, the empire could be conveniently bifurcated – split between a metropolitan home, where one was already seasoned to the climate, and a periphery where such seasoning took time and could potentially prove deadly. After the War, one does indeed see an anxiety, as Colley suggests, but it manifested as the sense that even 'home' could prove dangerous: one might well need time to become seasoned even within the British Isles. After the 1770s, such reflexive concerns would dissipate, and one begins to see a kind of medical nationalism, as authors increasingly cast warm climates as profoundly and completely foreign spaces, to be contrasted with the ideal environs of the metropole.

If Chapter 3 is thus concerned with the ways in which understandings of medicine in the periphery informed conceptions of empire, Chapter 4 is concerned with the inverse question. How did an 'imperial sensibility' come to inform British medicine in the eighteenth century? Material about the diseases of warmer climates is fairly rare in medical texts that were not primarily concerned with that topic before around 1700. From the 1720s, however, the periphery comes to take up a (admittedly small) part of many major works, with a larger place in those texts dedicated to medical meteorological analyses. As Harrison has shown, a sea change would occur in the 1750s, after the publication of John Pringle's *Observations of the Diseases of the Army* in 1752.[46] Carrying the logic of medical meteorology to its most extreme conclusion,

---

[45] Colley, *Britons: Forging the Nation, 1707–1837.*
[46] Harrison, *Medicine in an Age of Commerce and Empire: Britain and its Tropical Colonies, 1660–1830*, esp. Chapter 3.

Pringle would argue not only that the state of the air contributed to the production of the illnesses that plagued soldiers, but that it was by far the most important cause, eclipsing either diet or climate. And the most dangerous air was that rendered putrid by a variety of causes. Although putrefaction – in the sense of corruption – had been an important element in theories of disease since antiquity and had been emphasised by Pringle's teacher, the famed Hermann Boerhaave, one may identify in Pringle's text the source of what might be termed a 'putrefactive turn' in imperial medicine. While Pringle had largely been interested in the diseases of soldiers fighting in the low countries during the War of Austrian Succession, the association of putridity with warm weather quickly made his theories central to etiological analyses of the diseases of warm climates. And such analyses made their mark on metropolitan medicine and natural philosophy. The stakes of the debate between the English reverend and chemist, Joseph Priestley and the Edinburgh physician, William Alexander over 'the noxious quality of the effluvia of putrid marshes', I argue, were imperial ones. In questioning the ability of putrid air to cause putrid fevers, Alexander was not only challenging Pringle's logic – ensconced by the time of the debate in the mid-1770s – he was calling into question the logics governing the management of the military in the colonies.

Race

Chapters 5 and 7 take up the history of 'race-medicine', a term I have coined by way of analogy with 'race-science', first introduced by Nancy Stepan in the early 1980s.[47] Turning away from the emphasis, in most of the secondary literature, on questions of morphological structure and hence on racialised *anatomy* (questions shared between natural history and medicine), I ask instead about more specifically medical racial *physiologies* and, particularly, racial *pathologies*.[48] When, I ask most basically, does one find the first instances of diseases conceived of as 1) characteristic of a given race and 2) caused not by the same kinds of environmental factors that produced racial difference in the first place, but rather by racialised physical differences between (for example) black and

---

[47] Nancy Stepan, *The Idea of Race in Science: Great Britain, 1800–1960* (Hamden: Archon, 1982).
[48] Roxann Wheeler, *The Complexion of Race: Categories of Difference in Eighteenth-Century British Culture* (Philadelphia: University of Pennsylvania Press, 2000); Andrew S. Curran, *The Anatomy of Blackness: Science & Slavery in an Age of Enlightenment* (Baltimore: Johns Hopkins University Press, 2011). For a similar approach, in spite of its title, see Rana Asali Hogarth, 'Comparing Anatomies, Constructing Races: Medicine and Slavery in the Atlantic World, 1787–1838'. PhD Thesis (New Haven: Yale University, 2012). Among my inspirations for this turn are Warwick Anderson, *The Cultivation of Whiteness: Science, Health and Racial Destiny in Australia* (New York: Basic Books, 2003) and *Colonial Pathologies: American Tropical Medicine, Race, and Hygiene in the Philippines* (Durham, NC and London: Duke University Press, 2006).

white bodies? Or, to phrase this another way, when does race become a *cause* of illness, rather than (like most diseases of the period) an *effect* of climate, diet, and other environmental factors? The answer given in Chapter 5 is that this does not happen before at least mid-century. In at least partial distinction to sexual difference – which I discuss as a counter-point to and a flexible, mutually constitutive element of discourses concerning racial difference – race was not construed as an essential medical category for most of the eighteenth century. Focusing on the multiple and changing writings of the naval surgeon, John Atkins – perhaps the first author to introduce polygenist ideas (those positing a separate act of creation for different human races) in a medical text – I demonstrate that notions of racial fixity and the theoretical presuppositions of the medicine of warm climates did not mix. Atkins believed that blacks and whites were fundamentally different in their physical structures, and that neither diet nor climate could change this, but he made no arguments suggesting that such racial differences were the cause of the diseases he deemed characteristic of and peculiar to the Guinea Coast. Polygenism and medical environmentalism occupied different parts of the same text and little would change in Atkin's medical explanations when he recanted his unorthodox polygenetic views in the early 1740s.

In common with a number of historians, I date the turn towards hardening conceptions of race as part of a response to the abolitionist movement, beginning roughly in the 1760s.[49] The effect of anti-slavery propaganda was to politicise the very question of natural equality. 'It was one thing to entertain the possibility in the abstract', John Wood Sweet has wryly observed, 'It was quite another to confront it as a political challenge to immensely profitable colonial plantation regimes'.[50] Chapter 6 turns from race-medicine to race-science to explore the racial theories of Edward Long, author of a massive, three-volume *History of Jamaica* (1774), who first publicly espoused his polygenist views in response to the outcome of a court case in 1772 that appeared to support the anti-slavery cause. The chapter's aim is thus to situate debates about the origin of human races concretely in the context of responses to abolitionist critique. It is also, however, to draw attention to the difference that geographical

---

[49] The claim is of very long standing. In 1945, for example, Ashley Montagu argued, in a chapter on 'The Origin of the Concept of "Race"', that '[i]t was only when voices began to make themselves heard against the inhuman traffic in slaves and when these voices assumed the shape of influential men and organizations that, on the defensive, the supporters of slavery were forced to look about them for reasons of a new kind to controvert the dangerous arguments of their opponents'. Ashley Montagu, *Man's Most Dangerous Myth: The Fallacy of Race*, 2nd ed. (New York: Columbia University Press, 1945), 10. See also Seymour Drescher, 'The Ending of the Slave Trade and the Evolution of European Scientific Racism', *Social Science History* 14 (1990).

[50] John Wood Sweet, *Bodies Politic: Negotiating Race in the American North, 1730–1830* (Baltimore: Johns Hopkins University Press, 2003), 276.

specificity makes in the history of race, even when the focus is on anatomy rather than pathology. Race-science during the Enlightenment in the West Indies looks very different to metropolitan race-science in the same period, for reasons very specific to the location of its production. Long's polygenism also appears quite dissimilar to the kinds of rigid racialism with which we are more familiar from nineteenth-century sources. The reason for the differences is twofold. First, although Long was willing to buck biblical orthodoxy, he balked at materialism, a position that gained traction in racial studies following the successes of the phrenological movement in the early nineteenth century. Second, Long presents us with a (relatively rare) case of an eighteenth-century writer on 'race-science' with political sympathies toward a part of the world that was both outside the bounds of the European metropole and contained a majority black population. As a result, one finds a fundamental ambivalence in his writings on race, an ambivalence that stemmed directly from his desire to manage social relations and political systems in a slave society. Metropolitan figures who believed in the fixity of race (regardless of the question of origin) made a cornerstone of their position the essential identity of newly arrived African slaves and their descendants. For Long, however, the difference between 'salt-water' and 'creole' Negroes was to be the solution to the most pressing social problem of the sugar islands: slave insurrection. This understanding of the (potential) political and social differences between generations of slaves required a physical corollary: Long's polygenism presumed less fixity than the monogenism of a figure like Immanuel Kant.

Chapter 7, finally, returns to the history of race-medicine, picking up the thread from Chapter 5, as medicine begins to play a central role in debates about the end of the slave trade. I look first at critiques and defences of slavery that relied on medical experience and expertise, at tracts in which doctors and surgeons invoked their own histories and practices to point to ways that enslavement might be meliorated or – as some contended – that it already had been, in spite of the accusations of those who charged planters with neglect and brutal treatment. The chapter turns next to the questions of 'racialised' pathologies in the last decades of the century. Clear continuities to the earlier period may be traced: fixed physical characteristics were rarely invoked as explanations. And yet climate did not quite function in the same way that it once had. In the majority of earlier accounts, the diseases of non-Europeans had largely been examined as part of studies of the illnesses peculiar to non-European locations. Among the responses to abolitionist critiques, however, was greater attention paid to the illnesses of Afro-Caribbean slaves as explicitly compared to those of Europeans and white Creoles who inhabited the same geographical space. In situations where climate was essentially held in common, one finds increasing emphasis on diet, clothing, housing, and behaviour as explanations for health disparities between whites and blacks. If one does not find 'race' in these – still orthodox – writings, one does find more emphasis on the social and cultural differences that separated Northern Europeans from others. The final section of the chapter turns from the orthodox to the heterodox, looking at polygenist and rigidly racialist accounts in medical texts. Pathological and anatomical claims were to be found in particular abundance, I show, in discourses that asserted an innate capacity for Africans to labour under environmental conditions that putatively made it impossible for Europeans to take their place. And from the 1780s, one can locate precisely those claims that had been marked by their absence in the earlier period discussed in Chapter 5: claims that invoked physical variation as the *cause* of racialised medical differences. By the 1800s, race-medicine was beginning to take shape.

In the conclusion, I try to draw together two of the largest threads of the book, attempting to find common answers to two puzzles that have previously been seen as distinct. The last quarter of the eighteenth century saw the emergence of a growing agreement concerning human races. Where, as Nicholas Hudson has shown, one had previously spoken of near-innumerable 'nations' or 'peoples' in order to divide humanity into meaningful groupings, from the late 1700s, humankind was increasingly divided into a small number of races.[51] Many smaller differences had been elided to produce larger similitudes, to be contrasted with a few, now-large differences. Similarly, medical men had once found near-innumerable points of commonality between various points on the globe, noting, as Hans Sloane did in 1707, that parts of Jamaica were no warmer than Montpelier, and also noting multiple points of difference between even nearby locations, identifying 'micro-climates', in Katherine Johnston's account, as explanations for disease variation on the island of Jamaica.[52] By the 1780s, however, such small-scale differences were disappearing, as one begins to find accounts of 'tropical diseases', that bound the East and West Indies to each other and to locations in Africa. That growing similitude only made sense in the context of a larger difference: the distinction between the diseases of temperate and tropical climes. In discourses of race and discourses concerning the diseases of warm climates, then, one finds – at essentially the same time – a similar set of moves: smaller intra-regional differences ignored and inter-regional differences emphasised. That, I argue, is no mere coincidence. The emergence of modern conceptions of race, and the emergence of a category of tropical diseases were intertwined phenomena, to be explained by a history of medicine, race, slavery, and empire.

---

[51] Nicholas Hudson. 'From "Nation" to "Race": The Origin of Racial Classification in Eighteenth-Century Thought'. Eighteenth-Century Studies 29, no. 3 (1996): 246–64.

[52] Katherine Johnston, 'The Constitution of Empire: Place and Bodily Health in the Eighteenth-Century Atlantic', *Atlantic Studies* 10 (2013).

Part I

Locality

1 'The Same Diseases Here as in Europe'? Health and Locality Before 1700

Toward the end of January, 1686, the London doctor, Hans Sloane wrote to the naturalist John Ray, reporting to him (among other things) the ways that unscrupulous merchants were currently seeking to fool unwary purchasers of the febrifuge known as Jesuit's Bark. '[I]t being so good a drug, that they begin to adulterate it with black cherry and other barks dipped in a tincture of aloes, to make it bitter'. Sloane noted that anyone familiar with the substance might spot the trickery immediately, for 'the bitterness of the adulterated bark appears upon its first touch with the tongue, whereas the other is a pretty while in the mouth before it is tasted'.[1] The letter included news that suggested Sloane might soon have considerable use for the drug himself. 'I have talked a long while', he wrote, 'of going to Jamaica with the Duke of Albemarle as his physician, which, if I do, next to serving his grace and family in my profession, my business is to see what I can meet withal that is extraordinary in nature in those places. I hope to be able to send you some observations from thence, God Almighty granting life and strength to do what I design'.[2]

Although only twenty-six at the time, Sloane had already made a name for himself as a skilful collector of natural historical specimens.[3] Travelling through France while undertaking a medical degree (granted at the University of Orange in 1683), he spent a portion of his time gathering a sizeable collection of flora, which he then sent to Ray to make use of in his three-volume *History of Plants* (1686–1704). Sloane's previous work was on Ray's mind when he responded to the news that the young man might soon be working on an island that had only recently come into English possession. 'Were it not for the danger and hazard of so long a voyage', wrote Ray in April 1687, 'I would heartily wish such a person as yourself might travel to Jamaica, and search out

---

[1] Dr Hans Sloane to Mr Ray, Jan 29, 1686. In John Ray, *The Correspondence of John Ray: Consisting of Selections from the Philosophical Letters Published by Dr. Derham: And Original Letters of John Ray in the Collection of the British Museum / Edited by Edwin Lankester* (London: Printed for the Ray Society, 1848), 190.

[2] Ibid., 189.

[3] James Delbourgo, *Collecting the World: Hans Sloane and the Origins of the British Museum* (Cambridge, MA: Belknap Press, 2017).

and examine thoroughly the natural varieties of that island. Much light might be given to the history of the American plants, by one so well prepared for such an undertaking by a comprehensive knowledge of the European'.[4] In June, Ray got more detailed about the kinds of questions he hoped Sloane could answer. Great things were expected, 'no less than the resolving all our doubts about the names we meet with of plants in that part of America ... You may also please to observe whether there be any species of plants common to America and Europe'.[5] The largest number of specific queries derived from Ray's readings of a recent book by a Jamaican doctor, Thomas Trapham. Trapham's *Discourse of the State of Health in the Island of Jamaica* had appeared in 1679, and contained a number of natural historical observations.[6] Ray wanted the better-trained Sloane to determine the origin of ambergris (was it really the juice of a metal or aloe dropped into the sea?), the nature of the plant known as 'dumbcane', and precisely what Trapham meant when he described the 'shining barks of trees' that he had seen.[7]

Sloane had presumably already read Trapham's text, not least as preparation for the work expected of him as physician to Jamaica's new Governor.[8] Trapham's *Discourse* was the first English book written on the diseases of the West Indies. Indeed, today it is considered by some to be the first English monograph on tropical medicine more generally.[9] Sloane would soon meet Trapham in Jamaica, where the two butted heads over the Duke's medical treatment. The elite metropolitan physician was clearly irritated when Trapham was called in for a consultation as 'one who understood the country diseases having lived there several years'. By his own account, however, Sloane 'declined quarrelling with him. Thought my case hard enough in that I was blamed by some for want of success when his Grace would not take advice'.[10] Neither

[4] Mr Ray to Dr Hans Sloane, 1 April 1687. In Ray, 192.

[5] Mr Ray to Dr Hans Sloane (No date, presumably late June 1687). In ibid., 194–5.

[6] Thomas Trapham, *A Discourse of the State of Health in the Island of Jamaica with a Provision Therefore Calculated from the Air, the Place, and the Water, the Customs and Manner of Living &C* (London: Printed for R. Boulter, 1679).

[7] Ray, 195.

[8] The charge was not necessarily a promotion. '[King] James knew that Albemarle was a profligate and irresponsible man who had squandered his fortune in England', writes Dunn. '[H]e sent him to Jamaica to get rid of him. The duke, for his part, was eager to go because he had an interest in Caribbean treasure hunting'. The Duke's eventual death in 1688 was apparently tied to his profoundly immoderate celebrations following the announcement of the birth of the queen's son. Richard S. Dunn, *Sugar and Slaves: The Rise of the Planter Class in the English West Indies, 1624–1713* (Chapel Hill and London: University of North Carolina Press, 2000), 160.

[9] M. T. Ashcroft, 'Tercentenary of the First English Book on Tropical Medicine, by Thomas Trapham of Jamaica', *British Medical Journal* 2 (1979).

[10] This story derives from Estelle Frances Ward, *Christopher Monck, Duke of Albemarle* (London: J. Murray, 1915). Ward refers to the doctor as 'Traphan'. Sheridan notes the exchange in Richard B. Sheridan, 'The Doctor and the Buccaneer: Sir Hans Sloane's Case History of Sir Henry Morgan, Jamaica, 1688', *Journal of the History of Medicine and Allied Sciences* 41 (1986): 84.

doctor would achieve a great deal. The Duke died in October 1688, after which Sloane returned to England, having spent only fifteen months away.

Sloane's interactions with both Ray and Trapham would profoundly shape the most substantial product of his brief sojourn in the West Indies, his two-volume *Voyage to the Islands Madera, Barbados, Nieves, S. Christophers, and Jamaica* (1707 & 1725). Prior to this English-language work, in 1696 (by which time he had been elected secretary of the Royal Society), Sloane had published a Latin catalogue of Jamaican plant life. In writing a 'short account' of the catalogue at Sloane's request, Ray answered a number of the questions he had first posed a decade earlier.[11] Sloane, he noted 'hath informed us that the Dumb-cane so called, which being tasted, inflames the tongue and jaws in that manner, that, for awhile, it takes away the use of speech, is not properly any species of reed or cane, but of arum, or wake-robin'.[12] More generally, 'we are assured by his work that there are some plants common, not only to Europe and America, but even to England and Jamaica, notwithstanding the great distance of place, and difference both of longitude and climate'.[13] The import of this statement appeared in Sloane's *Preface* to the 1707 volume of his *Voyage*. Responding to the potential retort that his discoveries in the West Indies were hardly surprising, since one might imagine that all the plant life in such a foreign clime was novel, Sloane wrote, 'I answer it is not so ... I find a great many plants common to Spain, Portugal, and Jamaica, more common to Jamaica and the East-Indies, and most of all common to Jamaica and Guinea'. The natural history he was offering, he argued, could 'reasonably be suppos'd' to describe not only the botanical world of the Americas, but even of Guinea and the East Indies and thus 'to contribute to the more distinct knowledge of all those parts'.[14]

The argument that related plants in America to those in England was important to Sloane's overall purpose, which was, in part, to encourage a kind of trade of plant life between the Old and New Worlds. If one of Sloane's aims was to teach those who lived in or near Jamaica the uses of plants growing wild or in their gardens, another was to educate those in England about the virtues – particularly the therapeutic virtues – of the materials that he brought back. 'It may be objected', he suggested, 'that 'tis to no purpose to any in these Parts of the World, to look after such [Jamaican] Herbs, &c. because we never see them; I answer, that many of them and their several Parts have been brought over, and are used in Medicines every day, and more may, to the great Advantage of physicians and Patients, were People inquisitive enough to look

---

[11] Mr Ray to Dr Hans Sloane (no date). In Ray, 464.
[12] 'Preface by Mr Ray to Dr. Hans Sloane's Catalogue of Plants', in ibid., 465–8, on 67.
[13] Ibid., 468.
[14] Sloane, Preface, 12.

after them'.[15] As he made this argument, Sloane could, presumably, count on his readership calling to mind the efficacy of Jesuit's (or Peruvian) Bark.[16] Now medicinal and other plants were thriving throughout Europe: in England and Ireland, Holland, Germany, and Sweden.[17]

An argument about the similarity between Jamaica and Europe was also central to the medical portion of *Voyage*, which made up roughly 40 per cent of the 154-page Introduction to Volume I.[18] Before leaving with the Duke, Sloane narrated, 'I was told that the Diseases of this place were all different from what they are in Europe, and to be treated in a differing Method. This made me very uneasie, lest by ignorance I should kill instead of curing'. Sloane went on to inform the reader that his own experiences had shown that the notion that diseases in Europe and the West Indies were very different was false. '[A]bating some very few Diseases, Symptoms, &c. from the diversity of the Air, Meat, Drink &c. any person who has seen many sick people will find the same Diseases here as in *Europe*, and the same Method of Cure'. In fact, Sloane continued, in an oft-quoted sentence:

For my own part, I never saw a Disease in Jamaica which I had not met with in Europe, and that in People who never had been in either Indies, excepting one or two; and such instances happen to people practicing Physik in England, or anywhere else, that they may meet, amongst great number, with a singular disease, that they had never seen before, nor perhaps meet after with a parallel instance.[19]

Most scholars who have written about this aspect of Sloane's work have tended to take the author's statements at face value, seeing Sloane as an outlier largely because he portrayed himself as one. Thus, Harrison has argued that: 'A few European physicians, such as Sir Hans Sloane (1660–1753), expressed scepticism about the distinctiveness of diseases in the tropics, but such opinions (as Sloane himself noted) were at variance with both lay and professional opinion in the West Indies'.[20] Wendy Churchill, similarly, has read Sloane as offering a 'challenge to the developing notion that illness manifested

---

[15] Ibid., Preface, 11.

[16] On the history of the Peruvian bark, see Matthew Crawford, *The Andean Wonder Drug: Cinchona Bark and Imperial Science in the Spanish Atlantic, 1630–1800* (Pittsburgh: University of Pittsburgh Press, 2016).

[17] Sloane, Preface, 11.

[18] This section would later be translated into German and published as a work in its own right. Hans Sloane and Christoph L. Becker, *Johann Sloane ... von den Krankheiten, Welche er in Jamaika Beobachtet und Behandelt hat: aus dem Englischen Übersetzt und mit Einigen Zusätzen Begleitet* (Augsburg: Klett, 1784).

[19] Sloane, xc.

[20] Harrison, ' "The Tender Frame of Man": Disease, Climate and Racial Difference in India and the West Indies, 1760–1860', 70.

differently in different climates'.[21] It makes some intuitive sense to think of Sloane's as an unorthodox position, for it would seem to run counter to ideas dating back to antiquity that related climates and characteristic diseases. Andrew Wear, for example, has identified an early modern European tradition based on the Hippocratic text, *Airs, Waters, and Places*. That tradition, he has argued, 'contains both the constitution-shaping aspect of place and the belief that particular diseases reside in particular places' and 'acted in Europe as a conscious or unconscious template for views on the relationship between places, health, and disease'.[22] However, although it is clear that a Hippocratic lineage for eighteenth-century texts on diseases and places existed, one must also emphasise the fact that the lineage was neither continuous, straightforward, nor hegemonic.[23]

I argue in this chapter that Sloane's characterisation of medical understandings of the relationships between health and place were, if not wrong, at least rather selective. They served, at least in part, a particular set of social claims about the necessity, or not, for a doctor in Jamaica, to have expert, local knowledge of disease. Before making that case, however, it is necessary to capture the complexity of discourse about diseases and places prior to 1700. Section 2.1 explores the relative absence of references to *Airs, Waters, and Places* until the late sixteenth century, as well as the eventual deployment of the text in works such as Prosper Alpini's *De Medicina Aegyptiorum* (1591) and Jacobus Bontius' *De Medicina Indorum* (1645). Section 2.2 examines the flexibility and nuances of this neo-Hippocratic tradition from the seventeenth century onward, for Hippocrates' text was used as much to draw similarities between far-flung locations with common airs, waters, and places as it was to delineate differences. Far from solely being a resource for rote arguments about the peculiarity of afflictions in foreign locations (although it was this, too) the arguments of *Airs, Waters, and Places* could also be deployed to draw distant lands closer, allowing boosters for colonial settlement to cast new areas as new-found 'relations': sites seemingly designed for British settlement.[24] Different

---

[21] Wendy D. Churchill, 'Bodily Differences?: Gender, Race, and Class in Hans Sloane's Jamaican Medical Practice, 1687–1688', *Journal of the History of Medicine and Allied Sciences* 60, no. 4 (2005): 396.

[22] Andrew Wear, 'Place, Health, and Disease: The Airs, Waters, Places Tradition in Early Modern England and North America', *Journal of Medieval and Early Modern Studies* 38, no. 3 (2008): 445, 43. See also G. Miller, ' "Airs, Waters, and Places" in History', *Journal of the History of Medicine* 17 (1962).

[23] L. J. Jordanova, 'Earth Science and Environmental Medicine: The Synthesis of the Late Environment', in *Images of the Earth: Essays in the History of the Environmental Sciences*, ed. L. J. Jordanova and Roy Porter (London: British Society for the History of Science, 1979).

[24] 'The perfect agreement of English constitutions and American Air', Kupperman notes, 'was even urged as proof that God had intended North America for the English nation'. Karen

climates resulted in different diseases, to be sure. But we should be wary of ascribing our contemporary conceptions of the marked differences between the climates of the West Indies and of Britain (for example) to eighteenth-century actors, who also found many connections between the two sites.

With both the complexity and flexibility of the Hippocratic tradition in mind, then, Section 3.1 turns to the simple fact that it is difficult to find many texts about the West Indies that make the claim that Sloane insisted was the standard. Instead, therefore, of reading Sloane as a single figure rebutting a consensus position, I suggest that we see his claims as having emerged, at least partly, from his disputes with Trapham and other local physicians. As in the deadly dispute between Williams and Bennet, at stake was not, or not merely, the onto-logical question of the nature of diseases in different places, but also the epis-temological question of how one learned to diagnose and treat such diseases, and the social question – related to these others – of whom should be granted the authority and expertise to speak and act on such matters. When could local experience trump putatively generalisable scholarship and learning?

1.1   A Hippocratic Revival

By the early 1700s it was certainly not uncommon for medical works on the diseases of specific locations to invoke Hippocrates as their most illustrious classical forebear. Friedrich Hoffmann's 1705 *Dissertation on Endemial Diseases,* for example, opened by defining 'endemial' as 'an epithet of those Diseases which are peculiar to the Inhabitants of certain Nations, or Countries'. He then offered a long quotation (almost thirty lines) from the beginning of *Airs, Waters, and Places* to support his claim that 'With these diseases and their respective Natures the Physicians ought to well acquainted'.[25] Richard Towne, physician and author of *A Treatise of the Diseases Most Frequent in the West-Indies* (1726), was a world away from the illustrious Hoffmann, both geographically and professionally. The German was a professor at Halle, with an international reputation, while Towne – about whom we know little else – evidently had a medical practice in Barbados. Yet Towne too found it unproblematic to introduce his text by similarly suggesting that the idea that 'human Bodies are greatly influenced by the *Climate, Air, Soil, Diet &c.* of the

---

Kupperman, 'The Puzzle of the American Climate in the Early Colonial Period', *The American Historical Review* 87 (1982): 1283.

[25] Friedrich Hoffmann and Bernardino Ramazzini, *A Dissertation on Endemial Diseases or, Those Disorders Which Arise from Particular Climates, Situations, and Methods of Living; Together with a Treatise on the Diseases of Tradesmen ... The First by the Celebrated Frederick Hoffman ... The Second by Bern. Ramazini ... Newly Translated with a Preface and an Appendix by Dr. James* (London: Printed for Thomas Osborne and J. Hildyard at York, 1746), 1.

Places we inhabit, has been long ago judiciously and fully proved by the divine *Hippocrates* in his Book *de Aere, Aqua & Locis*'.[26]

Hippocrates was indeed a natural referent for those concerned with the relationship between environments and human health. His text admonished the physician to pay attention first to seasonality, then to winds, both hot and cold, distinguishing between those common in all places and those 'peculiar to each locality'. 'Whoever wishes to investigate medicine properly' needed to study the qualities of water – its taste and weight, whether it was marshy, soft or hard, whether it ran down from rocky heights, and if it was brackish and poorly suited for cooking. Was the soil well-watered or dry; locked within valleys or exposed on hilltops? Arriving in a city as a stranger the Hippocratic doctor needed to study its position relative to prevailing winds and the course of the sun. And the good physician must also be, in contemporary terms, something of an anthropologist, for he must consider 'the mode in which the inhabitants live, and what are their pursuits, whether they are fond of drinking and eating to excess, and given to indolence, or are fond of exercise and labour, and not given to excess in eating and drinking'.[27]

Most simply, certain locations gave rise to characteristic constitutions and illnesses. A city exposed to hot winds, but sheltered from cold, northern ones contained inhabitants with flabby bodies, who tended to eat and drink little, avoiding the excessive consumption of wine in particular. Women menstruated excessively, 'are unfruitful from disease, and not from nature', and suffered from frequent miscarriages. Children were prone to convulsions and asthma, men to 'dysentery, diarrhea, hepialus, chronic fevers in winter, of epinyctis, frequently, and of hemorrhoids about the anus'. On the other hand, they were largely spared diseases characteristic of cities with inverted exposure to prevailing winds: pleurisies, peripneumonies, ardent fevers, and acute diseases more generally.[28] Over all, Hippocrates' was a discourse concerned with differences, even small ones. A city that was turned to the rising sun was likely to be healthy, while one turned to the North would be less so, even if both were only a furlong from each other. Diseases in cities that lay to the east would be relatively rare and women would be both fecund and blessed with easy deliveries.[29] Climatic differences had even more profound effects. Asia and Europe, Hippocrates claimed, differed from one another 'in all respects'. Asia was much milder than Europe, its inhabitants concomitantly gentler, and its natural

[26] Richard Towne, *A Treatise of the Diseases Most Frequent in the West-Indies, and Herein More Particularly of Those Which Occur in Barbadoes* (London: J. Clarke, 1726), 1.

[27] Hippocrates. 'Airs, Waters, and Places', in *The Genuine Works of Hippocrates*, translated by Francis Adams (London: Printed for the Sydenham Society, 1849), 190.

[28] Ibid., 192.

[29] Ibid., 194–5.

products larger and more beautiful. The various seasons resembled one another in Asia, while in Europe, the year was marked by striking changes.[30] Asiatic equilibrium was not, however, to be envied. '[F]or a climate which is always the same induces indolence, but a changeable climate, laborious exertions both of body and mind; and from rest and indolence cowardice is engendered, and from laborious exertions and pains, courage'. If change – both temporal and spatial – mattered enormously in *Airs, Waters, and Places*, changeability mattered even more, the changes of the seasons being 'the strongest of the natural causes of difference'. Where the seasons changed little, as in Asia, one found comparatively little variation among peoples, so that Europeans, as well as being more warlike and hardier, were also more varied among themselves than their eastern counterparts.[31]

The arguments of *Airs, Waters, and Places* remained well known to both medical and lay audiences in the Islamic Middle Ages.[32] But the same was not true in Europe. Nancy Siraisi suggests that we should regard the text as essentially 'new' to Renaissance audiences until the early sixteenth century.[33] *Airs, Waters, and Places* was not included in printed editions of Hippocratic works until 1515 and it was not until the second half of the sixteenth century that one could begin properly to speak of a Hippocratic revival, one that involved a detailed, dedicated, and direct engagement with more than a few of Hippocrates' works.[34] This is not to suggest, of course, that healers in the Middle Ages or Renaissance were unaware of or unconcerned with the relationship between environments and health. Of the six Galenic 'non-naturals' – those factors over which patients had some control – two (air and diet) depended at least in part on location. What is perhaps more significant about Hippocrates' text was that it examined the relationship between environments and the health of *groups*. Galenic therapeutics, on the other hand, was more concerned with

---

[30] Ibid., 205–7. 'Given the author's preoccupation with a Europe/Asia divide', Denise Eileen McCoskey has written, 'one that insists on the superiority of the Europeans in both climatic and political terms, some have suggested that the text functions in part to help justify the recent Greek defeat of the Persians during the Persian Wars (499–479 BCE)'. Denise Eileen McCoskey, 'On Black Athena, Hippocratic Medicine, and Roman Imperial Edicts: Egyptians and the Problem of Race in Classical Antiquity', in *Race and Ethnicity: Across Time, Space, and Discipline*, ed. Rodney D. Coates (Leiden: Brill, 2004), 320.

[31] Hippocrates. 'Airs, Waters, and Places', 219, 221.

[32] Peter E. Pormann and Emilie Savage-Smith, *Medieval Islamic Medicine* (Washington, DC: Georgetown University Press, 2007), 45.

[33] 'Among the parts of the Hippocratic corpus that were in some sense "new" in the early sixteenth century – that were little or only partially or indirectly known in the Middle Ages, were not commented on by scholastic authors, and were not standard in university curricula – were two works of especial significance for the relation between medicine and history: the *Epidemics* and *Airs, Waters, Places*'. Nancy Siraisi, *History, Medicine, and the Traditions of Renaissance Learning* (Ann Arbor: University of Michigan Press, 2007), 73.

[34] Vivian Nutton, 'Hippocrates in the Renaissance', *Sudhoffs Archiv* 27 (1989). A more precise meaning of neo-Hippocratism in the eighteenth century is taken up in Chapter 2.

the particular history, constitution, diet, and behaviour of a given patient than the characteristic diseases of whole cities or even countries.[35]

If one can thus speak of a Hippocratic revival beginning in the universities in the mid-sixteenth century, it would be some time before tracts on health in foreign climes drew upon *Airs, Waters, and Places* as a resource. One finds, for example, little trace of a 'Hippocratic heritage' in Garcia d'Orta's *Colloquies on the simples and drugs of India* (1563), another text often cited as the first on 'tropical medicine'.[36] Born in Portugal around 1500, d'Orta studied in Spain before returning home in 1523 and receiving his medical qualifications in 1526. In 1530, he was appointed to a lectureship in natural history at the University of Lisbon and four years later sailed to Goa as personal physician to M. A. de Sousa, who would go on to become the Portuguese Viceroy in India. D'Orta remained in Goa until his death in 1568, penning his most famous work after almost thirty years of medical practice in India.

D'Orta's book is structured in the form of a series of dialogues between a character named for the author and a fictitious Spanish doctor named Ruano. Having known one another in their university days, the two meet again in Goa, as the newly arrived Ruano visits d'Orta and expresses his 'great desire to know about the medicinal drugs (such as are called the drugs of pharmacy in Portugal) and other medicines of the country, as well as the fruits and spices'.[37] Ruano continues with a longer list of his interests (and hence a fuller description of the contents of the non-fictitious d'Orta's book):

I further wish to learn of their names in different languages, and the trees or herbs from which they are taken. I also desire to know how the native physicians use them; and to learn what other plants and fruits there are belonging to this land, which are not medicinal; and what customs will be met with; for all such things may be described as having been seen by you or by other persons worthy of credit.[38]

---

[35] On the 'harnessing of the non-naturals to the "airs, waters, and places" approach' in the eighteenth century, see L. J. Jordanova, 'Earth Science and Environmental Medicine: The Synthesis of the Late Enlightenment', in *Images of the Earth: Essays in the History of the Environmental Sciences*, ed. L. J. Jordanova and Roy S. Porter (London: The British Society for the History of Science, 1979), 125.

[36] Harrison, *Medicine in an Age of Commerce and Empire: Britain and its Tropical Colonies, 1660–1830*, 33–4. Harrison notes that 'd'Orta had nothing to say about the effects of climate on European bodies', *Climates & Constitutions: Health, Race, Environment and British Imperialism in India, 1600–1850* (New Delhi and New York: Oxford University Press, 1999), 27.

[37] Garcia de Orta, Francisco Manuel de Melo Ficalho, and Clements R. Markham, *Colloquies on the Simples and Drugs of India* (London: H. Sotheran and Co., 1913), 1. Timothy Walker, 'Acquisition and Circulation of Medical Knowledge within the Early Modern Portuguese Colonial Empire', in *Science in the Spanish and Portuguese Empires, 1500–1800*, ed. Daniela Bleichmar, Paula De Vos, and Kristin Huffine (Stanford: Stanford University Press, 2008), 251–2.

[38] Orta, Ficalho, and Markham, 1–2.

The focus of the *Colloquies*, then – as with later works by Nicolás Monardes and Cristobál Acosta – was less on the distinctiveness of disease environments outside Europe and considerably more on the description of natural historical products that could be put to use in grappling with familiar ailments.[39] D'Orta's book is credited with offering the first Western description of the symptoms of Asiatic cholera, yet D'Orta himself made little of the disease's novelty, noting that it was known in the Latinate world as *Colerica Passio*, although the Indian form 'is more acute than in our country, for it generally kills in twenty-four hours'.[40] He offered no explanation for this difference and his discussion of the disease's aetiology made no mention of climatic differences between Goa and Europe. To Ruano's question: 'What men are most liable to take this disease, and at what time of the year is it most prevalent?', d'Orta's answer was as much moral as medical, pointing to excesses of the flesh:

Those who eat most, and those who consume most food. I knew a young priest here who died of eating cucumbers. Also those who have much intercourse with women. The disease is most prevalent in June and July, which is the winter in this country. As it is brought on by over-eating, the Indians call it MORXI, which means, according to them, a disease caused by much eating.[41]

Among the first physicians to write in what we should probably term a neo-Hippocratic *Airs, Waters, and Places* tradition was Prosper Alpini (1553–1616), who published a work on Egyptian medicine (*De Medicina Aegyptiorum*) in 1591. Alpini completed a medical degree at Padua in 1578. Two years later, after becoming physician to Giorgio Emo, Venetian Consul to Cairo, he accompanied Emo to Egypt, where he stayed for three years before returning to Venice. In 1603 he became Director of the botanical garden at Padua.[42] *De Medicina Aegyptiorum* was written, like D'Orta's book, as a dialogue between the author and a friend; in this case Alpini's master at Padua and a former director of the Botanical Garden, Melchior Guilandino. An introduction detailed Alpini's adventures with Emo on their way to Alexandria. (As a nineteenth-century commentator noted, dryly: 'When a man undertakes a voyage, and afterward writes a book, one may be pretty sure that he meets with a storm in which he is

---

[39] On Monardes' *Historia medicinal de las cosas que se traen de nuestras Indias Occidentales que sirven en medicina* (1565–74), see Daniela Bleichmar, 'Books, Bodies, and Fields: Sixteenth-Century Transatlantic Encounters with New World Materia Medica', in *Colonial Botany: Science, Commerce, and Politics in the Early Modern World*, ed. Londa Schiebinger and Claudia Swan (Philadelphia: University of Pennsylvania Press, 2005). Cook describes Acosta's (1578) *Trata de las drogas y medicinas de las Indias Orientales* as 'almost entirely derivative of Orta'. Harold J. Cook, *Matters of Exchange: Commerce, Medicine, and Science in the Dutch Golden Age* (New Haven and London: Yale University Press, 2007), 200.

[40] Orta, Ficalho, and Markham, 155.

[41] Ibid., 158.

[42] Jerry Stannard, 'Alpini, Prospero', in *Complete Dictionary of Scientific Biography* (Detroit: Charles Scribner's Sons, 2008).

nearly shipwrecked. Alpinus forms no exception to the general rule.')[43] Of the four books into which the main text was broken, the latter three were largely concerned with a description of Egyptian medical practices. Alpini was, for the most part, a critical witness, believing, for example, that Egyptian physicians bled too much and too often. In the first book, however, he described the climate and characteristic diseases of the country. To Guilandino's question as to whether there were many diseases 'which the Greeks call endemic',[44] Alpini answered that there were, and proceeded to offer a long list, including 'what the Greeks call ophthalmia' (caused by a local 'nitrous dust' that inflamed the eyes); leprosy (explained by an Egyptian diet that involved, he claimed, the consumption of salted and rotten fish); and elephantiasis (another illness the physician ascribed to dietary causes, brought on by the consumption of local fish, by bad water, and by vegetables like yams and cabbages, which Alpini argued generated a thick and viscous phlegm that gravitated to the feet, producing the malady's characteristic tumours.)[45] Among the most oft-referenced parts of Alpini's text was his discussion of the plague, which he claimed had taken half a million lives in Cairo alone in the year he arrived. The physician sought to refute common notions about the disease, which had killed so many in Europe, first in the fourteenth century and intermittently thereafter. It was a very rare occurrence, Alpini argued, for the plague to be produced in Egypt itself. Such an event required unusually large flooding of the Nile. Certainly, the disease was neither produced nor reproduced in the country every seven years, as some had claimed. Instead, it spread contagiously from Greece, Syria, and the Barbary Coast.[46] For European readers with much more than an academic interest in questions of the origin and means of transmission of the plague, Alpini's views remained points of reference and contention well into the nineteenth century.

Alpini's was, of course, a scholarly medical text, filled with learned references to classical sources. But the association between places and diseases was accepted far beyond the university's walls. Travelling through the Middle East in 1596–7, Fynes Moryson encountered an area on the road toward Constantinople where a 'Fenny Plaine lies, and the mountains, though more remote, doe barre the sight of the Sunne, and the boggy earth yielding ill vapours makes Sanderona infamous for the death of Christians'.[47] At roughly

[43] Joseph Ince, 'Prosper Alpinus, de Medicina Aegyptiorum Libri Quatuor. A. D. 1591', *Pharmaceutical Journal and Transactions* II (1860): 368.

[44] Prosper Alpinus and Jacobus Bontius, *Prosperi Alpini, Medicina Aegyptiorum ... Ut Et Jacobi Bontii, Medicina Indorum* (Apud Lugduni Batavorum: Gerardum Potvliet, 1745), 49; Prosper Alpini, *La Médicine Des Egyptiens*, trans. R. de Fenoyl (Paris: Institut français d'archéologie orientale, 1980), 87.

[45] Alpini, *La Médicine Des Egyptiens*, 93, 99.

[46] Ibid., 104–24.

[47] Wear, 445.

the same time, 'G.W'. – identified in the 1915 reproduction of his 1598 text as 'the poet and swashbuckler, George Whetstone' – penned a work on *The Cures of the Diseased in Forraine Attempts of the English Nation*.[48] The dedication, to Queen Elizabeth, mentions Whetstone's 'iniust imprisonment in *Spayne*', the illness he contracted, and his cure 'by an especiall Phisition of that King', from whom he learned 'his methode for the same, and such other Diseases, as have perished your Maiesties people in the *Southerne* parts'. The same disease that had laid him low, Whetstone claimed, was the means by which 'whole Kingdomes in both the *Indias* have been depopulated'.[49] One finds no reference to Hippocrates, Galen, or any other medical writers in the short work, but the force of the *Airs, Waters, and Places* tradition seems clear in afflictions such as the 'Erizipila', 'a Disease very much raigning in those Countries, the rather proceeding of the unwholesome aires and vapours, that hot Climates doo yield, whereof many people doo perish'.[50]

It does seem to me, however, that it requires too much of a stretch to associate all comments that relate health to location with the arguments in *Airs, Waters, and Places*. Where the Hippocratic text was concerned with the relationship between specific afflictions and the locations in which they were found, much of the non-medical discourse – unsurprisingly, since it was often written by explorers, current or prospective settlers, or those more interested in geography than the physician's arts – seems concerned with the more general and rather simpler question of whether particular sites were healthy or not. More specific and widespread references to this specific Hippocratic work would appear to be the product of the mid-seventeenth century onward. We should also be wary of assuming that even such weakly Hippocratic ideas were uncontested. Among early modern sailors seeking to circumnavigate the globe, for example, the insistence on the differences between lands took a back seat to the more profound distinction between the earth's terrestrial and aqueous surfaces. They believed, Chaplin has argued, 'that all humans suffered from being removed from land and that any land was sufficient to recover them; this was an especially strong countercurrent against the airs, waters, places tradition, and at odds with other beliefs that differentiated among human bodies in place-specific ways'.[51]

This maritime counter-narrative lasted until at least the mid-eighteenth century. From that point sailors' beliefs that any land – and only land – could cure

---

[48] G. W., 'The Cures of the Diseased in Forraine Attempts of the English Nation, London, 1598. Reproduced in Facsimile', ed. Charles Joseph Singer (Oxford: Clarendon Press, 1915), 'Introduction', 5.

[49] Ibid., 10.

[50] Ibid., 17.

[51] Joyce E. Chaplin, 'Earthsickness: Circumnavigation and the Terrestrial Human Body, 1520–1800', *Bulletin of the History of Medicine* 86, no. 4 (2012): 517.

scurvy, that classic naval disease, came under increasing criticism. A belief in 'earthsickness' (a need and longing for the land that paralleled homesickness) seems to have faded quickly in the wake of James Cook's voyages and his much popularised cures for scorbutic illnesses. Considerably before that, of course, the age of exploration had given way to the age of empire, and for the majority of those who concerned themselves with events beyond the bounds of Europe, Hippocrates' text increasingly provided a template for new ways of discussing novel locations for trade and conquest. In 1645, slightly more than fifty years after its first appearance, Alpini's book was republished, bound together with a work on the diseases of the East Indies: Jacob Bontius' *De Medicina Indorum*.[52]

Born in 1591, the son of the first professor of medicine at the University of Leiden, Bontius obtained his medical degree in 1614 and began to try and build a practice. By the mid-1620s, however (as he later noted in a letter to his brother), he had decided that the competition in his native land was too great. 'The profits of physic were small on account of the multitude of medicasters', he wrote, acknowledging the perspicacity of his sibling's counsel to 'make for the fertile plains of Java, where, to speak ingenuously, virtue is held in some higher esteem'.[53] In 1627 he sailed with his family to the East Indies. Bontius was, however, to be no mere physician. He was appointed to oversee all the medical operations of the Dutch East India Company, tasked with running the hospital in Batavia, supervising the medical outfitting of the Company's ships, inspecting the settlement's physicians and surgeons, and providing medical care for the most eminent men in the Company's service.[54]

Apart from these many medical duties, Bontius was also expected to provide a natural history of Holland's oriental holdings. He seems to have revelled in this latter task. As soon as he arrived in the East Indies, he wrote to his brother, 'I applied myself not only to attain a knowledge of the herbs growing here in Java, but likewise to acquire a more perfect idea of the aromatics in which our part of the country is the most fruitful'.[55] Illness plagued his family's first few years. He lost his first wife before he reached the Indies, his second in 1630 (less than three years after their marriage), and his eldest son in 1631. Bontius himself had fallen dangerously ill twice, both times while Batavia was being (unsuccessfully) besieged by Sultan Agung, king of the Mataram Sultanate.

---

[52] Prosper Alpinus and Jacobus Bontius, *P. Alpini, De Medicina Aegyptiorum & Jacobus Bontii, De Medicina Indorum* (Paris: Nicalaus Redelichuysen, 1645).

[53] James Bontius, *An Account of the Diseases, Natural History, and Medicines of the East Indies* (London: John Donaldson, 1776), 169.

[54] Harold J. Cook, 'Global Economies and Local Knowledge in the East Indies: Jacobus Bontius Learns the Facts of Nature', in *Colonial Botany: Science, Commerce, and Politics in the Early Modern World*, ed. Londa Schiebinger and Claudia Swan (Philadelphia: University of Pennsylvania Press, 2005).

[55] Bontius, 167.

Botany apparently occupied his mind even through his afflictions. '[W]ould to God', he wrote in 1629, 'that the disease, by which I have been confined these four months, still permitted me, as for long after I arrived here, to roam thro' the delightful circumambient woods of Java, and attain a more perfect knowledge of the many noble herbs which are to be met with in this country'.[56]

As with earlier writers about the New World, Bontius was very explicit about the connection between his medical and natural historical interests. Where diseases were endemial, he noted, 'there the bountiful hand of nature has profusely planted herbs whose virtues are adapted to counteract them'.[57] These endemial diseases were many; so profuse in fact that Bontius claimed that his discussion was limited only to those maladies whose manifestation or cure was different to that known in Europe. Like Alpini, he placed great stress on certain climates' capacities to promote putrefaction. At pains to refute the notion that the air in this part of the 'torrid zone' was hot and dry, Bontius argued that the island's warm and moist atmosphere was the principal cause of the cholera morbus, a potentially deadly disease, aggravated by locals' excessive consumption of fruit.[58] The airs, waters, and places of the country, that is, had a profound effect on its characteristic illnesses. How strongly indebted Bontius was to a neo-Hippocratic tradition may be seen from the following long discussion of the fever known as 'Tymorenses, peculiar to the Indies'.

This fever arises from various causes, of which the principal are these: the smell of the saunders tree when newly felled; which (on the testimony of the inhabitants of the country) sends out from its bark some vapours of I know not what poisonous quality, and noxious to the brain ... Besides, the constitution of the air is thick, and extremely heavy: for, the dwellings of the inhabitants are on the highest mountains, where on account of the situation, clouds and watery vapours prevail. The cold, likewise, is sometimes as severe as in Holland: all which concur to produce thick humours and turbid spirits. Add to these several causes, the custom, in this country, of eating a great deal of fruits, which as they are for the most part green, and on account of their moisture, obnoxious to putrefaction, generate bad juices in people whose constitutions have been altered by the sea, hard labour, gross diet, and intemperature of the air.[59]

This is a Hippocratic litany: local plants, the patient's geographic and altitudinal situation, the temperature of their surroundings, their diet, and habits.

1.2   The Flexibility of the Hippocratic Tradition

And yet, even in this passage, one also sees the problem in associating Hippocratic ideas with the notion of which Sloane was apparently critical: that

---

[56] Ibid., 24.
[57] Ibid., 27.
[58] Ibid., 52.
[59] Ibid., 66–7.

diseases were all different in different places. For, as often as not, *De Medicina Indorum* sought to draw parallels between European nations and the Indies. One might note above that one of the causes of the Tymorenses was not, in fact, the humid climate for which Java was famed, but rather the cold of its mountains, which was 'sometimes as severe as in Holland'. Indeed, the passage quoted above continued with a longer comparison:

I had almost omitted to subjoin, as another cause, the sudden change of air which our people experience when they descend from the cold mountains to the shore and the ships, where they are scorched with heat ... What are also greatly to be guarded against, are the winds which blow from the mountains after midnight, in Java and the circumadjacent islands: just as in some of the southern parts of France and Italy, especially in the kingdom of Naples, and the territory of the Pope, the cold wind which blows from the hills, and is called the serene, produces pleurisies, peripneumonies, and other acute disorders.[60]

Nor are these invocations of similarity solely to be found in discussion of cold-weather afflictions. The consumption of fruit, Bontius argued, contributed greatly toward the production of dysentery. Were a person incautious, eating the local produce 'without rice, or bread, or a little salt, he scarcely can escape the disorder'. Yet, the same thing happened in France and Spain, 'where people, who eat much grapes without bread, are immediately seized with a Diarrheoea or Dysentery'.[61] The myriad constructions of both similarity and difference in fact follow from the logic of Hippocrates' own text. To be sure, where climates were diametrically opposed, one found radically different diseases. But such oppositional climates were largely abstractions. 'It is not everywhere the same with regard to Asia',[62] Hippocrates acknowledged of Europe's counterpart. Indeed, the opposition between a uniform East and a changeable West might be read as much as pedagogic as literally descriptive, for *Airs, Waters, and Places* concluded by noting that the text had largely concerned itself with extremes: 'Thus it is with regard to the most opposite natures and shapes; drawing conclusions from them, you may judge of the rest without any risk of error'.[63]

This flexible aspect of the Hippocratic tradition in fact proved to be of crucial importance in the discussion of the New World. Few writers in British North America, for example, had an interest as portraying their climate as antithetical, and hence potentially inimical, to that found at home. Colonists

---

[60] Ibid.
[61] Ibid., 15. Harrison suggests that '[t]his mention of France and Spain – both Catholic countries – is perhaps significant, in as much as the Dutch Protestant Bontius may be equating dietary indulgence with the supposed laxity of these nations'. Harrison, *Climates & Constitutions: Health, Race, Environment and British Imperialism in India, 1600–1850*, 49.
[62] Hippocrates. 'Airs, Waters, and Places', 206.
[63] Ibid., 222.

declared America to be England's sister or mother, and emphasised those parts of each country that lay within the same latitudinal bounds. George Peckham, describing America's appearance on Mercator's map, claimed that the 'Counterey dooth (as it were with arme advaunced) above the climats both of Spayne and Fraunce, stretche out it selfe towards England onlie'.[64] For some, America's climate was not only not detrimental, it was positively salutary for the sons and daughters of Albion. For Francis Higginson, in 1630, 'the Temper of the Aire in *New-England* is one speciall thing that commends this place. Experience doth manifest that there is hardly a more healthfull place to be found in the World that agreeth better with our English Bodyes'.[65] A 'sup' of this air, he suggested, 'is better than a whole draft of old England's ale'.[66] *Airs, Waters, and Places* certainly suggested that different diseases were to be found in different climates. But there was considerable disagreement over whether climates in very different geographical locations were, in fact, radically distinct.

One found fewer defenders of the climate in Africa, where discussions turned on the slave trade rather than settlement. If Asia had been Europe's foil for Hippocrates, Africa increasingly took on that role after the discovery of the New World. In the late seventeenth century, Willem Bosman spent more than a dozen years as Chief Factor for the Dutch on the Guinea Coast. In 1704 he wrote a description of that time in the form of a series of letters to a physician friend (now identified as Dr Havart, who had served as a surgeon in the service of the Dutch West India Company).[67] The book was rapidly translated into other European languages: English and French in 1705; German in 1708; Italian in 1752. The book's popularity presumably stemmed from the fact that Bosman was largely correct in declaring that:

[T]he Coast of Guinea, which is part of Africa, is for the most part unknown, not only to the Dutch, but to all Europeans, and no particular description of it is yet come to light; nor indeed any thing, but a few scraps, scattered in books written upon other subjects, most of which are contrary to truth, and afford but a sorry sketch of Guinea.[68]

---

[64] Joyce E. Chaplin, *Subject Matter: Technology, the Body, and Science on the Anglo-American Frontier, 1500–1676* (Cambridge, MA: Harvard University Press, 2001), 134.

[65] Ibid., 154.

[66] Wear, 454.

[67] Willem Bosman, *A New and Accurate Description of the Coast of Guinea, Divided into the Gold, the Slave, and the Ivory Coasts ... Illustrated with Several Cutts. Written Originally in Dutch by William Bosman ... To Which Is Prefix'd, an Exact Map of the Whole Coast of Guinea* (London: Printed for James Knapton, and Dan. Midwinter, 1705). Albert Van Dantzig, 'Willem Bosman's "New and Accurate Description of the Coast of Guinea"· How Accurate Is It?', *History in Africa* 1 (1974). I use the English edition in the discussion below, but see: 'English Bosman and Dutch Bosman: A Comparison of Texts', *History in Africa* 2 (1975).

[68] Bosman, Preface, 1.

Few who read the text could envy Bosman his time in the region. With rare exceptions – and most of those in the past – the country was described as unwholesome and deadly. Better care and cultivation might improve it, but at present Guinea bore a 'dreadful mortal name'.[69] The Isle of St Thomé, he claimed, was known in Europe as 'the Dutch Church-Yard', and even the Portuguese, to whom the Dutch had ceded the island, were, 'tho' more used to this scorching Air', dying in huge numbers.[70] The first time Bosman visited the Kingdom of Benin, he noted, 'we lost half our men'.[71] He wrote to Havart during his second voyage there, observing that an equal number of men were now dead, that most of the rest were sick, and that this had 'struck such general terrour into the Sailors, that the oldest of them is afraid of his life'. The problem was the place itself. Sudden changes between the heat of the day and the cold of the night induced diseases in European bodies. Even worse was the 'thick, stinking, and sulphurous' mist which spread through the valleys. '[I]f this odious Mixture of noisome stenches very much affects the state of health here', wrote Bosman, 'it is not to be wondered, since 'tis next to impossibility, not only for new Comers, but those who have long continued here, to preserve themselves intirely from its malign Effects'. The only people to be spared the ravages of the destructive mist were the 'Natives', since they were 'bred up in the Stench' and hence, presumably, were unaffected by it.[72] Yet they had their own diseases, in particular small pox and the worm named for the region. Worst for their health were their moral sensibilities, about which Bosman was vicious. 'The Negroes are all without exception, Crafty, Villanous, and Fraudulent, and very seldom to be trusted', and their 'too early and excessive venery' was given as the reason that, despite otherwise healthy lives, natives 'seldom arrive to a great Age'.[73]

The difference between this early eighteenth-century description of the disease environment of Africa, and those given of the West Indies at the same time is striking. Clearly no sense of a disease environment common to the tropics yet existed. But perhaps nothing makes clearer the relative health of the two parts of the world in European eyes than the changing claims about the origins of a disease that had been associated with the Americas almost since the time of Columbus: syphilis. By the 1530s, the new disease was laid at the feet of America's Indians, a new people who were unfamiliar with the word of Christ and who were portrayed as without any moral restraint. 'They have as many wives as they desire', wrote Amerigo Vespucci, 'they live in promiscuity without regard to blood relations; mothers lie with sons, brothers with sisters;

[69] Ibid., 17.
[70] Ibid., 414.
[71] Ibid., 429.
[72] Ibid., 105–6, 108.
[73] Ibid., 117, 10.

they satisfy their desires as they occur to their libidos as beasts do'.[74] Against this orthodoxy, however, Daniel Turner, in a 1717 text on the disease, noted that no less a figure than Thomas Sydenham (soon to become known as the English Hippocrates) denied the New World origin of syphilis.[75] Sydenham acknowledged the (by then) common explanation, which traced the disease from the West Indies to Europe the year after Columbus' discovery: 'But it seems rather to me', he argued, 'to have taken its rise from some Region of the Blacks near *Guinea*, for I have learn'd from many of our People of good Credit, who live in the *Caribbee-Islands*, that the Slaves brought from *Guinea*, even before they land, and also those that live there, have this Disease without impure Copulation'.[76] As we will see in Chapter 2, the idea that it was African slaves who were ultimately responsible for many virulent West Indian diseases, and not the country's own climate, would become a central trope from the mid-eighteenth century onwards.

Like America and unlike Guinea, the West Indies had many settlers who served as boosters and propagandists, unwilling to have the islands dismissed as intrinsically unhealthy. And, perhaps more generally, as Bontius' example shows, writers had become somewhat leery of classical distinctions, particularly those among the frigid (or polar), temperate, and torrid (or tropical) zones. From the late fifteenth century, scholars and explorers had argued that there was clearly a problem in the division between a habitable 'temperate' region below the Polar Circle and above the Tropic of Cancer and the uninhabitable areas that were supposed to bound it.[77] As Tomaso Giunti noted in 1563: '[I]t is clearly able to be understood that this entire earthly globe is marvelously inhabited, nor is there any part of it empty, neither by heat nor by cold deprived of inhabitants'.[78] Increasingly, the areas between the Tropics were portrayed not

---

[74] Anna Foa, 'The New and the Old: The Spread of Syphilis (1494–1530)', in *Sex and Gender in Historical Perspective*, ed. Edward Muir and Guido Ruggiero (Baltimore: Johns Hopkins University Press, 1990), 31–2.

[75] Daniel Turner, *Syphilis. A Practical Dissertation on the Venereal Disease … In Two Parts* (London: Printed for R. Bonwicke, Tim. Goodwin, J. Walthoe, M. Wotton, S. Manship, Richard Wilkin, Benj. Tooke, R. Smith, and Tho. Ward, 1717).

[76] Sydenham continued: 'It seems therefore probable to me, that the *Spaniards*, that first brought the Disease into *Europe*, were infected with it by the Contagion of the Blacks bought in *Africa*, to some Nation whereof it may be Endemial; for there are many People that border upon *Guinea*, among whom that barbarous Custom of changing Men for Ware prevails'. Thomas Sydenham, *The Whole Works of That Excellent Practical Physician, Dr. Thomas Sydenham Wherein Not Only the History and Cures of Acute Diseases Are Treated Of … But Also the Shortest and Fastest Way of Curing Most Chronical Diseases*, 9th ed. (London: Printed for J. Darby, A. Bettesworth, and F. Clay, in trust for Richard, James, and Bethel Wellington, 1729), 247–8.

[77] See, in general, Nicolás Wey Gómez, *The Tropics of Empire: Why Columbus Sailed South to the Indies* (Cambridge, MA: MIT Press, 2008).

[78] Quoted in John M. Headley, 'The Sixteenth Century Venetian Celebration of the Earth's Total Habitability: The Issue of the Fully Habitable World for Renaissance Europe', *Journal of World History* 8, no. 1 (1997): 3.

as searing deserts, but as seasonally constant versions of climates with which Europeans were familiar. The Bermudas were, for the poet Edmund Waller in 1645 (playing on the name of the company that had held the charter for the islands at the time) the 'summer isles'. Switching seasons in the main text, he contrasted the idyllic region – 'so moderate the clime' – with England: 'For the kind Spring which but salutes us here/Inhabits there and courts them all the year'.[79] In 1682, Abraham Cowley lyricised about the 'temprate summer' to be found in the tropics: 'More rich than Autumn and the Spring more fair'.[80] Nor was this merely a poetic trope. In 1679, the Jamaican doctor, Thomas Trapham described Jamaica approvingly as 'a summer country' with a 'whole summer year'.[81]

It should be noted, of course, that although such claims demonstrated a cosmopolitan enthusiasm for places beyond one's home, they were not devoid of Eurocentrism. For their effect was to render England, in particular, a microcosm for the globe. The seasons experienced over the course of a year in Britain were mapped on to the climates of other parts of the world, at all times. The analogy between European seasons and foreign climates had been in Hippocrates. Asia, it was claimed in *Airs, Waters, and Places* 'both as regards its constitution and mildness of the seasons, may be said to bear a close resemblance to the spring'.[82] The point was much more systematically enunciated, however, in the late seventeenth and early eighteenth centuries: indeed, almost precisely at the same time that Sloane published the first volume of his *Voyage*. In 1696, William Cockburn related 'hotter constitutions, hot Countries, or a warmer Season'.[83] A dozen years later, in 1708, John Polus Lecaan published a work purporting to offer advice to aid English forces in southern Europe, and 'all other hot Climates, as our Plantations in the West Indies, &c'. 'If then the difference of Season produces in our Bodies different Effects', he wrote, 'no

---

[79] 'The Battel of the *Summer-Islands*' in Edmund Waller, *The Works of Edmund Waller, Esq., in Verse and Prose: Published by Mr. Fenton* (London: J. and R. Tonton and S. Draper, 1744), 52–4.

[80] Abraham Cowley, *The Poetical Works of Abraham Cowley in Four Volumes* (Edinburgh: Apollo Press, 1784), 203.

[81] Trapham, 3 & 59. 'Drawing upon the early Spanish promotion of the Caribbean', Parrish notes, 'writers promoting the British "Sugar-Isles" painted a world always green and fertile while ignoring the more distempered facts of earthquakes and hurricanes'. Parrish, *American Curiosity*, 32.

[82] Hippocrates. 'Airs, Waters, and Places', 206. In this, Asia was, therefore, also like an East facing city, which 'resembles the spring as to moderation between heat and cold', 194.

[83] W. Cockburn, *An Account of the Nature, Causes, Symptoms, and Cure of the Distempers that are Incident to Seafaring People with Observations on the Diet of the Sea-Men in His Majesty's Navy: Illustrated with Some Remarkable Instances of the Sickness of the Fleet During the Last Summer, Historically Related* (London: Hugh Newman, 1696), 51. Cf. 109–10: 'These, by the bye, are the fatal, but almost perpetual, consequences of a diaphoretical practice in Fevers; especially on young people, in a hot season of the year, or a warm climate'.

doubt but the Difference of Climate, and Change of Diet, will likewise alter our Constitutions'.[84] Earlier, he had made a similar point in more detail:

As in other countries the Differences of Seasons produce different Effects in our Bodies; for by the more or less Heat the Pores of our Bodies are more or less open, the Air more or less pure, Food more or less spirituous; so without doubt great Difference of Climate, or of Heat or Cold, is very prejudicial to all Strangers, and the cause of numerous Distempers, especially to the *English*, who are very Irregular and Careless in their way of Living.[85]

The following year, J. Christie, in his *Abstract of Some Years Observations Concerning such General and Unperceived Occasions of Sickliness in Fleets and Ships of War*, was considerably less prolix, both in title and text: 'as the Season or Climate are varied', he stated simply, 'so do all our Distempers vary to the very same kinds'.[86]

1.3   Local Knowledge and Medical Expertise

The analogy between seasons and climates had a rather clear corollary. If the West Indies were, like other warm climates, just like Europe in a given season, it should follow that the diseases found in such climates should be similar to seasonal distempers in Europe. That is – even as a good Hippocratic – one would not necessarily expect to find that diseases were, as Sloane intimated he had been told, 'all different from what they are in Europe'. Richard Ligon's brief remarks in his *True and Exact History of the Island of Barbadoes* might function as one example, although it is not quite clear whether he regarded the differences between the diseases of England and Barbados as those of degree or kind. '[S]icknesses are there more grievous', he wrote, 'and mortality greater by far, than in *England*, and these diseases many times contagious'. In terms of treatment, Ligon encouraged physicians to learn about the 'simples' to be found in the Caribbean: 'For certainly every Climate produces Simples more proper to cure the diseases that are bred there, than those that are transported

---

[84] John Polus Lecaan, *Advice to the Gentlemen of the Army of Her Majesty's Forces in Spain and Portugal: With a Short Method How to Preserve Their Health; and Some Observations Upon Several Distempers Incident to Those Countries, and All Other Hot Climates, as Our Plantations in the West-Indies, &C. To Which Are Added the Medicinal Virtues of Many Peculiar Plants Growing Naturally in Those Parts, and Not Wild in England.* (London: P. Varenne, 1708), 20.

[85] Ibid., 4.

[86] J. Christie, *An Abstract of Some Years Observations Concerning Such General and Unperceived Occasions of Sickliness in Fleets and Ships of War* (1709), 3. See also Stubbes: 'in hot Countreys, as well as in hot seasons, the rule of *Hippoc.* takes place'. Henry Stubbes, 'An Enlargement of the Observations, Formerly Publisht Numb. 27, Made and Generously Imparted by That Learn'd and Inquisitive Physician, Dr. Stubbes', *Philosophical Transactions* 3 (1668): 709.

from any other part of the world: such care the great Physitian to mankind takes for our convenience'.[87] It is worth noting, however, that Sloane knew of at least one major source (and the number of such sources was small)[88] in large agreement with his own position, namely that the diseases of the West Indies were essentially the same as those familiar to a European physician.[89] The text was Hickeringill's *Jamaica Viewed*, which had appeared first in 1661. A new edition of the work, of which Sloane owned a copy, was published in 1705.[90] The discussion of the disease environment in the West Indies was short, but one suspects that the following passage, rich with analogies to the growth of plants, would have caught Sloane's eye:

That though *Infant-Settlements*, like *Infant-Years*, are usually most fatal; yet their *Blossoms* once set, are not so easily *Blasted*. Happily experimented in *Jamaica*, whose blooming hopes now thrive so well, and their Stocks so well *Rooted*, that they are not easily *Routed*. The Major part of the Inhabitants being old *West-Indians*, who, now *Naturalized* to the Country, grow better by their *Transplantation*, and flourish in Health equivalently comparable to that of their *Mother-Soil*. For which I need not beg Credit, since there is no *Country Disease* (as at *Virginia* and *Surinam*) endemically raging throughout the Isle; nor any new and unheard of Distempers that want a *name*.[91]

Given how few sources were available at the time on diseases in Jamaica, and given that they clearly do not all argue that the diseases there were all different to those found in Europe, it seems likely that Sloane had something rather specific in mind when he sought to counter this claim. Indeed, I would

[87] Richard Ligon, *A True and Exact History of the Island of Barbados* (London: Humphrey Moseley, 1657), 117, 18. The idea that cures of local afflictions were to be found nearby was common enough that it was often referenced through a Latin tag: *ubi morbus, ibi remedium*. See James Lind, *A Treatise of the Scurvy. In Three Parts. Containing an Inquiry into the Nature, Causes, and Cure of That Disease. Together with a Critical and Chronological View of What Has Been Published on the Subject* (London: A. Millar, 1753), 263.

[88] It was not merely that the number of *medical* writings about the West Indies was small. '[T]he island colonists', notes Dunn, 'publicized their doings very little. Back in the Elizabethan era, when English sailors knew the Antilles far better than the North American coast, reports from the New World centered on the Caribbean. But after 1607 the focus shifted decisively north … None of the islands boasted a printing press, nor did the islanders use the London presses. During the entire course of the century eight or ten promotional tracts designed to lure immigrants to the Caribbean colonies were issued in England, whereas the Virginia Company sponsored some twenty propaganda pieces in the period from 1609 to 1612 alone'. Dunn, *Sugar and Slaves: The Rise of the Planter Class in the English West Indies, 1624–1713*, 23–4.

[89] Stubbes does not suggest that there are diseases peculiar to the West Indies in his Henry Stubbes, 'Observations Made by a Curious and Learned Person, Sailing from England, to the Caribe-Islands', *Philosophical Transactions* 2 (1666); 'An Enlargement of the Observations, Formerly Publisht Numb. 27, Made and Generously Imparted by That Learn'd and Inquisitive Physician, Dr. Stubbes'.

[90] Churchill, 398.

[91] Edmund Hickeringill, *Jamaica Viewed with All the Ports, Harbours, and Their Several Soundings, Towns, and Settlements Thereunto Belonging.*, 3rd ed. (London: Printed and sold by B. Bragg, 1705), 41–2. Cf. Churchill, 427–8.

suggest that we do not read Sloane's claims as transparent descriptions of the medical consensus in the late seventeenth century, but rather as a fairly pointed response to another text: Trapham's. For Trapham had made the argument that Sloane opposed very clearly in his *Discourse*. Due to its climate, Trapham claimed, Jamaica was a much more salubrious country than England, being largely free of many of the diseases that plagued the colder country. 'As for diseases usually found here', he suggested:

they are far short of the long beadrowl [beadroll] which infest our native country: No small Pox or very rarely, saving sometimes brought from *Guinny* by Negroes, terrify or remark us; no Scurvy that almost universal contagion of our native country is got here, or continued if brought; no depopulating Plague that ere I have heard of in the West *Indies*; Consumption nothing so frequent, and when, never so piningly tedious. As for Venereal Affects their symptoms are all lessened, and their discharge more easy far than in colder climes[.][92]

And just as local conditions affected the manifestations of diseases, they also affected their treatment.

For that the place alters much the cure of the Disease, I question not; wherefore Holland which is cold and moist requires a double dose generally of that Physick, whereof in France single will well work and serve the turn. And in a confirmed Pox, they generally remove from one to the other place, from heavier phlegmatick low Countries to the more brisk and drier Air of *France*, placing much of cure in the nature of the Region. And ours of Jamaica being so sweatingly warm, and the air from its Nitre piercingly cleansing, assists much our ready cure[.][93]

Reading Sloane against Trapham opens the text to a much more natural interpretation than is commonly accorded it. For Sloane's claim was *not* that climate had no effect on disease. As a protégé of the famed London physician, Thomas Sydenham, such a position would be profoundly odd. Indeed, to determine what Sloane's argument was, it is useful to keep the dicta of Sydenham in mind, as we will see below.

We should, I think, take both seriously and literally Sloane's clear claim that he encountered virtually no *new* diseases in Jamaica. As Churchill has shown, more than a third of the 128 case histories that made up the section of *Voyage* entitled 'Of the Diseases I observed in Jamaica, and the Method by which I used to cure them', are made up of three kinds of illness then all too familiar to the European doctor: twenty-six intermittent fevers, nine cases of 'belly-ach', and eleven of venereal afflictions.[94] One reads of 'tertians', 'dropsies',

---

[92] A beadroll was, originally, 'a list of persons to be specially prayed for', and hence, later, 'a list or string of names'. The OED gives the first usage with this latter meaning in 1529. Trapham, 68–9.

[93] Ibid., 122–3.

[94] Churchill, 407.

and lethargy; of miscarriages and attempted abortions; of 'hectics' and 'fluxes' and the effects of excessive alcohol consumption. Sloane includes only one disease seemingly peculiar to 'Blacks' on the Island, a flesh-eating illness that appeared to be governed by the phases of the moon:

The virulency of the Humour was such, as that after it had eaten into the Bone, the joints of the fingers and toes would drop off, and they die, as I have been assur'd by those who have lost several Negros of this Disease, I was assur'd was peculiar to Blacks ... So soon as this Disease again appear'd, I thought, that perhaps this was proper to Blacks, and so might come from some peculiar indisposition of their Black skin ... This was a very strange Disease not only in itself, but that it followed very regularly the Full and New Moon.[95]

Even here, however, one suspects that Sloane, who – generally, in this text – downplayed any physiological differences between Blacks, Indians, and Europeans, might well have placed this 'strange Disease' into the category of those 'singular disease[s]' that one encountered even in England.[96]

Overall, Sloane was greatly loath to ascribe any oddities in diseases to general climatic causes. Thus, discussing a fever that lasted less than a day, but caused a degree of weakness that one normally associated with illnesses that lasted months, he wrote: 'This was, I think, peculiar to this Fever, though at first I suspected it was to all diseases here, by reason of the hot climate, but I found all other diseases accompanied with the same symptoms as in Europe, and therefore look on this symptom as a thing particular to this fever, and such uncommon symptoms now and then attend Endemic diseases everywhere'.[97] Without mentioning him by name, Sloane rather pointedly refuted Trapham's claim that venereal diseases were more easily treated in the West Indies. 'It is generally believed in Europe', he claimed, 'that Gonorrhea and the Pox are with more ease and sooner, cured in Jamaica and hot countries than in Europe'. Sloane admitted that he himself 'was of the opinion of the

---

[95] Sloane, cvi–cvii.

[96] As Cristina Malcolmson has recently shown, Sloane's views on race were complex. While it is generally true, as Churchill has argued, that Sloane 'transgressed categories of gender and race' in the *Voyage*, the same was not true in material presented to the Royal Society. For the Society in the 1690s, Malcolmson shows, members were interested in skin colour generally and the skin of 'Negroes' particularly. In their discussions, Sloane spearheaded the drive to investigate the possibility of race-difference as he attacked the climate theory. At a meeting in March, 1690, Sloane argued that there was a 'Specifick Difference' between 'Negrow' and white skin, which made curing skin diseases and ulcers in the former more difficult than the latter. Sloane also claimed that 'woolly' hair was another characteristic of 'the Negro race of Mankind' and suggested that there were racial differences between skulls, although this latter point seems to have been met with little enthusiasm among the Society's members. Cristina Malcolmson, *Studies of Skin Color in the Early Royal Society: Boyle, Cavendish, Swift* (Farnham: Ashgate, 2013), 65, 76, 7. Sloane's complex and even contradictory positions are elegantly summarised on 189–90.

[97] Sloane, xcvii.

generality of the world when I went to Jamaica'. But he found himself mistaken: Gonorrheas 'have the same symptoms as in Europe ... [I] found as the Disease was propagated there the same way and had the same symptoms and course among Europeans, Indians, and Negroes, so it requir'd the same remedies and time to be cur'd'.[98]

Yet, that one found almost no novel diseases in Jamaica did not mean that one found there all the diseases commonly treated in London, and certainly not that they were as prevalent in a warm climate as a cold one. Such a claim would, in fact, be very peculiar for a follower of Sydenham, who had insisted on the *seasonality* of diseases.[99] If Sloane argued with Trapham's claims about venereal diseases he was notably silent about Trapham's observations concerning the virtual absence of small pox, scurvy ('that almost universal contagion of our native country'), and plague. Small Pox is mentioned once amongst Sloane's cases (and not as the current affliction of the patient being treated);[100] scurvy and the plague not at all. All three of these were commonly associated with cold weather and, in general, winter afflictions are notably absent from Sloane's cases.[101] In a number of cases, in fact, where patients exhibited the symptoms of common cold-weather afflictions, Sloane made a point of explaining their occurrence. Thus, for example, the case of Sir Francis Watson, who suffered from asthma. Sloane pointed out that Watson lived in a location known as 'the Seven Plantations'. 'This place is cooler than the town of St Jago de la Vega and Sir Francis Watson, who lived here used to be more troubled with the *Asthma* than when in town. For this purpose, he had made a chimney in one of the rooms of his house, which was the only one I ever saw on this Island, except in Kitchens'.[102] Elsewhere, Sloane noted the oddity of having to treat patients for consumption in such a sultry climate: 'Although this Climate be very hot, some of these were troubled with true Consumptions, for which I ordered them some easie Opiates, and other Medicines. I have

---

[98] Ibid., cxxviii.

[99] 'Lastly, the seasons of the year that principally promote any particular kind of diseases, are to be carefully remarked. I own that some happen indiscriminately at any time, whilst many others, by a secret tendency of nature, follow the seasons of the year with as much certainty, as some birds and plants. And indeed, I have often wondered, that this tendency of some distempers, which is very obvious, has been hitherto observed but by a few ... [C]ertain it is that knowledge of the seasons in which diseases ordinarily arise is of great use to a physician towards uncovering the species of the disease, as well as the method of curing it; and that the consequence of slighting this piece of knowledge is ill success in both'. 'The Author's Preface' in Thomas Sydenham and Benjamin Rush, *The Works of Thomas Sydenham, M.D., on Acute and Chronic Diseases with Their Histories and Modes of Cure: With Notes, Intended to Accommodate Them to the Present State of Medicine, and to the Climate and Diseases of the United States* (Philadelphia: B. & T. Kite, 1815), xxvi.

[100] A patient's mother notes that the ulcers and other symptoms with which her daughter was currently afflicted 'had come on after the small pox'. Sloane, cxx.

[101] Sloane notes the seasonality of small pox in ibid., l.

[102] Ibid., lx.

observed the same disease about Montpelier, among the Inhabitants of that Place, though the air be esteemed a remedy for it'.[103]

This reference to the warm weather and concomitant diseases that one might experience in Europe was telling, for part of Sloane's overarching argument was that the climates of Jamaica and parts of Europe were not as different as might be imagined. Hence, presumably, the similarity of plant life between the West Indies and 'the South Parts of France'. Sloane took some pains to note that, although Jamaica lay in the 'torrid zone' between the tropics of Cancer and the Equator, 'yet the air of it may very well be affirm'd temperate, in that the heat of the days is qualified by the length of the nights'.[104] Indeed, 'I never found more heat here than as in some valleys near *Montpelier* where the situation of the Hills in their neighbourhood occasioned excessive heat'.[105] On this point one finds Sloane echoing Hickeringill once again. The self-styled 'Jolly Captain' could find little to criticise in Jamaica's weather, claiming that 'I have found the air as sulphurous and hot in *England*, in the months of *June, July, and August* ... as in the hottest seasons in *Jamaica*'.[106] Indeed, for Hickeringill, it was Jamaica that deserved the title 'temperate' more than any location in the Old World: 'Yet as the extremities of cold in these Regions betwixt the *Tropicks* are indisputably more remiss than in *England*, and the rest of *Europe*, so the Heat qualified with the benefit of Breezes, more justly styles them *Temperate*, than those *Climates* that have already falsly, (tho' with vulgar consent) *usurp'd* the title'.[107] Throughout his text, Sloane similarly sprinkled comments that, 'notwithstanding the heat', downplayed the environmental and atmospheric differences between Europe and the West Indies. Hence, for example, 'The Rainbow here is as frequent as any where in times of Rain';[108] 'Falling stars are as common as elsewhere', and thunder had the same effects as in Europe.[109]

It could not be gainsaid, however, that the island's heat had medically significant effects. Those who travelled there from colder climes needed to be seasoned to higher temperatures. It is worth noting, in fact, that while Trapham used neither the term nor the concept of seasoning, Sloane devoted no small amount of attention to it. One suspects that for Trapham, a discussion of the ill effects that might greet a newcomer's arrival would have gone against the boosterism that pervades most of his text. Thus, while he did acknowledge that

---

[103] Ibid., 14.

[104] Ibid., vii. Cf. Hickeringill.

[105] Ibid., ix. In making this point, Sloane was in agreement with Trapham, for both regarded the climate of Jamaica as a very salubrious one. 'The air here', Sloane wrote, 'notwithstanding the heat, is very healthy. I have known Blacks one hundred and twenty years of age, and one hundred years old is very common amongst temperate livers', ibid., ix.

[106] Hickeringill, 2.

[107] Ibid., 4.

[108] Sloane, xxxii.

[109] Ibid., xlv.

those who were newly come to Jamaica might wish to avoid the area around
the port for some time, he also suggested that they regard the diarrhoea or flux
that they were likely to experience as 'a friendly rather than injurious motion
of Nature, caused either by a new sort of Drink & Diet, which falls out in most
places more or less, the which ceaseth without prejudice or any other remedy
than a little time; or else the same may arise from rejoicing intemperance,
too often welcoming the new arrivers'.[110] Sloane had his own criticisms of
the intemperate, but in describing the afflictions of newcomers to Jamaica, he
tended to stress the direct effect of the action of a blazing sun.[111] Furthermore,
whatever the discomfort felt, the body's response was a salutary one.[112]

I did not at all doubt that these eruptions were the effect of the Sun Beams, which
throwing into our blood some fiery parts, put it into brisker motion, whereby it was
purg'd of those *heterogenous* and unaccustom's Particles it had from the warm sun, and
perhaps by that fermentation was likewise clear'd of some other parts might be hurtful
to it ...[113]

The climate of Jamaica, then, was indeed different from that found in Europe –
different enough that those coming from squally England needed to undergo an
uncomfortable seasoning in order to inure them to a warmer part of the globe. One
might expect – and indeed, found – that the winter diseases of cold climates were
relatively or entirely absent. But it was not so bizarrely and extremely different
that profoundly different disease environments might be expected. The key point
for Sloane was that when diseases manifested themselves, they were to be identified and cured in precisely the same ways as they were in Europe. Intermittent
fevers, to take merely one example, did not exhibit one variety in the temperate
zone and another between the tropics and hence did not require different cures
in each place. This was a claim at once ontological and social. Ontologically,
one may note its similarity to doctrines espoused by Sydenham. 'Every specific disease', he wrote, 'arises from a specific exaltation, or peculiar quality of

---

[110] Trapham, 71. Trapham is one of the few authors I have come across who reverses the logic of
seasoning, suggesting that new arrivals from chilly Europe might be *better off* than locals: 'It
may not be improper to remark that those Brezes of the night do less injury to new comers from
the colder Europe than to the more antient inhabitants, whose pores being as it were moulded
into the bore of the Indian Air, are of larger size and more receptive of the chilling Brezes than
such as come from the northern parts: hence also such as pass directly out of Europe hither
are not so easily assaulted with fevorish attracts as those from the *Carib* Isles: for those little
tracts of land of *Barbadoes, Nevis, Monserat &c* being well opened, and therefore affording
nothing so much of night Brezes as the large woody mountains of Jamica do, hath not inured
them thereto, while their greater diurnal heat hath sufficiently disposed them to a most ready
reception of the night cold Invaders', ibid., 10–11.

[111] On the case of a 'Captain Nowel' and his excessive drinking, see James Delbourgo, 'Slavery in
the Cabinet of Curiosities: Hans Sloane's Atlantic World', www.britishmuseum.org/research/
news/hans_sloanes_atlantic_world.aspx (2007), last accessed 15 Jan. 2018.

[112] Sloane, xciv–xcv.

[113] Ibid., 25.

some humour contained in a living body'. Diseases were not, that is, merely the 'confused and irregular operations of disordered and debilitated nature'. Instead, they arose when humours were retained in the body too long, either because Nature could not remove them, because of atmospheric effects, or because they had been infected by some sort of poison. By these, or related causes:

these humours are worked up into a substantial form or species, that discovers itself by particular symptoms, agreeable to its peculiar essence; and these symptoms, notwithstanding they may, for want of attention, seem to arise either from the nature of the part in which the humour is lodged, or from the humour itself before it assumed this species, are in reality disorders that proceed from the essence of the species, newly raised to this pitch[.][114]

This specificity in the *cause* of diseases led to a specificity of both symptoms and methods of cure. Although Sydenham was willing to acknowledge that the age or constitution of a patient might cause some minor variations in the appearance of a given disease, he made no mention at all of differences that might be due to race or (perhaps more tellingly) geographic location. 'The same disease appears attended with the like symptoms in different subjects; so that those which were observed in Socrates, in his illness, may generally be applied to any other person afflicted with the same disease'.[115] Sloane appears to have had the same idea, for although he might often have mentioned the age or humoural constitution of a patient in his case notes, he rarely notes their location (even within the West Indies) except to suggest an environmental explanation for the manifestation of a disease seemingly out of season.

The social or professional significance of Sloane's arguments flows from this insistence on a common ontology for diseases in Jamaica and England. For if diseases differed due to climate, requiring distinct dosages according to place, as Trapham argued, then it would seem to follow that those, like Trapham, who possessed local knowledge, would be at an advantage in curing local manifestations of illnesses. Despite his connections, his training, and his experience in Europe, Sloane could be considered at a disadvantage, since he did not understand 'the country diseases having lived there several years'. Where diseases were identical in both places, however, Sloane's status could be deservedly transferred from England to the West Indies. Sloane's was not at all an argument that denied that Jamaica and Europe were different disease environments. It was an argument, rather, that insisted that the opinions of a high-status metropolitan doctor trumped the views of a Jamaican physician, however much the latter knew of local conditions.[116]

---

[114] Sydenham and Rush, xxx.
[115] Ibid., xxvii.
[116] One can see that this kind of argument would be particularly devastating to any knowledge claims made by local, non-European practitioners.

Again, despite Sloane's (rhetorically powerful) claims to the contrary, he was hardly alone in his views. The debate between those who claimed a kind of universal, or at least easily transferrable, medical knowledge and those claiming superior, locally-based empirical and experiential skills was one that shaped medical practice and socio-professional life throughout the growing empire. We have seen that the debate continued until at least 1750, when it culminated in a duel between two Jamaican physicians. One finds it in print, however, even before Sloane's *Voyage* was published, in a text with which he was probably familiar. In 1696, William Cockburn, a Baronet who would be elected a Fellow to the Royal Society the following year, published the first edition of his *An Account of the Nature, Causes, Symptoms, and Cure of the Distempers that are Incident to Seafaring People.* The work was based on his experiences, beginning in 1694, as one of the first physicians to an English naval fleet. Its aims were, in his words, 'to discover such sicknesses as may be peculiar to people that use our narrow Seas' and to distinguish these both from illnesses on land and those more common closer to the Equator.[117]

While such sicknesses might be peculiar, however, Cockburn concluded that the physician needed to know comparatively little that was new in order to practice in foreign climes: 'the reasoning will hold somewhere else'. After all, a sailor's diet was similar in most places, and diseases that followed from 'victualling' might therefore be supposed to be familiar. The main difference would lie in the air 'which we know is more serene and warm in those places' near the equator. That said, the physician familiar with the mechanical philosophy could determine the effects of this air on the human frame without stirring from his chair. '[B]ecause of its gravity (which is always greatest in a serene Air)', Cockburn opined, 'the blood and all that's carried along in it, are more minutely broken and divided in the lungs ... and therefore is more apt to separate its small and fine parts, and so to have a greater motion and all the consequences that follow upon that'.[118] The second edition of the work appeared under an altered title in 1706, but Cockburn had not changed his views on the ease with which a suitably trained metropolitan physician might diagnose and treat tropical diseases from a distance.[119] So confident of his own analysis was he, that he declared himself 'convinced that this matter does admit of such certainty, as such Surgeons of an indifferent Education might be able to Practise in those

---

[117] Cockburn, 3.

[118] Ibid., 72–3. On Cockburn and his circle of 'Tory Newtonians', see Anita Guerrini, 'Archibald Pitcairne and Newtonian Medicine', *Medical History* 31 (1987); 'The Tory Newtonians: Gregory, Pitcairne, and Their Circle', *Journal of British Studies* 25 (1986); 'James Keill, George Cheyne, and Newtonian Physiology, 1690–1740', *Journal of the History of Biology* 8 (1985); Theodore M. Brown, 'Medicine in the Shadow of the Principia', *Journal of the History of Ideas* 48, no. 4 (1987).

[119] William Cockburn, *Sea Diseases: Or, a Treatise of Their Nature, Causes, and Cure. Also, an Essay on Bleeding in Fevers; Shewing, the Quantities of Blood to Be Let, in Any of Their Periods. The Second Edition Corrected and Much Improved* (London: Geo. Strahan, 1706).

Fevers, in the E. and W. Indies with as great success, as Physicians commonly have in *England* and other temperate Countries'.[120]

As Harold Cook has shown, arguments like Cockburn's were increasingly common within the British armed forces after the Glorious Revolution. In the larger army and navy after 1688, what was prized was a form of medicine that was 'more universalistic and empirical, less individualistic and learned'.[121] This contrasted with the more traditional and scholarly methods of the Royal College of Physicians, resulting in heated debates between the College and the Admiralty. 'A crucial difference in attitudes towards medicine itself divided the two groups', Cook writes. 'The military wanted quick and efficacious cures for specific diseases that would be good for any soldier or sailor in any cir-cumstance, while the learned physicians wished to maintain the importance of learned physic, with its emphasis on the individual'.[122] Part of this latter emphasis, of course, involved knowledge about location. It was thus perhaps inevitable that Cockburn's attempts to operationalise his insights met with limited success, precisely because leading medical men in England found it difficult to accept that greater personal knowledge of the particulars of practice in the Indies might not be useful. Cockburn had conceived of a plan whereby surgeons overseas might produce a more easily standardised record, so that 'by their having a good number of Orderly Observations, it might be easy for any one to find the right method of these Fevers in the W. Indies'. Cockburn laid the scheme before the Admiralty, who were apparently enthusiastic, but proposed forwarding the matter for the approval of the College of Physicians. Protesting that this was unnecessary, Cockburn, somewhat disingenuously, sought to por-tray his proposal as one that had little to do with his own views: 'because I did not direct any particular Method to be followed, but only foretold the different success of each method in general use'. The College failed to come to a con-clusion on the matter, but their reasons for doing so were illuminating. 'I per-ceive they were at a loss what Judgment to make of those Particularities which differ from our practice in these Parts of the World', wrote Thomas Millington, the College President, 'As being perfect Strangers to what does, or does not succeed in the *West Indies*'.[123]

One can see from Cockburn's failure to convince members of the College that Hippocratic arguments were a two-edged sword. What social work they might do depended upon location. In the metropole, elite physicians might insist on the applicability of the arguments of *Airs, Waters, and Places* in the

[120] Ibid., 105.
[121] Harold J. Cook, 'Practical Medicine and the British Armed Forces after the "Glorious Revolution"', *Medical History* 34 (1990): 26. See, similarly, Alsop, 30.
[122] Cook, 'Practical Medicine and the British Armed Forces after the "Glorious Revolution"', 14.
[123] All quotations, including that from Millington's letter in Cockburn, *Sea Diseases: Or, a Treatise of Their Nature, Causes, and Cure. Also, an Essay on Bleeding in Fevers; Shewing, the Quantities of Blood to Be Let, in Any of Their Periods. The Second Edition Corrected and Much Improved*, Preface.

face of claims that sidelined or rejected their scholarly expertise in favour of an emphasis on simplicity, universality, and efficacy. For Sloane in the West Indies, however, the practice that flowed from Hippocratic logics gave the advantage to those who were *not* metropolitan elites. Thus, in spite of the fact that Richard Towne dedicated *A Treatise of the Diseases Most Frequent in the West-Indies* to Sloane, one suspects that on this issue, at least, his sympathies were with Trapham. When the text appeared in 1726, one year after the publication of the second volume of Sloane's *Voyage*, Towne could boast of 'seven years practice' in Barbados.[124] The introduction to his short book was well crafted, showing Towne to be well-versed in current mechanical theories, but more committed to located empiricism. 'I have introduced no more Philosophy into this Treatise', he noted, 'than what was necessary to explain the Reasonableness of the Practice, and to guide those into a right Application of it, for whose Use it was principally calculated'.[125] And from the outset, although Towne did not acknowledge the point explicitly (indeed, he implicitly sought to play it down) the text was framed in opposition to Sloane's, arguing that the same diseases manifested differently in different places, and that illnesses existed in the West Indies that had never been seen in Europe.

It is no wonder then that the *Alterations* made in our *Constitutions* should be conformable to the Causes from whence they arise, and consequently that *Diseases* should be in some Places more or less frequent than they are in others, and attended with Symptoms as different as the *Qualities* of the *Countries* where they are produced. This Variety in the Degrees of *Violence*, and Diversity of *Types*, by which Distempers are distinguished from each other, must necessarily require the peculiar Attention of the Physician in his Management of them, and therefore no one *Methodus Medendi* can be framed so general and absolute as to tally with every *Climate*.[126]

Few of Towne's readers could have perused this last sentence without thinking of Sloane, who only the year before had defended his decision to publish the names of his patients when describing their case histories by suggesting that he only did so 'to prove that the Diseases there were the same as in *England*'. But Towne took some of the sting out of his implied criticism of Sloane's 'one method fits all' approach to the practice of medicine in warm climates by suggesting that Sloane himself had been interested, like Towne, in the particularities of place. Both men were, Towne claimed, part of a lineage of 'learned Physicians' that included Alpinus, William Piso, and Bontius, all of whom had 'employ[ed] their Pens upon such Diseases as are *endemic* or *popular*, in those Places where their Practice afforded them the greatest Opportunity for *Observation*'.[127]

---

[124] Towne, 3.
[125] Ibid.
[126] Ibid., 1 2.
[127] Ibid., 2–3.

In spite of this effort to construct a commonality with a powerful patron, it nonetheless seems clear that Towne, like Trapham and unlike Sloane, saw the diseases of the West Indies as entities different to those found in Europe and hence requiring treatment modified to local conditions.[128] Towne, in fact, even identified two illnesses 'to which the blacks are no strangers, but as far as I can be informed they are utterly unknown in Europe: I mean the Elefantiasis under the circumstances it occurs in the West Indies, and a distemper called there the *Joint-Evil*'.[129] For those whose careers were to be made in the colonies, an emphasis on geographical specificity played to their strengths. For the sojourning Sloane, lack of local knowledge was a potential liability, one to be removed by rejecting the putatively Hippocratic premise of his opponents.

Conclusion

In a now-classic article about the ways that the 'torrid zone' functioned within the European imaginary, Karen Kupperman offered a valuable periodisation. Whereas before the seventeenth century, English would-be travellers to the southern parts of North America 'expressed profound anxiety over the effect hot climates would have on them', from the 1630s, 'propagandists for southern colonies' began to argue that their regions provided an ideal middle zone between extremes of cold and heat.[130] A number of scholars have since nuanced the first part of this claim, pointing to both positive and negative responses to America, even in the earliest periods of its European exploration and settlement.[131] But most have tended to affirm the second part, stressing the strategic importance of promotional attitudes to imperial desires. Portraits of fecundity, verdancy, and the peacefulness of native inhabitants, Susan Parrish has noted, 'had everything to do with attracting settlement and investment in the face of negative reports of starvation, disease, hurricanes, intemperate weather, and Indian massacres'.[132] I believe we can assume a similar periodisation for the West Indies, although their later dates of English settlement (1627 for

---

[128] In terms of diagnosis, for example, one could not rely on an examination of the urine as one could in Europe. The warm weather changed the fluid too dramatically, so that 'Prognosticks taken from an examination of the urine are much more precarious here than in Europe'. 61–2. In terms of treatment, Towne called attention to the practice of Paracenthesis or 'tapping': 'How frightful soever this Undertaking may appear in Europe, yet it is practiced almost every day in Barbadoes with good success', 135.

[129] Towne, 184.

[130] Karen Kupperman, 'Fear of Hot Climates in the Anglo-American Experience', *William and Mary Quarterly* 41 (1984): 213–40, 213, 217.

[131] Chaplin, *Subject Matter: Technology, the Body, and Science on the Anglo-American Frontier, 1500–1676*. Parrish. Jan Golinski, 'American Climate and the Civilization of Nature', in *Science and Empire in the Atlantic World*, ed. James Delbourgo and Nicholas Dew (New York and London: Routledge, 2008).

[132] Parrish, 33.

Barbados; 1655 for Jamaica) suggest that periods in which attitudes about their climates were negative would have been short. Certainly, by 1679, Trapham was serving as a booster for a climate he and others were happy to portray as eminently suitable for British bodies. Eight years later, Richard Blome's *Present State of His Majesty's Isles and Territories in America*, declared that 'it is confirmed by a long experience, that there is no such antipathy betwixt our *Britanick* Temper and the Climate of Jamaica, as to necessitate them to any Distemper upon their arrival there, or occasion Diseases to prove mortal or contagious more than in other parts'.[133] It is possible, then, that Sloane – if he had been thinking of specific works when he claimed to have been led to believe that diseases were all different in Jamaica – had considerably older texts in mind. More up-to-date volumes, as we have seen, all tended to portray the West Indies as a summer version of England, and hence as a location that possessed many of the same diseases as England, and very few completely new ones. Where Trapham and Sloane disagreed – publicly – was not over diagnosis, but over therapeutics. And there, Sloane was indeed in a minority, at least among civilians, in insisting that what he had learned in Britain and France could be transferred directly to Jamaica.

In terms of the history of medicine, the stakes involved in not taking Sloane as simply a faithful barometer of medical opinion concerning the diseases of the New World are high. Among the tasks of this book is the attempt to explain how it came to be believed to be a fact that the latitudes between the tropics contained radically different disease environments compared to northern Europe. If Sloane accurately captured the tenor of the times, then the problem for the historian involves explaining how such attitudes spread from the West Indies to other imperial holdings where such understandings of fundamental difference were not common.[134] If Sloane's claims are to be nuanced in the ways I have suggested, the task is a different one. It amounts to asking about eighteenth-century events and processes that led to the *emergence* of conceptions both of similarity within the tropics and conceptions of difference between the tropics and the so-called temperate zones. It is to this latter question that we turn in subsequent chapters, beginning in the next with the emergence of a belief that we saw traces of in Trapham's writings: the notion that the movement of peoples via the slave trade was *producing* a disease environment in the West Indies resembling that in Africa, where no such commonality had existed before.

---

[133] Quoted in ibid., 87.

[134] As we shall see, geographical specification is required here. West Africa had a much poorer reputation as a disease environment than the East Indies in the early eighteenth century. Curtin, ' "The White Man's Grave": Image and Reality, 1780–1850'; 'Epidemiology and the Slave Trade'; *The Image of Africa: British Ideas and Action, 1780–1850*.

2   Changes in the Air: William Hillary and English Medicine in the West Indies, 1720–1760

In 1759, William Hillary, a physician who had kept a practice in the West Indies for the preceding dozen years, published a book on the diseases of Barbados.[1] Early reviews tended to be positive. Reviewers griped, not unreasonably, at the doctor's repetitive style and his often unnecessary displays of erudition, yet they lauded his judgement and attention to detail.[2] 'Reading his description', one claimed, 'is almost equivalent to seeing the patient, and differs only as a copy from the original ... [I]n this particular', the reviewer continued, offering perhaps the highest praise possible, 'he is little inferior to the *British Hippocrates, Sydenham*'.[3] In 1762, Solomon de Monchy, City Physician of Rotterdam and author of a prize-winning essay answering a question about the 'causes of the usual diseases among seamen in voyages to the West Indies', offered a list of British physicians upon whom he was relying.[4] The authors he cited were 'Mead, Pringle, Huxham, Lind, Watson, Bisset, Hillary', placing the last-mentioned author in illustrious company only three years after his text's first printing.[5] In 1766, Hillary's work appeared, unaltered, in a second edition. Benjamin Rush would be responsible for the publication of a third in 1811.[6] It would be a rare work on the diseases of the Caribbean in the last decades of the eighteenth century that did not cite Hillary's *Observations*.

In this chapter I aim to offer the first detailed intellectual history of Hillary's medical writings, a history that will simultaneously provide a description of

---

[1] William Hillary, *Observations on the Changes of the Air and the Concomitant Epidemical Diseases, in the Island of Barbados. To Which Is Added a Treatise on the Putrid Bilious Fever, Commonly Called the Yellow Fever; and Such Other Diseases as Are Indigenous or Endemial, in the West India Islands, or in the Torrid Zone* (London: C. Hitch and L. Hawes, 1759).

[2] *The Monthly Review, or Literary Journal* (November, 1759): 369–81; *The Critical Review, or Annals of Literature* 7 (1759): 520–29.

[3] *The Critical Review*, 521.

[4] de Monchy, iv.

[5] Ibid., v.

[6] William Hillary and Benjamin Rush, *Observations on the Changes of the Air, and the Concomitant Epidemical Diseases in the Island of Barbados: To Which Is Added, a Treatise on the Putrid Bilious Fever, Commonly Called the Yellow Fever; and Such Other Diseases As Are Indigenous or Endemial, in the West India Islands, or in the Torrid Zone* (Philadelphia: B. & T. Kite, 1811).

the medical landscape relevant to work on the diseases of warm climates from the 1720s to the 1760s.[7] Recovering the resources necessary for Hillary's theorising will allow us to track the complex interrelations between different forms of medicine informed by the mechanical philosophy, as well as the roles played by medical meteorology, theories of contagion, and notions of environmental causation in understanding the diseases of the 'torrid zone'. To this empirical or descriptive base, I add two further argumentative layers. Each relies on the structure of Hillary's text for its explication.

The volume was divided into two fairly distinct parts. The first – *Observations on the Changes of the Air and the Concomitant Epidemical Diseases, in the Island of Barbados* – was a diary of the weather on the island, correlated with descriptions of the diseases observed by Hillary in his practice over a period of several years in the 1750s. The second half – *A Treatise on the Putrid Bilious Fever, Commonly Called the Yellow Fever; and such Other Diseases as are Indigenous or Endemial, in the West India Islands, or in the Torrid Zone* – involved a description of diseases that were commonly found in the West Indies but would be unfamiliar to most physicians in England. In the terminology of the day, the first half of the book was concerned with *epidemical*, the second half with *endemial* diseases.

As we saw in the last chapter, by the seventeenth century the touchstone for works on diseases peculiar to a given part of the world was Hippocrates' *Airs, Waters, and Places*. Chapter 1 spent some time describing a 'Hippocratic revival' based around the text, as it was increasingly used to understand the distempers characteristic of lands between the Tropics. The study of epidemics and their relationship to the seasons also had a Hippocratic root. Those who produced a medico-meteorological diary in the early eighteenth century cited the Hippocratic works *Epidemics I* and *III* almost without fail.[8] Many of Hillary's contemporaries who vaunted Hippocrates for his empiricist method tended not to distinguish between these three texts, seeing in each examples of the author's attention to data rather than 'sterile' theory, as well as a common and characteristic emphasis on the relationship between human health and the weather. Historians, similarly, have often been more interested in the methodological differences between neo-Hippocratics and other medical sects (Galenists and chemists, for example) than the more seemingly narrow

---

[7] For shorter accounts, see Frederick Sargent, *Hippocratic Heritage: A History of Ideas About Weather and Human Health* (New York: Pergamon Press, 1982), 224–8; Sheridan, *Doctors and Slaves: A Medical and Demographic History of Slavery in the British West Indies, 1680–1834*, 22–4; Harrison, *Medicine in an Age of Commerce and Empire: Britain and its Tropical Colonies, 1660–1830*, 53–60.

[8] Hippocrates, 'Epidemics I', in *The Genuine Works of Hippocrates*, translated from the Greek by Francis Adams, with a Preliminary Discourse and Annotations. In Two Volumes, Vol. 1, 352–382 (London: Sydenham Society, 1849). Hippocrates, 'Epidemics III', Ibid., 388–420.

differences, in theory and practice, among neo-Hippocratics. In any case, if one is concerned with the *production* of the Hippocratic texts, treating the three texts together makes sense. It was assumed, in the eighteenth century, based on the language and logic of each work, that the same person authored both *Epidemics I* and *III* and *Airs, Waters, and Places*. And one might note that all three texts are quintessentially Hippocratic in that they examine collective diseases, rather than those of individual patients.

As can be seen from Hillary's volume, however, the *audiences* for new works based on each text were rather different. Hillary concluded his weather diary on 30 May 1758 when he returned to England. He published his observations, he claimed 'for the Benefit of the Inhabitants of that Island, and sincerely with that they may be of Service to them and all theirs'.[9] By contrast, in the preface to the part of the work on endemial diseases, Hillary declared that 'I principally write and publish these for the Good of the Inhabitants, and the Benefit of those who commonly practice in the West-India Islands'.[10] The two halves of the book were involved in two largely, if not completely, different conversations. In the first half, Hillary cited and engaged with metropolitan authors, such as Boerhaave and John Huxham. In the second, he argued with West Indian physicians – Towne and Warren, for example – and others who had treated diseases in the torrid zone.

My first argument, then, is that historians seeking to understand 'the' Hippocratic revival would do well to pay attention to the geographic location of those vaunting the physician from Cos. Speaking broadly, one might, indeed, be better off speaking of at least two, interacting, revivals – one more metropolitan and dealing with epidemic diseases, the other more colonial and dealing with endemic distempers. The point is an important one, given this book's emphasis on the history of 'difference-making', for *Epidemics* and *Airs, Waters, and Places*, in spite of many similarities, draw the attention to two rather different differences. *Airs, Waters, and Places*, of course, was concerned with the diseases characteristic of different regions and climates. *Epidemics*, on the other hand, opened with a discussion of the diseases found in a given year – broken down by seasons – in the town of Thasus. Subsequent sections described the 'constitutions' of successive years in the same place. If *Airs, Waters, and Places* was thus focused on spatial difference, *Epidemics* was concerned with temporal changes; the first compared climates, the second constitutions. A physician relying on *Epidemics* could, in fact, pay almost no attention to the question of how a different location might change their analysis. Sydenham's account of epidemic constitutions in London, for example, was resolutely local, a fact that drew criticisms from James Lind, a leading

---

[9] Hillary, 136.
[10] Ibid., Preface, unnumbered, 142.

naval physician and author of *An Essay on Diseases Incidental to Europeans in Hot Climates* (1768), a work solidly in the tradition of *Airs, Waters, and Places*. According to Lind, the reason that Sydenham found phlebotomy such a universal remedy for almost all fevers was because of his limited geographical experience. Had the 'eminent physician' practiced even a few miles from the metropolis, in the low marshy areas outside London, Lind opined, he would probably have changed his mind. Had he ventured even farther forth, yet more of his ideas would have been altered. Knowledge of the autumnal fever that one finds in Europe, or 'of the great mortality produced by its rage in hot climates' – precisely the information Lind supplied in his treatise – would have led Sydenham to retract the idea that a continual fever was 'the most constant and primary fever of nature'.[11]

Medical writers, like Sydenham, who used *Epidemics* as a model tended implicitly to downplay the differences made by geography and to emphasise those induced by seasonality. During a period in which Britain's imperial holdings and trading interests were growing, use of *Epidemics* to discuss the relationship between environment and health drew distant lands closer to the metropole, while use of *Airs, Waters, and Places* tended to stress the differences of foreign climes. As we shall see, Hillary's medico-meteorological diary made the West Indies seem familiar, his account of the diseases peculiar to Barbados made the entire torrid zone seem distinctive.

The second main argument I make in this chapter serves as part of an answer to the question posed at the end of the last. When and why did medical practitioners begin to conceive of the West Indies in particular and the tropics more generally as distinct disease environments, different from England and other northern countries not merely in degree, but in kind? Historians Kenneth Kiple and Kriemhild Ornelas have pointed to Hillary's text as 'the first to report a significantly different disease environment in the West Indies from that of Europe'.[12] In the next chapter, I suggest that naval medical texts served as a principal source for a new conception of tropical disease environments as *sui generis*, and point to British military engagements in the Caribbean in the late 1730s and 1740s as moments in which a broader English populace became aware of the dangers posed to 'unseasoned' soldiers in climates far from home. In the second half of the present chapter, however, my concern is with Hillary's

---

[11] James Lind, *An Essay on Diseases Incidental to Europeans in Hot Climates: With the Method of Preventing Their Fatal Consequences. To Which Is Added, an Appendix Concerning Intermittent Fevers* (London: T. Becket and P. A. de Hondt, 1768), 68.

[12] Kenneth F. Kiple and Kriemhild Coneé Ornelas, 'Race, War, and Tropical Medicine in the Eighteenth-Century Caribbean', in *Warm Climates and Western Medicine: The Emergence of Tropical Medicine, 1500–1900*, ed. David Arnold (Amsterdam and Atlanta: Rodopi, 1996). See also Kenneth F. Kiple, *The Caribbean Slave: A Biological History* (Cambridge: Cambridge University Press, 1984).

formulation of the medical distinctiveness of hot climates. His own explanation for this distinctiveness made almost no explicit use of military texts or
mention of military campaigns.

As befits a figure writing in a transitional period – between the early eighteenth century when all climates were regarded as possessing both similarities
and differences and the late eighteenth century, when disease environments had
begun to harden into geographically determined zones – Hillary's arguments were
both fascinating and complex. It is true that he described a good many diseases
common to the 'torrid zone' and largely unknown in England, yet the reasons
given for both similarities and differences varied. Yellow fever, for example, was
a characteristic affliction in Barbados and one induced by the climate. For it, and
perhaps it alone, Hillary associated its cause not merely with a warm climate, but
with a specifically *tropical* one. Indeed, Hillary's yellow fever may be the first
explicitly identified tropical disease. However, for other afflictions (yaws and elephantiasis, for example) he balked at equating geographical location and disease
environment. The West Indies was not home to diseases common to countries
with warm climates solely by virtue of its position between the tropics. It was
not nature that connected the Guinea Coast to Barbados, but human action. The
slave trade *made* the West Indies like parts of Africa and unlike England. The
West Indian disease environment might have been distinctive to Hillary, but for
the most part its difference was to be explained not by geography, but by history.

2.1   A Rational and Mechanical Essay

Born in 1698, Hillary began his medical career at 18, with an apprenticeship to
an apothecary. His university training began roughly five years later, in Leiden,
where his status as a religious dissenter did not prevent his attendance, as was
the case at Oxford or Cambridge. There he studied under Hermann Boerhaave
and completed his thesis, on intermittent fevers, towards the middle of 1722.
Around a year later, he moved back to Yorkshire, establishing a practice in the
town of Ripon, where he stayed for more than a decade before moving to Bath.
The shift was a dramatic one. Ripon was a small country town, while Bath –
famous since Roman times – had become not merely a site for water cures,
but for aristocratic entertainment; where 'the cream of English Society …
divert[ed] itself with the waters, conversation, music, dancing, the theatre, and
the pleasure of being seen in the company of the most distinguished people in
the land'.[13] The rather dour Quaker clearly found that his relocation required
some adjustment, as one can see from the two editions of his first publication,

[13] C. C. Booth, 'William Hillary: A Pupil of Boerhaave', *Medical History* 7, no. 4 (1963): 304;
William Addison, *English Spas* (London: B. T. Batsford Ltd., 1951), 58–73. On medicine
in spa towns, see Roy Porter, ed. *The Medical History of Waters and Spas, Medical History
Supplement 10* (London: Wellcome Institute for the History of Medicine, 1990).

an essay on the smallpox. The first was completed at Ripon, its Preface dated May 1732, although it was not published until 1735. Hillary suggested that smallpox's frequency and mortality 'particularly to several Families of the first Rank' was the main impetus for his attempts to divine a better cure for the disease. That may have endeared him somewhat to leading local figures, yet his explanation for why it would be elites that seemed to suffer so much from the affliction nowadays cannot have been so appealing:

[Their] Educations and manner of living, do dispose their Constitutions to be more severely afflicted with this Disease, than those who are brought up with a more plain, simple Diet, and a hardier manner of Life; for I cannot but very much blame the Luxury of the present Age, for the fatal Advances which this, and some other Diseases, have of late Years made.[14]

The Preface to the second edition, completed in Bath and published in 1740, was shorter, with passages about several topics trimmed and omitted. Particularly striking, however, was the removal of his former criticisms of aristocratic lifestyles. Hillary now needed to make his living not from hardy farm folk, but from the coddled upper classes and if he still disapproved, he made efforts to hide it.[15]

In medical terms, the treatise on smallpox was thoroughly indebted, as Hillary noted, to the 'sagacious and learned Dr. Boerhaave', who was credited as the inventor of the cure for the disease promoted in the text (a cooling, 'antiphlogistic' regimen and repeated bloodletting).[16] In the early eighteenth century, Leiden was the centre for medical learning in Europe and Boerhaave was its leading light. More than 1900 students matriculated at Leiden between 1701 and 1738, with a third of these coming from England, Scotland, Ireland, and the British colonies. And more students studied directly with Boerhaave than any other medical professor at the university. In the 29 years he served as professor, he 'promoted' 178 students, of whom 43 came from English speaking countries.[17]

---

[14] William Hillary, *A Rational and Mechanical Essay on the Small-Pox: Wherein the Cause, Nature, and Diathesis of That Disease, Its Symptoms, Their Causes, and Manner of Production, Are Explained ... With the Diagnostic and Prognostic Symptoms ... To Which is Prefixed, a Short History of the First Rise and Progress of That Disease; and an Essay on a New Method of Curing It, as We Do Other Inflammatory Diseases* (London: G. Strahan, 1735), iv, v.

[15] '[O]nly those with sufficient leisure and capital could devote time to personal wellbeing', Guerrini has observed in her study of George Cheyne, another physician who sought to make a second career in Bath. 'The interface between the new culture of leisure and its relationship to health was especially evident in the new spa towns'. Anita Guerrini, *Obesity and Depression in the Enlightenment: The Life and Times of George Cheyne* (Norman: University of Oklahoma Press, 2000), 101.

[16] Hillary, 1735, xiv.

[17] G. A. Lindeboom, *Hermann Boerhaave: The Man and His Work* (London: Methuen, 1968), 356–7.

As one of these students Hillary imbibed his master's emphasis on the body as a machine, albeit more of a 'hydraulico-pneumatical engine' than the clockwork imagined by many earlier proponents of the mechanical philosophy.[18] One of Boerhaave's earliest orations at Leiden had been entitled 'On the Use of Rational Mechanics in Medicine' (1703). The first edition of Hillary's work bore the self-consciously similar title 'A Rational and Mechanical Essay on the Smallpox'. In his preface, Hillary declared that 'a human Body is (as much as it is the Object of Medicine) a Machine' and that 'Diseases are nothing but Defects and Irregularities of those actions, Motions, and Properties, produced in this wonderful Human Machine'.[19] Smallpox, he argued, was a disease that was both epidemical and contagious. Epidemical in that it proceeded from a common cause, afflicted the majority of people in a given region, and did so in a definite space of time; contagious in that it was passed from one patient to another via the air, which carried 'infectious Miasmata' from person to person.[20] The particles that made up this dangerous miasma were too minute to be directly perceived, but from their effects, Hillary concluded that they must affect both the solid and fluid parts of the body. By virtue of their sizes, either individually or through the production of larger molecules via mutual attraction, they must be able both to form obstructions in 'the ultimate minute subcuticular Arteries' – and hence allow the production and accumulation of putrid pus – and to stimulate the body's nervous solids to produce both stronger and more frequent contractions, driving fluids more rapidly and with more force throughout the body. The result, Hillary concluded, would be 'a violent Inflammatory Fever, with all its dangerous, and too often fatal, Consequences'.[21]

The focus of the essay would change substantially in the second edition, even if the contents would not. Gone were the encomiums to the wondrous human machine. In their place were blander materialist pronouncements: 'The *Agent* and *Patient* both being *Matter*, are subject to the same unalterable

---

[18] On Boerhaave as an iatrophysicist, see ibid., esp. 61–7, 272–4. The term 'hydraulico-pneumatical engine' was Robert Boyle's. See Barbara Orland, 'The Fluid Mechanics of Nutrition: Herman Boerhaave's Synthesis of Seventeenth-Century Circulation Physiology', *Studies in History and Philosophy of Biological and Biomedical Sciences* 43 (2012): 365. Orland offers a superb summary of Boerhaave's model on 364. For a helpful overview of medicine in this period, see Lester S. King, *The Philosophy of Medicine: The Early Eighteenth Century* (Cambridge, MA: Harvard University Press, 1978).

[19] Hillary, *A Rational and Mechanical Essay on the Small-Pox: Wherein the Cause, Nature, and Diathesis of That Disease, Its Symptoms, Their Causes, and Manner of Production, Are Explained ... With the Diagnostic and Prognostic Symptoms ... To Which Is Prefixed, a Short History of the First Rise and Progress of That Disease; and an Essay on a New Method of Curing It, as We Do Other Inflammatory Diseases*, vii.

[20] Ibid., 32.

[21] Ibid., 38.

Laws which *Matter* in general is'.[22] The title changed, so that it was now a 'Practical Essay' rather than a 'Rational and Mechanical' one. The mechanical explanation for the effect of the smallpox contagion on the human system remained, but it was now moved from the first section following the historical introduction to chapter five of eight. Perhaps the decision to emphasise more his novel treatment was occasioned by criticisms of some of the more theoretical elements of Hillary's arguments. That, at least, would explain the somewhat petulant tone the author adopted in his new preface, as he defended theory against its detractors. 'It would be highly obliging to Mankind in general', he wrote sarcastically, 'if those Gentlemen who declaim so much against Theories, would shew us some more effectual Methods (if such there are) of improving our Knowledge in Physic and Diseases'.[23] Whatever he thought of theory, however, Hillary downplayed it in his revisions. The subtitle of the first edition emphasised the causes of the disease, that of the second its prevention and cure.

The timing for the publication of the rational and mechanical essay was perhaps not optimal. The last decade of the seventeenth and the first three decades of the eighteenth centuries saw the rise of several mechanical theories of human health and disease, put forward by 'Newton-struck' British physicians.[24] Hillary cited two of these 'Tory Newtonians' – Archibald Pitcairn and John Freind – as 'Ornaments of the Faculty' of medicine, adding Boerhaave to them to complete the triumvirate of those who so supported his therapeutic venesection for those afflicted by the disease.[25] In fact, Boerhaave had attended Pitcairn's lectures when the latter had served as professor at Leiden in the early 1690s. Newton himself loaned his credibility and gave his patronage to these followers, so that to be a Newtonian physician (though this could mean many things) in the 1710s was to be almost assured of professional success.[26]

---

[22] *A Practical Essay on the Small-Pox: Wherein a Method of Preparing the Body before the Disease Comes on, and of Deriving the Variolous Matter from the Vital to the Remote Parts of the Body after the Accession ...; to Which Is Added, an Account of the Principal Variations of the Weather, and the Concomitant Epidemic Diseases, as They Appeared at Rippon ... From the Year 1726, to the End of 1734*, 2nd ed. (London: C. Hitch and J. Leake, 1740), vi.

[23] Ibid., v, vi–vii.

[24] Theodore M. Brown, 'Medicine in the Shadow of the Principia', *Journal of the History of Ideas* 48, no. 4 (1987). Brown uses the term 'Newton-struck' on 630.

[25] Hillary, *A Practical Essay on the Small-Pox: Wherein a Method of Preparing the Body before the Disease Comes on, and of Deriving the Variolous Matter from the Vital to the Remote Parts of the Body after the Accession ... to Which Is Added, an Account of the Principal Variations of the Weather, and the Concomitant Epidemic Diseases, as They Appeared at Rippon ... From the Year 1726, to the End of 1734*, 24. On Tory Newtonianism, see Guerrini, 'James Keill, George Cheyne, and Newtonian Physiology, 1690–1740'; 'The Tory Newtonians: Gregory, Pitcairne, and Their Circle'.

[26] 'The Tory Newtonians: Gregory, Pitcairne, and Their Circle', 310. On the many meanings of Newtonianism, see *Obesity and Depression in the Enlightenment: The Life and Times of George Cheyne*, 38.

Hillary's model for the effect of the smallpox contagion on the body was solidly 'Newtonian', with its focus on attracting particles that blocked the body's tiniest arteries, causing obstructions that led to increased pressure through the remaining vessels.[27]

By the 1740s, it has been argued, Newtonian physiology was under threat on multiple fronts,[28] strict mechanism increasingly being supplemented by an attention to Hippocratic environmentalism. Where Pitcairne in 1688 had been critical of Hippocrates for lacking knowledge of science's true method – geometry – John Arburthnot captured the tenor of the new combination in 1733, while describing the logic of his *Essay Concerning the Effects of Air*.[29] 'I have ventur'd to explain the Philosophy of this Sagacious old Man [Hippocrates], by mechanical Causes arising from the properties and Qualities of the Air'.[30] Where an earlier mechanical medicine had focused on the body as a machine, the newer form turned increasingly towards a mechanical understanding of the environment around the body. In his essay on the smallpox, as in his later work, Hillary was something of a bell-weather, for the same text that saw him change his focus away from theory to therapy also saw his turn towards the systematic study of diseases, air, and seasonality.

2.2   Weathering Epidemics

Hillary opened his account of the smallpox by arguing that the disease had not always troubled humanity. Variations across both time and space mattered. Human bodies had not changed over time, but the distempers that afflicted those bodies had.[31] Hillary seemed conflicted over whether the disease, once

---

[27] Hillary, *A Rational and Mechanical Essay on the Small-Pox: Wherein the Cause, Nature, and Diathesis of That Disease, Its Symptoms, Their Causes, and Manner of Production, Are Explained ... With the Diagnostic and Prognostic Symptoms ... To Which Is Prefixed, a Short History of the First Rise and Progress of That Disease; and an Essay on a New Method of Curing It, as We Do Other Inflammatory Diseases*, 36. In common with other Newtonians, like Pitcairne, largely Hillary eschewed a Cartesian concern with the shape of the corpuscles involved. For Pitcairne's model and his critiques of Cartesianism, see Andrew Cunningham, 'Sydenham Versus Newton: The Edinburgh Fever Dispute of the 1690s between Andrew Brown and Archibald Pitcairne', *Medical History, Supplement* 1 (1981): 88–90.

[28] Anita Guerrini, 'Isaac Newton, George Cheyne, and the "Principia Medicinae"', in *The Medical Revolution of the Seventeenth Century*, ed. Roger French and Andrew Wear (Cambridge: Cambridge University Press, 1989), 222–3.

[29] 'Archibald Pitcairne and Newtonian Medicine', 72; John Arbuthnot, *An Essay Concerning the Effects of Air on Human Bodies* (London: Printed for J. Tonson, 1733).

[30] Quoted in Andrea A. Rusnock, 'Hippocrates, Bacon, and Medical Meteorology at the Royal Society, 1700–1750', in *Reinventing Hippocrates*, ed. David Cantor (Burlington: Ashgate, 2001), 146.

[31] Cf. the Preface: 'not only new Species of Disease, but new Symptoms attending the same ancient known Diseases, do frequently arise, either from the different Constitutions of Years, changes of Air, the variety of Men's Constitutions, their Inventions of Luxury, and Errors in the six Non-Naturals, or from some other accidental Causes', Hillary, *A Rational and*

it had appeared in Arabia, as he claimed, and moved from thence to the rest of the world, manifested in the same way. On the one hand, he observed that in the Islamic world of the eighth century, smallpox 'appeared with much the same symptoms then in their warm Climate, as it does now in ours'.[32] On the other, the disease seemed both 'more violent and fatal' in Britain than its neighbours, 'probably from our different manner of living, and different Qualities of the Air of our Island'. Yet whatever might be said of its symptomatology, there was no denying that *treatments* needed to be altered according to climate. The English physician had been informed of the successes of inoculation against smallpox by a native of Constantinople, but he remained unconvinced of its efficacy closer to home.[33] Hillary had little doubt over whether to closely follow Arabian physicians in their cures. Avicenna's advice, for example, to treat measles by submerging the patient in cold water was not to be followed. The practice might work in the climate in which the prince of physicians had worked, but it would be 'dangerous and imprudent' in Britain.[34]

If his historical survey led Hillary to attend to the effects of geography on the manifestation and treatment of disease, so too did the nature of smallpox itself. Smallpox was, for Hillary, an epidemic disease and as a result the physician needed to approach its aetiology in a way radically different to that of a distemper that afflicted only individuals. He would make the point explicit in an addendum to the second edition of his *Essay*. To understand epidemics, one needed to turn away from Galenic medicine, with its focus on the missteps of a single patient, towards Hippocratic medicine, with its attention to the shared environments in which many lived at once.

'Tis well known that many Diseases owe their Rise to Intemperance, and the irregular Use of the Non-naturals; but as these only affect particular Persons, they can't be the Cause of epidemic Diseases, these affecting People in general, whose Ages, Constitutions, and Way of Life is sometimes very different, and they must therefore proceed from more general Causes.[35]

Mechanical Essay on the Small-Pox: Wherein the Cause, Nature, and Diathesis of That Disease, Its Symptoms, Their Causes, and Manner of Production, Are Explained ... With the Diagnostic and Prognostic Symptoms ... To Which Is Prefixed, a Short History of the First Rise and Progress of That Disease; and an Essay on a New Method of Curing It, as We Do Other Inflammatory Diseases, vi, 1.

[32] Ibid., 12.

[33] Ibid., xviii.

[34] Ibid., 16. The problem, it should be noted, was not with the medical theories and practices of Arabian physicians *per se*. Hillary was hardly parochial in these matters, and tended to have more sympathy with the medical writers of the Islamic Middle Ages than with many of their Christian successors: 'it would have been a great Happiness to their Patients, if the *European* Physicians, their Successors, had more strictly followed them therein, (with some small Allowance for the change of Climate)'. Ibid., 19.

[35] 'An Account of the Principal Variations of the Weather, and the Concomitant Epidemic Diseases, as They Appeared in Rippon, and the Circumjacent Parts of Yorkshire, from the

The most likely general cause was the air, which could itself be malign and filled with harmful effluvia, or could be the vehicle by which miasmatic exhalations were carried from patient to patient. Thus the logic of the weather diary, which one might use to track the relationships between the emergence of particular diseases and the 'Changes of the Air and Weather' that preceded, accompanied, and followed them.[36]

Although he bemoaned the fact that 'so few beside the great Hippocrates, have thought such Inquiries worth their Notice', Hillary was not the first to produce such a medico-meteorological diary.[37] To his chagrin, he was not even the first to do so in Yorkshire.[38] By the 1720s and 1730s, such diaries had become something of a fad, but forms of them had a longer history. In 1663, Robert Hooke had called for a 'History of the Weather', one to be constructed using a variety of the new instruments then available (the thermometer and barometer chief among them), as well as observations of the diseases most rife in particular seasons and meteorological conditions. The latter, medical part of the call was not taken up to any great extent, but weather diaries were being published already by the end of the seventeenth century, when one could find preprinted forms circulating among observers.[39]

The weather diary became genuinely popular after 1723, when the physician and secretary of the Royal Society, James Jurin, published an invitation to observers around the world, asking for their participation in a global project to produce a 'compleat Theory of the Weather'.[40] Jurin offered explicit instructions for how to both make and record observations, supplying a sample table to encourage the production of more standardised results. Andrea Rusnock has noted, however, that standardisation remained a serious problem in a period where even different cities might use different measures. To avoid the difficulties posed by uncalibrated instruments, Jurin convinced the Royal Society Council to send thermometers built by the renowned instrument maker Francis Hauksbee to specific observers, particularly those 'in more distant

---

Year 1726 to the End of 1734', in *A Practical Essay on the Small-Pox* (London: C. Hitch and J. Leake, 1740), viii. The 'Account' begins on page 162 of Hillary's *Practical Essay*, but is separately paginated.

[36] Ibid., vii.

[37] Ibid., iv.

[38] Ibid., viii.

[39] Jan Golinski, *British Weather and the Climate of Enlightenment* (Chicago: University of Chicago Press, 2007), 54–5. The barometer quickly became a symbol of Enlightenment and a luxury object: 'few gentlemen [are] without one', noted Richard Neve, author of the *Baroscopologia*, in 1708. Ibid., 108–36, Neve quoted on 21. Sloane travelled to Jamaica with one in the 1680s, though he seems not to have used it in producing his 'Journal of the Weather' for St Jago de la Vega. Sloane, Vol. 1, ix, xxxiii–xlii.

[40] Quoted in Andrea A. Rusnock, *Vital Accounts: Quantifying Health and Population in Eighteenth-Century England and France* (Cambridge: Cambridge University Press, 2002), 113.

Regions'.[41] Results poured in from throughout Great Britain, Europe, and even America. In 1726, Jurin published a second edition of his Invitation, which added a call for information about the relationships between diseases and the weather, in the hope, as Jurin noted in a letter, that this 'may give us some light into ye obscure Theory of Epidemical Distempers'.[42] Hillary began his medico-meteorological diary that year.

He kept the diary in Ripon from the summer of 1726 to the fall of 1734, when he heard of the death of a leading physician in Bath and decided to leave behind both the 'fatigue' of a country practice and his daily record-keeping. Of course, a diary might be kept anywhere: the issue had more to do with the details of Hillary's practice than its location. He suggested that 'acute epidemical Diseases so seldom appear, that I could not pursue these Observations', but the point was surely less that Ripon was more sickly than Bath, and more that upper class visitors were more likely to suffer from chronic illnesses – hence their journey to partake of the waters – than epidemic outbreaks.[43] It has been argued that it was Sydenham's practice among the poor of London that led him to the study of epidemics that so many after him emulated. 'Without an extensive practice amongst the poor', Andrew Cunningham has written, 'such a topic would have been impossible and indeed unthinkable'.[44] One begins to see from this why so many medico-meteorological diaries were produced in peripheral locations – both outside England and within it – for it was there that even successful physicians treated a number and variety of patients unlikely in elite metropolitan settings.

2.3   From Bath to Barbados

One cannot imagine that Hillary had originally intended to practise medicine in the West Indies. When he travelled to Barbados in 1747, he was nearly 50 years old, and had uprooted himself once already in the move away from Yorkshire. The shift to Bath had originally seemed promising. As recently as 1744, John Fothergill, a prominent English physician and, like Hillary a Quaker, had written to his brother Alexander reporting that 'Dr. Hillary was well; he has pretty good business'.[45] But only two years later, matters were considerably worse. Hillary was contemplating a trip to Jamaica when news arrived of 'the

---

[41] Ibid., 114.

[42] Quoted in ibid., 122.

[43] Hillary, 'An Account of the Principal Variations of the Weather, and the Concomitant Epidemic Diseases, as They Appeared in Rippon, and the Circumjacent Parts of Yorkshire, from the Year 1726 to the End of 1734', 62.

[44] Andrew Cunningham, 'Thomas Sydenham: Epidemics, Experiment, and the "Good Old Cause"', in The Medical Revolution of the Seventeenth Century, ed. Roger French and Andrew Wear (Cambridge: Cambridge University Press, 1989), 176.

[45] Booth, 305.

Death of the only Physician at Barbados'.[46] Fothergill had recommended the position. 'His relations I doubt not will be averse to him leaving England at any rate', he acknowledged, yet 'his situation at Bath is not the most agreeable nor the prospect very pleasing'. Fothergill evinced no great enthusiasm for Jamaica, but Barbados was another question:

at Barbados there are several meetings, the Island pleasant and healthy: the people much more humane and polite than any where else with a prospect of good employ: I have been far from urging him to go to either, yet was I in the like situation, I own I should be strongly drawn to the last place ... The galling situation he is in at present, I see renders life a burthen to him, but this betwixt ourselves.[47]

Hillary's 'galling situation' had apparently arisen as a result of speculation. In 1737, a cooper named Milsom had discovered two springs just outside Bath. Hillary analysed the spring water and declared it to possess salutary properties, publishing a short book in 1742 entitled *An Inquiry into the Contents and Medicinal Virtues of Lincomb Spaw Water*.[48] Seeing the opportunity to dramatically expand his practice, Hillary partnered with Milsom to quickly construct a building suitable for the reception of patients with chronic conditions. Yet preparing the ground for construction appears to have destroyed the spa, leaving the investors without any return for the 1,500 pounds they had spent.[49] No doubt one of the appeals of a sojourn in Barbados was the fact that he could leave the Lindcomb debacle well behind him.[50]

Although there were fairly few medical practitioners in the West Indies for much of the eighteenth century, the medical marketplace could still be difficult to negotiate. A clear hierarchy existed, one that distinguished, for example, between surgeons who might tend to slaves on plantations and those who served whites in towns or military settings.[51] Above these surgeons were ranked doctors, 'generally one or two eminent Men', Charles Leslie claimed in *A New History of Jamaica* (1740), 'who have the Employment, and soon get to be rich'.[52] Wealth was indeed a possibility, if less of a certainty than Leslie made it

---

[46] Ibid., 306. The word eminent is missing in the letter published in Fothergill's letters.

[47] Ibid.

[48] William Hillary, *An Inquiry into the Contents and Medicinal Virtues of Lincomb Spaw Water, near Bath. By William Hillary, M.D* (London: Printed for J. Leake, in Bath; and sold by C. Hitch [London], 1742).

[49] The failure of a spa was not unusual. Addison notes that this was the likely outcome of at least 99 per cent of such ventures. Addison, 121. See also Hamlin on the cut-throat world of spa promotion: Christopher Hamlin, 'Chemistry, Medicine, and the Legitimization of English Spas, 1740–1840', *Medical History. Supplement* 10 (1990): 69.

[50] William Tyte, *Bath in the Eighteenth Century: Its Progress and Life Described*. Bath: 'Chronicle' Office, 1903. 47–8.

[51] Chakrabarti, 155.

[52] Cited in ibid. Charles Leslie, *A New History of Jamaica: From the Earliest Accounts, to the Taking of Porto Bello by Vice-Admiral Vernon. In Thirteen Letters from a Gentleman to His Friend.* (London: Printed for J. Hodges, 1740), 50.

seem. Having established a medical practice in Kingston in the seventeen teens, Dr John Cochrane had enough money on hand to be able to send his brother, Dr William Cochrane £500 in 1735.[53] Dr John Lettsom claimed to have made £2,000 in six months on Tortola and neighbouring islands in the 1760s.[54] Not all were so fortunate. Outfitting costs were higher for private practitioners than those serving in the army or navy.[55] At least Hillary, with his prestigious degree and links to the local Quaker community, would have had an easier entrée than those with fewer qualifications and connections. As in Britain, looking and sounding the part helped matters considerably. 'No body, and especially Surgeons in Jamaica are respected', wrote Cochrane in 1714, 'unless they go handsome in their Cloaths – this is not vanity but meer Necessity'.[56] It has been suggested that it was Hans Sloane's confident bedside manner, as much as his medical talents, that helped convince wary Jamaican patients. 'One wrote that Sloane's presence "was very much wanted", while commenting of a rival that "I never much beleave much of his Doctorin"'.[57] Hillary's long career in Barbados would seem to make clear that he had possessed similar capacities.

Given the paucity of physicians in the British Caribbean in this period, we can make a well-informed guess as to the identity of the unnamed physician whose death opened the space that Hillary would soon fill.[58] Of the elite doctors on the island, the best known outside the West Indies was probably Henry Warren, whose short book on the yellow fever became one of the standard references on the disease soon after its publication.[59] Warren had studied at Dublin and Leiden, where he had received his degree. We remain unsure about the date of his demise, but he would have been 57 in 1746 and while one finds occasional mention of him in various sources before that date, I can find none afterward.[60]

---

[53] Sheridan, *Doctors and Slaves: A Medical and Demographic History of Slavery in the British West Indies, 1680–1834*, 46.

[54] Ibid., 63.

[55] Ibid., 43.

[56] Quoted in ibid.

[57] Miles Ogborn, 'Talking Plants: Botany and Speech in Eighteenth-Century Jamaica', *History of Science* 51 (2013): 268.

[58] Numbers were usually low, but could rise sharply during, and just after, wartime. 'Doctors who were difficult to recruit for private practice in the colonies in wartime were generally in surplus at the conclusion of a European war ... Several years after Dr. Wright came to Jamaica [after Seven Years War], the widow of a doctor who had practiced in the island wrote concerning her son who wished to follow in his father's footsteps. She warned that if he intended to settle in Jamaica the medical profession would "not afford him bread"'. Sheridan, *Doctors and Slaves: A Medical and Demographic History of Slavery in the British West Indies, 1680–1834*, 44–5.

[59] Henry Warren, *A Treatise Concerning the Malignant Fever in Barbados: And the Neighbouring Islands: with an Account of the Seasons There, from the Year 1734 to 1738. in u Letter to Dr. Mead. by Henry Warren* (London: Printed for Fletcher Gyles, 1740).

[60] P. J. Wallis and R. V. Wallis, *Eighteenth Century Medics (Subscriptions, Licences, Apprenticeships)*, 2nd ed. (Newcastle Upon Tyne: Project for Historical Bibliography,

Were it indeed Warren who Hillary succeeded, the symmetry would be elegant. The author of the most-cited account of yellow fever in the West Indies for the 1740s and 1750s would be replaced by the author of the definitive account of the disease for at least the next two decades.

One advantage of Hillary's removal from Bath was that he could once again take up his habit of maintaining a medico-meteorological diary. This he did, and in spite of the fact that the publication dates of the two diaries were separated by almost two decades, the main bodies of the texts were remarkably similar, being largely concerned with descriptive correlations between weather and disease. 'The Season continuing very wet', Hillary noted toward the end of 1729, for example, 'and the Wind generally in the Southern Points; about the Middle of November an Epidemical Cough seiz'd almost every body'. In broad strokes, this is not markedly different from the following comments from October, 1752: 'The Weather continuing to be wet and cool, several were seized with an irregular, ingeminated, intermitting, quotidian Fever'.[61] The later diary had both more – and more numerical – meteorological information, exemplifying the growth of what has been termed the 'quantifying spirit' of the eighteenth century.[62] Hillary now owned a hygrometer, though he ceased recording its results, finding 'its Variations to be so immaterial ... as to not be worth recording'. He had waited to begin his observations until he possessed a barometer, the last having been lost through an accident. After making regular observations with the replacement, however, he lamented the delay, for much the same reason he had abandoned measuring the air's humidity: 'the greatest Variation in [the air pressure], in six Years time, was never more than four Tenths of an Inch'. His diary in Ripon had only noted the heaviness of precipitation in general terms. In Barbados a friend nearby supplied him with rainfall data, precise to the tenth of an inch, at least until the instrument broke in January 1757. And in the West Indies he now possessed a 'Fahrenheit's Mercurial Thermometer, made at Amsterdam', with which he could make numerical measures of the temperature, replacing the relative measures – 'cold', 'very cold' – used in his earlier diary.

In both texts etiological understandings were offered in addenda. In the Ripon diary, a collection of 'aphorisms' and 'remarks' – written by an

---

1988), 629. Wallis and Wallis list Warren's dates as 1689–a1740. He was, however, presumably still alive when Dale Ingram dedicated a book to him in 1744. Dale Ingram, *Essay on the Nature, Cause, and Seat of Dysentery's, in a Letter to Dr. Henry Warren of Barbados* (Barbados: William Beeby, 1744).

61 Hillary, *Observations on the Changes of the Air and the Concomitant Epidemical Diseases, in the Island of Barbados. To Which Is Added a Treatise on the Putrid Bilious Fever, Commonly Called the Yellow Fever; and Such Other Diseases as are Indigenous or Endemial, in the West India Islands, or in the Torrid Zone*, 22.

62 Tore Frängsmyr, J. L. Heilbron, and Robin E. Rider, *The Quantifying Spirit in the Eighteenth Century* (Berkeley: University of California Press, 1990).

'ingenious Acquaintance' – were supplied at the end. The author of these provided mechanical, but not, it should be noted, Newtonian explanations for various afflictions. The body was composed of fluids and fibres, but no mention was made of attracting particles or molecules. According to Hillary's 'acquaintance', to take one example, warm and dry seasons induce inflammatory diseases affecting the head because heat causes the thinner parts of the body's fluids to be lost, leaving behind a thicker portion that flows less easily through the body, with obstructions, inflammations and fevers as the result. The 'delicate Texture of the Blood Vessels of the Head', it was argued, are even more greatly affected by such obstruction than other parts of the body, hence the onset of melancholia and hypochondriac disorders.[63] In the Barbados diary, the explanations were Hillary's, proffered in footnotes phrased as numbered queries and thus styled after Newton's *Opticks*. None of the etiological claims made in these queries were specific to the climate of Barbados. Like Newton's queries, they made general causal claims (phrased as questions) and most followed the same logics invoked in Hillary's earlier work. The first query thus sought to explain why, when the summer of 1752 turned from hot and dry at the beginning of June to hot and wet for the rest of the summer, 'Dysenteries became very frequent and epidemical', and '[m]any Children were seized with an Aphthous Fever'.

Query. Was not both the Dysentery and this Aphthous Fever, caused by the falling of so much Rain, and rendering the Air cooler, by which the great Perspiration and Sweating, caused and continued by the long continued Driness and Heat before being suddenly abated and stopped; were they not now turned upon the Bowels, and the Humours being rendered acrid by that Heat, so produced these Diseases?[64]

Befitting the part of the text Hillary intended to contribute to metropolitan discussions, the conclusions were thus not phrased as being about West Indian weather and West Indian diseases, but rather about universal relationships between weather and disease, as informed by observations made in the West Indies.

Aetiology, of course, is not the entirety of medicine, and where climate made a difference in the diary (albeit a fairly small one) was in Hillary's medical practice. The introduction to his text noted his intention to describe those

---

[63] Hillary, *A Practical Essay on the Small-Pox: Wherein a Method of Preparing the Body before the Disease Comes on, and of Deriving the Variolous Matter from the Vital to the Remote Parts of the Body after the Accession ... to Which Is Added, an Account of the Principal Variations of the Weather, and the Concomitant Epidemic Diseases, as They Appeared at Rippon ... From the Year 1726, to the End of 1734*, 64.

[64] Hillary, *Observations on the Changes of the Air and the Concomitant Epidemical Diseases, in the Island of Barbados. To Which Is Added a Treatise on the Putrid Bilious Fever, Commonly Called the Yellow Fever; and Such Other Diseases as Are Indigenous or Endemial, in the West India Islands, or in the Torrid Zone*, Note, 18–19.

situations where the diseases he had observed differed from English afflictions due to the heat or other climatic variations, as well as the changes he had made to his methods or medicines.[65] Yet while a number of prescriptions were included (detailed, he suggested, for Barbadian residents), there were only a small handful of times where Hillary explicitly noted the ways in which diseases or cures changed substantially from the English norm. Intermitting fevers, he observed, were rarer on the island than they had been in the past, and it was difficult for the physician to induce a remitting fever to intermit, as was the practice and customary outcome in England.[66] The physician could learn little from studying the urine in the West Indies, despite its utility in England, and Hillary was forced to find a substitute for the usual cordial waters found in the shops. In Barbados these heated and inflamed the blood too much.[67] On the other hand, a number of diseases were completely unchanged – the climate having no effect at all. One October saw several afflicted with a continued remitting fever, but this changed soon to an 'ingeminated Quotidian, with all the Symptoms of that Fever, as usual in England'.[68] Inflammatory rheumatisms were common in Britain but not in the Indies, yet one year they appeared in Barbados just as they usually did in England.[69] In March 1754, an epidemic of slow nervous Fever broke out, but the physician aware of metropolitan discussions of the disease and its treatment required no new information:

And the Fever now put on and appeared in this warm Climate, with all the same Symptoms as it usually does in England; and as they are accurately described by that learned and able Physician Dr. Huxham in the cooler Climate of Plymouth, which therefore I need not here repeat.[70]

Almost all the diseases whose description fills page after page would be utterly familiar to an English audience: dropsies and dysentery; smallpox, catarrhs, and peripneumonies. The diseases of warm seasons in England predominated, but the overall sense is one of fundamental similarity. For the most part, only occasional mention was made of diseases specific to warm climates, like the prickly heat or one that seemed to have no name, but was characterised by the

---

[65] Ibid., xiii.
[66] Hillary associated the decline in the occurrence of intermitting fevers with the growing clearing and cultivation of land in Barbados. Ibid., 23, 125. On the difficulty in getting a remitting fever to intermit 'as it frequently uses to do in England', see ibid., 65, 126.
[67] Ibid., 92, 36. Towne made a similar argument about the problems involved in studying the urine in the warm climate. 'Prognosticks taken from an Inspection of the Urine are much more precarious here than in Europe'. Towne, 61–2.
[68] Hillary, Observations on the Changes of the Air and the Concomitant Epidemical Diseases, in the Island of Barbados. To Which Is Added a Treatise on the Putrid Bilious Fever, Commonly Called the Yellow Fever; and Such Other Diseases as Are Indigenous or Endemial, in the West India Islands, or in the Torrid Zone, 22.
[69] Ibid., 41.
[70] Ibid., 56.

gangrenescent boils with which it afflicted children.[71] The only exception was an illness that recurred in almost every year and with which Hillary opened the second section of his book: the yellow fever.

2.4   Yellow Fever

We will take up Hillary's theory of yellow fever in a moment. First, however, we need to understand its predecessors, not least because Hillary himself framed his discussion as a response to Warren's *Treatise*, published two decades earlier. Warren, in turn, expressed his desire to correct Towne's comments on the affliction. Both earlier physicians had denied the disease the status of something entirely new. For Towne, yellow fever was simply a type of ardent fever, to be understood in clear parallel to other forms of the disease as they were familiar to European physicians. The Barbadian climate, with its humidity and the salinity of its air, contributed to the production of the disease, but Towne made no generalisation about 'tropical' climates and drew no analogies between this warm weather distemper and those found elsewhere at similar latitudes. For Warren, the yellow fever was not even originally produced in Barbados. It was a contagious disease bred in the Levant, which made its way to the otherwise healthy island through the movements of goods and people. It was thus precisely the same disease that afflicted others in Europe. Insofar as the West Indian climate mattered for the spread of yellow fever, then, its most important attribute was its difference to the climate in Palestine.

Born in 1690, Towne was probably the first person to publish a description of yellow fever in the West Indies. Like both Hillary and Warren (with the last of whom he may have overlapped), he was a graduate of Leiden and, like Hillary again, Towne's medical writing shows the marks of his training, with regular citations to Freind, Pitcairne, and Boerhaave, among others. The explanation he offered for the cause of many of Barbados' illnesses was largely mechanical. The moist warm air tended to relax the body's fibres and increase the viscidity of the blood while decreasing the air's capacity to expand the pulmonary vessels. The salt from the sea air stimulated the heart and organs, so that the blood pumped faster, but the thickened blood became less able to make its way through the secretory glands. The result was obstructions and stagnation. One particular outcome of such obstructions was fever, the heat arising from the 'unusually strong rubbing', according to Boerhaave, of the fluid Parts among each other, against the Vessels, and the Vessels against the liquid'.[72] Towne quoted the entirety of one of Boerhaave's aphorisms to

---

[71] Ibid., 129.

[72] Hermann Boerhaave, *Boerhaave's Aphorisms: Concerning the Knowledge and Cure of Diseases. Translated from the Last Edition Printed in Latin at Leyden, 1715. With Useful Observations and Explanations, by J. Delacoste, M.D.* (London: Printed for B. Cowse and W. Innys, 1725), Aphorism 675, 156.

describe the effect of the heating of the body that accompanied one particularly dangerous fever 'which so endemically rages in these *Parts*', and which he termed a *Febris Ardens Biliosa*, a particular kind of ardent fever.[73] That the fever was a *bilious* one seemed obvious to Towne, given that roughly three days after the first symptoms the surface of the body was suffused with that humour, giving the patient that 'Saffron Tincture' characteristic of the disease.[74] Drawing attention to his own local knowledge and expertise, Towne observed that those unfamiliar with the West Indies were sometimes confused. 'I have known some ingenious Practitioners', Towne wrote, 'upon their first coming strangely surprised at the Novelty of the *Appearances* they have met with, in this Island, even to so great a degree, that they have mistaken the *Yellowness* of the Skin in a Fever of no more than twenty four Hours standing, for a confirmed and inveterate Jaundice'.[75] Towne's book was aimed, in part, to help prevent the newcomer from making such dangerous errors. Once properly diagnosed, treatment followed along lines surely familiar to most physicians, whether newcomers or old hands, involving immediate and then repeated bloodletting to cool the body and relieve it of its surfeit of blood, followed by emetics to break up and remove the excess bile (blisters served this purpose, too), and cooling, subacid drinks.

Writing thirteen years later, Warren found this analysis preposterous. Without naming Towne, he sharply rebuked the author of a 'Treatise published a few years ago, concerning the Distempers of *Barbados*; which, I fear, has misled many unwary Practitioners into a false notion of the Distemper, and so into a wrong Method of Practice, full of Danger and pregnant of Errors'.[76] In the unlikely event that readers were unaware of Warren's precise target, all confusion would have been removed when he lambasted his unnamed opponent for introducing the term *Febris Ardens Biliosa* to describe the disease that he denoted as the 'malignant fever' of Barbados.

At the crux of Warren's disagreement with Towne was the question of yellow fever's aetiology. Warren believed it was contagious – and hence brought to the island from elsewhere – while Towne, of course, believed it to be a disease indigenous to the West Indies. Both men were loath to convey the impression

---

[73] Towne, 201. Boerhaave, 158. '689. Heat increased doth dissipate the most liquid parts out of our Blood, that is, the Water, Spirits, Salts, and subtilest Oils; it drieth the remaining Mass, thickens it; causes it to run together into an unmoveable and not resolvable Matter: it freeth the Salts and Oils, attenuates and makes 'em sharper, exhales and moves 'em; consequently it wears the smallest Vessels out and breaks 'em; dries the Fibres, makes 'em stiff and shrivell'd; hence produces suddenly many, quick, dangerous and mortal Diseases; which may easily be accounted for, and derived from the first effect of heat mention'd here'. 158. Quoted in Latin in Towne, Note, 24–5.

[74] · Towne, 23.

[75] Ibid., 4.

[76] Henry Warren, *A Treatise Concerning the Malignant Fever in Barbados and the Neighbouring Islands: With an Account of the Seasons There, from the Year 1734 to 1738. In a Letter to Dr. Mead.* (London: Printed for Fletcher Gyles against Grays-Inn in Holborn, 1740), 2.

that Barbados, in spite of the presence of dangerous diseases, was an unsalu-
brious spot. Towne assured his readers that the diseases he described in his
book were not necessary consequences of travelling to the island from Europe.
To insinuate such would be 'doing an unpardonable Act of Injustice to one of
the most delightful *Countries* in the Creation'.[77] Yet Warren took this defence
one step further, by arguing that there were 'no Malignant Distempers truly
Indigenous, or Natives of this Island; and that such have always been brought
in among us from some other infected places'.[78] The last time the disease made
its appearance, Warren claimed, was 1733, when it had been introduced from
Martinique. Yet it was no more a native of Martinique than Barbados, having
made its way to the Americas on a ship from Marseilles, which was carrying
goods from the Levant. The distemper, in its essence, was of an '*Asiatic
Extract*'.[79]

   One of Warren's best arguments in favour of his case turned on the problem
of seasoning. Why did yellow fever disproportionately strike newcomers and
not natives? Towne cited Sydenham's observation that fevers make up two-
thirds of all chronic illnesses, suggesting that 'in the West Indies (especially
with regard to strangers) the proportion runs much higher'.[80] Most people, he
claimed, 'how wary soever they may be in their conduct, are obliged to undergo
what the inhabitants call a *Seasoning*'.[81] Warren, similarly, noted that the fever
the French called *La Maladie de Siam* or *La Fievre Matelotte* ('because Sea-
Faring People and New-comers are chiefly obnoxious to it'),[82] upon its arrival
in Barbados 'soon swept away a Multitude of People, especially New-comers,
and Sea-faring persons, such as had purer Blood, and probably less adust than
that of the Natives; or of those whose Constitutions had been for many Years
fitted and habituated to the Climate'.[83] For Warren, however, the fact that the
disease struck harder those who had cleaner fluids seemed to make a mockery
of Towne's explanation, which relied on the effect of the climate on people's

---

[77] Towne, 15.
[78] Warren, 1.
[79] Ibid., 5.
[80] Towne, 19.
[81] Ibid., 19–20.
[82] Warren, 3–4. The connection to Siam seems to have been erroneous. 'In 1690', wrote Carter,
   'began in Martinique an epidemic of which we have a full account by Père Labat (1722). It
   was brought quite certainly from Recife to Martinique by the *Oriflamme*, a French war vessel
   which had cleared from Bangkok, but had touched at Pernambuco. Because of this origin,
   the epidemic, which spread generally over the West Indies and the continental shores of the
   Caribbean, became known as the "epidemic of the *Oriflamme*", or the "*mal de Siam*". Indeed,
   it gave the latter name "*mal de Siam*" to the disease for a long time and over a wide area, much
   of which was infected from other sources and with a fever absolutely unknown to Siam'. Henry
   Rose Carter, *Yellow Fever: An Epidemiological and Historical Study of Its Place of Origin*
   (Baltimore: The Williams and Wilkins Company, 1931), 196.
[83] Warren, 5.

fluids and fibres, producing, in sickness, 'a *bilious*, adust, overfermented *Blood*'.[84] Why, Warren asked, should those who had spent the least time in the warm, saline, moist atmosphere be the most likely to suffer?

For how then comes it that Strangers and New-comers, whose blood is purest and least impregnated with exalted Oils and Salts, should be most liable to this Disease? How comes it that the Natives of the *Torrid Zone*, whose juices we may reasonably suppose to be more acrid and alcalescent, are however much less obnoxious to it, if the malignant Symptoms proceeded merely from a Suffusion of Bile? How comes it that all Sorts and Conditions of the People, who live in the same Island, nay, in the same Town and Air, shall never receive the Infection, provided they keep themselves a little out of its Reach, and at a sufficient Distance from infected Persons and Places?[85]

Warren claimed this critique was so salient that it even persuaded Towne. 'I had the Pleasure', he explained (with none to contradict him), 'of convincing him of those Mistakes and I must do him the Justice to declare that he frankly retracted his opinion before he died, and would willingly have called in the Copies, could he have found Means of doing it'.[86]

Whether Towne had been convinced or not, Hillary would have none of this in his *Observations*. Yet Warren was attempting to draw upon powerful allies. He had composed his treatise as a letter and dedicated it to Richard Mead, Fellow of the Royal Society and personal physician to George II. Warren's work relied heavily on the logic Mead had used in his enormously popular *Short Discourse Concerning Pestilential Contagion*.[87] First published in 1720, seven editions appeared within a year, with the ninth published in 1744. The work was inspired by the outbreak of plague in Marseilles in 1720 and the subsequent British panic about its spread.[88] Together with Sloane and John Arbuthnot, Mead played a significant role on producing the Quarantine Act of 1721. Quarantine made sense, Mead claimed, because the plague was not native to England: avoid contagious goods and people and the disease itself could be avoided.

If England were 'innocent' of inflicting this affliction on the world, however, from where did it spring? Mead pointed his finger firmly in the

[84] Towne, 33.
[85] 'How comes it that the *Negroes*', continued Warren, 'whose Food is mostly rancid Fish or Flesh, nay often the Flesh of Dogs, Cats, Asses, Horses, Rats &c, and who mostly lead very intemperate Lives, and who are always worse clad, and most exposed to Surfeits, Heats, Colds, and all the Injuries of the Air, are so little subject to this Danger?', Warren, 13–14.
[86] Ibid., 15.
[87] Richard Mead, *A Short Discourse Concerning Pestilential Contagion and the Methods to Be Used to Prevent It.* (London: Printed [by William Bowyer] for Sam Buckley, and Ralph Smith, 1720). The first seven editions would remain unchanged. Although the point is mentioned in the first edition, it is the eighth that offered a detailed discussion of the origin of the illness and the mode of its production in Africa.
[88] Arnold Zuckerman, 'Plague and Contagionism in Eighteenth-Century England', *Bulletin of the History of Medicine* 78, no. 2 (2004).

direction of Africa, guilty of breeding not only this disease but others as well. '[T]he *Plague* has always the same Original', he wrote, 'and is brought from *Africa*, the Country which has entail'd upon us two other infectious Distempers, the *Small-Pox* and *Measles*'. Epidemics might arise in any nation – particularly in spaces such as military camps or jails – and could spread like a pestilence. Yet the 'true' plague, claimed Mead, found its origin in Ethiopia or Egypt 'and the *Infection* of it carried by Trade into the other Parts of the World'.[89]

In essence, Warren would transfer Mead's arguments from England to the West Indies. Both men offered a dichotomous understanding of diseases across the globe. Many earlier authors, like Hoffmann, had avoided charging any one part of the world with producing worse afflictions than any other. Following the logic of *Airs, Waters, and Places,* each region simply had a number of diseases characteristic of it. For Warren and Mead, however, the globe could be divided in two: those regions responsible for the production of certain foul and pestilential afflictions and those who were the blameless victims of contagion. According to Mead, England was not only not the home of the plague, the measles, and smallpox, it was not even the origin for a disease known as the *Sudor Anglicus* (English Sweat) or *Febris Ephemera Britannica*. This was 'most probably of a foreign Original', and the English had in fact, 'by the salutary Influence of our Climate' reduced its malignity.[90] The habit of blaming foreign climes for the introduction of a given disease had a venerable history, but Mead and Warren had taken it one step further, by arguing that their locations were to be blamed for no particularly malign disorders at all. Warren would thus make a dual move, producing both difference and similarity, but it was an unusual coupling, one that joined the West Indies to England and opposed both to Asia and Africa.

Hillary was unimpressed. 'I cannot conceive', he wrote, 'what were the Motives which induced a late ingenious Author to think that this Fever was first brought from Palestine to Marseilles, and from thence to Martinique, and so to Barbadoes, about thirty seven Years since'. The disease, he argued, was rarely contagious and had, in any case, been observed on the island before the 1730s. Far from being a foreign import, it was 'indigenous to the West-India Islands, and the Continent of America which is situated between, or near to the Tropics, and most probably to all other Countries within the Torrid Zone'. If the disease was not new to the West Indies, however, it was new to European physicians. Hillary claimed to find no mention of it in any classical sources – 'none of them has ever mentioned, or probably ever seen this Disease' – or even those of

---

[89] Richard Mead, *A Short Discourse Concerning Pestilential Contagion and the Methods to Be Used to Prevent It.*, Eighth, with large Additions ed. (London. Sam. Buckley, 1722), 20–1.

[90] Ibid., 64.

the Arab world 'who lived and practiced in the hot climate'.[91] Word of it came
from contemporary observers in the Spanish Americas, or from the French in
Siam, a kingdom, Hillary informed the reader, 'which is situated between the
Tropicks, near the same Latitude with the West India Islands'.[92] In Hillary's
hands, yellow fever may have been the first tropical disease, an affliction native
neither to only one particular country or place nor to warm climates in general,
but rather to precisely the region between the Tropics of Cancer and Capricorn.

The disease's aetiology was also suitably tropical. Noting that the illness
'most commonly seizes Strangers' Hillary nonetheless ignored Warren's
criticisms of a climatic explanation of seasoning.[93] The yellow fever, he
argued – drawing upon and altering Towne's formulation – was a putrid bilious
fever. Somewhat disingenuously, Hillary put forward two options for the fever's
proximate cause: it was either occasioned by infectious miasmata, or else by
the 'great Heat of the Air, and Water, and the Putrefaction of our Fluids etc.
from thence'.[94] Since he had earlier spent a good deal of time dismissing the
notion that the illness was infectious, this left the warm and humid Barbadian
atmosphere as the remaining culprit. The body rotted from within.

As befitted a novel disease, Hillary's explanation was new as well. Almost
all other afflictions described in his *Treatise* could be explained using a fairly
mechanical and dyadic logic. The body in illness had consisted either of fibres
too tense and rigid, accompanied by dense, viscid blood, or else fibres too
lax and blood too weak and thin. Health was to be found in the balance. For
the putrid bilious fever, however, Hillary closely followed John Huxham in
his 1750 *Essay on Fevers* (the theoretical counterpart to his two volumes on
Observations of the Air), in introducing a third state of the blood 'of more dangerous Consequence than either; I mean a state of it, that more immediately
tends to *Dissolution* and *Putrefaction*'.[95] After the introduction to the blood
of a 'bilious putrefying Diathesis', all the humours, but particularly the bile,
became 'inquinated with a putrid bilious Acrimony', which broke the larger
globules of blood that were characteristic of the body in health into smaller
parts, allowing them then to pass through ducts intended for excretion. In
time, even the brain was affected and 'all the Humours of the Body are almost

[91] Hillary, *Observations on the Changes of the Air and the Concomitant Epidemical Diseases, in
the Island of Barbados. To Which Is Added a Treatise on the Putrid Bilious Fever, Commonly
Called the Yellow Fever; and Such Other Diseases as Are Indigenous or Endemial, in the West
India Islands, or in the Torrid Zone*, 144, 155.

[92] Ibid., 143.

[93] Ibid., 146.

[94] Ibid., 153.

[95] John Huxham, *An Essay on Fevers, and Their Various Kinds, as Depending on Different
Constitutions of the Blood: With Dissertations on Slow Nervous Fevers; on Putrid, Pestilential,
Spotted Fevers; on the Small-Pox; and on Pleurisies and Peripneumonies* (London: S. Austen,
1750), 41.

changed into a putrescent lethiferous Ichor'.[96] If not rapidly prevented, the inevitable result was death.

Huxham had discussed a number of means by which such a putrefactive state might be achieved, but for Hillary's analysis of yellow fever, they came down to only one: climate.[97] To be sure, climate had mattered for Towne's and Warren's accounts, too. For Warren, Barbados was warm enough to promote the spread of contagion once it reached the island, but the West Indies could not be the disease's original home. Like England, the West Indies was a victim, not a culprit. For Towne, the warmth, humidity, and salinity of the air affected the body's fluids and fibres, inducing an ardent fever. Yet where Towne and Warren both took time to defend the Barbadian climate against its detractors, Hillary made little such effort. For Hillary, yellow fever was a marker of the island's peculiarity, its commonality with the rest of the Torrid Zone and its difference from Europe. Putrefaction evoked not merely the relative differences of laxity and viscidity, but the fundamental difference of life and death.

2.5   Slavery, Nativity, and the Production of Similarity

Hillary's discussion of yellow fever came in a section concerned with *acute* endemial diseases, those 'not so frequently seen in most parts of Europe'.[98] It was, in fact, an outlier in its novelty for the European reader. Most of the other diseases considered alongside it were more or less familiar to metropolitan physicians.[99] The Dry Belly Ache, for example, frequently afflicted those in the West Indies, but it had been known to seize patients in England and parts of Europe; dysentery was all too common in England; tetany was a disease associated with warm but not necessarily tropical climates and was well known to the ancient Greeks; and rabies was 'neither new, nor endemial or epidemical to Mankind', though it might be endemic to dogs in hot countries.[100]

Quite different were the illnesses considered in the second part of the book – *chronic* endemial diseases – which Hillary declared to be 'unknown and never seen but in the hot climates, except when they are carried by the

---

[96] Hillary, *Observations on the Changes of the Air and the Concomitant Epidemical Diseases, in the Island of Barbados. To Which Is Added a Treatise on the Putrid Bilious Fever, Commonly Called the Yellow Fever; and Such Other Diseases as Are Indigenous or Endemial, in the West India Islands, or in the Torrid Zone*, 153–4.

[97] On Huxham and the 'putrefactive paradigm', see Chapter 4.

[98] Hillary, *Observations on the Changes of the Air and the Concomitant Epidemical Diseases, in the Island of Barbados. To Which Is Added a Treatise on the Putrid Bilious Fever, Commonly Called the Yellow Fever; and Such Other Diseases as Are Indigenous or Endemial, in the West India Islands, or in the Torrid Zone*, 276.

[99] The exception was a disease that had neither been seen nor described by earlier physicians, which Hillary termed *Apthoides Chronica*. See ibid., 277.

[100] Ibid., 182, 201, 20, 45.

Sick into the colder Countries'.[101] Nyctalopia, Elephantiasis, Guinea Worm, Yaws, and other illnesses joined the putrid bilious fever as distempers that made Barbados a disease environment very different from Europe's and much like that of warmer lands. According to Kiple and Ornelas, Hillary's medical perception of the West India islands as fundamentally dissimilar to England's arose due to important shifts in the demography of the West Indies since 1700. To that date, they point out, the number of imported slaves to Jamaica and Barbados had been relatively small, with 60 per cent of the 220,000 slaves sent to Barbados. 'Indeed, 50 years earlier, Barbados was the only English Island importing slaves, and it was there, where the still mostly white populations had achieved a density of some 200 per square mile, that yellow fever made its first known epidemic appearance in the Western Hemisphere'.[102] Kiple and Ornelas plausibly suggest that Hillary's medical treatment of the huge numbers of those who suffered from the disease inspired his belief that he was working in a radically new disease environment.

One can certainly not deny the importance of demographic changes on the islands. Looking at Jamaica, it has been estimated that roughly 88,000 slaves were imported in the 46 years after British wrested control of the island from the Spanish in 1655. Almost three-and-a-half times this number (302,859) were imported in the period from 1702 to 1750, and more than five times the number (457,816) from 1751 to 1800.[103] Benjamin Moseley, writing in 1799, offered statistics on 'white' and 'black' populations on the same island across the eighteenth century. In 1698, he reported, the ratio of the black to the white population was 5.4 to 1 (40,000 blacks to 7,365 whites); in 1741, it was 10 to 1 (100,000 blacks to 10,000 whites); and in 1787, 11.1 to 1 (255,780 blacks to 23,000 whites).[104] Doctors on either Barbados or Jamaica thus saw a spectacular increase in the slave population in the middle of the eighteenth century, compared to the early 1700s.

This demographic explosion in the numbers of enslaved peoples was tied directly to the needs of the sugar trade. Sugar cultivation and production was both labour and capital intensive, considerably more so than cacao or indigo.[105] Between the 1680s and 1720, planters adopted an 'integrated' model for their plantations, one that combined both the growth of sugarcane and the transformation of the pressed juice into sugar crystals. To supply the necessary labour force, colonists imported increasing numbers of slaves, bought first

[101] Ibid., 276.
[102] Kiple and Ornelas, 68.
[103] Sheridan, *Doctors and Slaves: A Medical and Demographic History of Slavery in the British West Indies, 1680–1834*, 102.
[104] Benjamin Moseley, *A Treatise on Sugar* (London: Printed for G. G. and J. Robinson, 1799), 157.
[105] Dunn, 168.

from the Royal African Company, and then, after the Company lost its monopoly in 1698, from private slave traders. In the first years of the eighteenth century, Africans were being shipped to Jamaica at a rate of 4,500 a year, three times as fast as in the 1670s.[106] By the 1720s, most slaves worked in labour forces of one hundred or more people, arranged into gangs according to their stamina, with women in Jamaica and elsewhere making up the majority of field hands.[107] The economic success of such moves could not be gainsaid. Sugar output from Jamaica alone increased eightfold between 1700 and 1774, from 5,000 to 40,000 tons a year.[108] Barbadians who shifted from growing tobacco to growing sugar became rich almost overnight, so that they were already by 1680 the wealthiest men in British America.[109] The trend continued in the eighteenth century. Vincent Brown notes that the average net worth of a person in England or Wales in 1774 was £42, while that of free whites in the American colonies was roughly twice this (£89) and that of a free white person in the British West Indies was a staggering £1,042 sterling.[110]

Such financial success came at the expense of the lives of the enslaved, whose living and working conditions worsened with their rising numbers. 'Slavery had always been brutal in British America', observe Trevor Burnard and John Garrigus, 'but the violence exercised against Africans dramatically increased as the slave population grew'.[111] In 1740, Charles Leslie claimed of the Jamaican planters that 'No Country excels them in barbarous Treatment of Slaves, or in the cruel Methods they put them to death'.[112] Labour conditions were incredibly harsh, made even worse with shifts towards sugar monoculture.[113] Land that could have provided pasture for animals was instead turned to a more profitable crop. Ploughing that might have been performed by animals

---

[106] Ibid., 165.
[107] Trevor Burnard and John Garrigus, *The Plantation Machine: Atlantic Capitalism in French Saint-Domingue and British Jamaica* (Philadelphia: University of Pennsylvania Press, 2016), 41; Sheridan, *Doctors and Slaves: A Medical and Demographic History of Slavery in the British West Indies, 1680–1834*, 141–5; Richard S. Dunn, 'Sugar Production and Slave Women in Jamaica', in *Cultivation and Culture: Labor and the Shaping of Slave Life in the Americas*, ed. Ira Berlin and Philip D. Morgan (Charlottesville and London: University Press of Virginia, 1993); Barbara Bush, *Slave Women in Caribbean Society* (Bloomington: Indiana University Press, 1990); Barbara Bush-Slimani, 'Hard Labour: Women, Childbirth, and Resistance in British Caribbean Slave Societies', *History Workshop Journal* 36 (1993).
[108] Burnard and Garrigus, 38.
[109] Dunn, *Sugar and Slaves: The Rise of the Planter Class in the English West Indies, 1624–1713*, 85.
[110] Vincent Brown, *The Reaper's Garden: Death and Power in the World of Atlantic Slavery* (Cambridge, MA: Harvard University Press, 2008), 16.
[111] Burnard and Garrigus, 39.
[112] Leslie. Quoted in Burnard and Garrigus, 40.
[113] On labour conditions under slavery in the Americas, see in general Ira Berlin and Philip D. Morgan, eds., *Cultivation and Culture: Labor and the Shaping of Slave Life in the Americas* (Charlottesville and London: University Press of Virginia, 1993).

was instead carried out by slaves, who had the added burden of collecting grass after their work in the sugar fields was complete, in order to feed what cattle the islands could support.[114] Workdays lasted for twelve hours, although this number could increase during crop time, when the mill ran all night and planters feared the canes would spoil if they were not ground quickly enough.[115] Slaves were expected to supplement the rations supplied them by their masters by working on their own provision grounds when not in the fields.[116] As Sheridan notes, however, it seems likely that the typical Jamaican slave was 'underfed and overworked', with substantial dietetic deficiencies in protein and fat in particular.[117] As a point of comparison, it might be noted that slaves ate much less well than contemporary English agricultural labourers.[118] The effect of these conditions can be seen in the marked failure of slave populations in the Sugar Islands to reproduce themselves. Slave numbers may have risen dramatically across the eighteenth century, but this increase was due entirely to the importation of new enslaved peoples. By 1750, the enslaved population across the British Caribbean was somewhat less than 300,000 souls, despite the fact that, to that date, roughly 800,000 slaves had been imported.[119] The population density of slaves was rising, in other words, and slaves were 'highly stressed,

---

[114] Elsa V. Goveia, *Slave Society in the British Leeward Islands at the End of the Eighteenth Century* (New Haven and London: Yale University Press, 1965), 116–17.

[115] Ibid., 130.

[116] 'At Prospect Estate in the developing Parish of Portland, slaves worked 12 hours a day for an average of 272 days, with 60 days off. Illness or other problems stopped work for 33 days. During their days off, enslaved people produced their own food, constructed their own housing, and attended to the needs of themselves and their children'. Burnard and Garrigus, 42. On provision grounds, see also Sheridan, *Doctors and Slaves: A Medical and Demographic History of Slavery in the British West Indies, 1680–1834*, 164–9; Woodville K. Marshall, 'Provision Ground and Plantation Labor in Four Windward Islands: Competition for Resources During Slavery', in *Cultivation and Culture: Labor and the Shaping of Slave Life in the Americas*, eds. Ira Berlin and Philip D. Morgan (Charlottesville and London: University Press of Virginia, 1993).

[117] Sheridan, *Doctors and Slaves: A Medical and Demographic History of Slavery in the British West Indies, 1680–1834*, 171; Kiple; Jerome S. Handler, 'Diseases and Medical Disabilities of Enslaved Barbadians, from the Seventeenth Century to around 1838 (Part I)', *The Journal of Caribbean History* 40 (2006); 'Diseases and Medical Disabilities of Enslaved Barbadians, from the Seventeenth Century to around 1838 (Part II)', *The Journal of Caribbean History* 40 (2006).

[118] Dunn, *Sugar and Slaves: The Rise of the Planter Class in the English West Indies, 1624–1713*, 278.

[119] Philip D. Morgan, 'The Black Experience and the British Empire, 1680–1810', in *Black Experience and the Empire*, eds. Philip D. Morgan and Sean Hawkins (Oxford: Oxford University Press, 2006), 90. 'Sugar cultivation consumed enslaved labor', writes David Richardson, 'in most British sugar colonies deaths of slaves consistently exceeded births, some by as much as 4% a year'. David Richardson, 'Through a Looking Glass: Olaudah Equiano and African Experiences of the British Atlantic Slave Trade', ibid., 78. For contemporary debates over what Sheridan, *Doctors and Slaves: A Medical and Demographic History of Slavery in the British West Indies, 1680–1834*, 222–48. calls 'the problem of reproduction', see Chapter 7.

prone to disease, and likely to die'.[120] Hillary had clearly seen nothing like these conditions before his arrival in the New World.

One should be cautious nonetheless in seeing demography as a transparent explanation, for neither population increases nor the yellow fever outbreaks of the 1720s and 1730s are sufficient to explain Hillary's position. After all, Warren's arguments had been based on observations made on the island from 1734 to 1738, a period that saw striking demographic changes and outbreaks of the malignant fever.[121] Indeed, Warren claimed that in the six years after the most recent outbreak of the disease in 1733, the British crown had lost 'upwards of Twenty-Thousand very useful subjects, the much greatest part of whom were Sea-Faring People'.[122] Yet, unlike Hillary, Warren did not claim that Barbados constituted a novel disease environment, nor did he attempt to draw the West Indies into a larger complex of tropical countries.

To some extent, the seeming idiosyncrasy of West Indian diseases in the second half of Hillary's *Observations* was an artefact of the genre to which he was contributing. Writing about epidemic distempers in the first half of the text, as we have seen, Hillary had pointed to multiple similarities between the diseases in England and Barbados. Writing about endemial diseases, however, such similarities – while acknowledged – were then to be ignored. Inflammations of the bowels, various forms of colic, and multiple kinds of diarrhoea were all common to both parts of the world and were, 'with some Allowances for the Warmth of the Climate', to be managed in much the same manner. 'But as these last are all judiciously treated on by several learned and able Physicians in Europe, it is not necessary to say any thing on them here, since they should be treated here, much in the same manner as they are there'.[123] The effect, then, was to remove discussion of the illnesses that both affected the largest number of patients and were similar in both Europe and the West Indies and to focus discussions on those diseases that were 'indigenous and endemial in the West-India Islands, or peculiar to the Torrid Zone; and are seldom or never seen in the colder European Nations'.[124]

The very fact that Hillary's aim was to describe peculiar and endemic diseases thus tended to over-emphasise differences due to geographic location and under-emphasise the many similarities. That said, he was still able to list more than a dozen diseases likely to be unfamiliar (in practice, if not in theory)

---

[120] Burnard and Garrigus, 230.

[121] Warren.

[122] Ibid., 73–4.

[123] Hillary, *Observations on the Changes of the Air and the Concomitant Epidemical Diseases, in the Island of Barbados. To Which Is Added a Treatise on the Putrid Bilious Fever, Commonly Called the Yellow Fever; and Such Other Diseases as Are Indigenous or Endemial, in the West India Islands, or in the Torrid Zone*, 201–2.

[124] Ibid., 140.

to European physicians. From what causes did these illnesses arise? To a large extent, that question could be reduced to another: what was the geographical origin of each disease? Was the affliction *indigenous, endemial,* or both? Were the disease indigenous, the climate was the likely cause; were it endemial, but not indigenous, then it must have reached the West Indies by some set of movements.

For Hillary it was clear that many diseases – such as Elephantiasis, the *Lepra Arabum*, Leprosy of the Joints, and the Yaws – were not native to the West Indies, however much they might flourish on the islands now. Both Mead and Warren had pointed to trade as the cause for the increasing spread of contagious diseases. Hillary was rather more specific, pointing (like Kiple and Ornelas) to the slave trade in particular as the mechanism by which a once-healthy part of the New World had become a haven for disease.[125] In the past, Hillary claimed, 'we do not find that they had any of the before described diseases, which are indigenous to Africa, and have been imported with the African Negroes from thence, to these Western parts of the World; though these parts are as warm as Africa is'.[126] One can hear in the last part of this sentence an echo of Mead's arguments: a warm climate was necessary, but not sufficient for the first creation of many distempers. Hillary also clearly shared Mead's distaste for the African disease environment. Barbados was not as blessed as 'the happy Climate of England, which is totally a Stranger to this [the *Lepra Arabum*], and some other miserable diseases',[127] but it had been vastly more fortunate than Africa, where so many of the worst afflictions were native.

Adamant that Africa was and Barbados was not the origin for multiple distempers, Hillary was less clear on whether there was a rather more general climatic aetiology at work. Although he would argue that many diseases were common throughout the Torrid Zone, he hedged his bets on the reason for the commonality. Elephantiasis was 'a disease which is *either* indigenous or endemial to such countries as are within the Torrid Zone';[128] Nyctalopia, similarly 'may justly be deemed an indigenous or endemial disease in the Torrid Zone; though it is but very rarely seen in England, or in the other parts of Europe'.[129] His position was a complex one. A distinction of kind and not merely degree could be maintained between the disease environments of the temperate and torrid zones: disease environments defined by both geography

---

[125] Curtin, 'Epidemiology and the Slave Trade'. Sheridan, *Doctors and Slaves: A Medical and Demographic History of Slavery in the British West Indies, 1680–1834.*

[126] Hillary, *Observations on the Changes of the Air and the Concomitant Epidemical Diseases, in the Island of Barbados. To Which Is Added a Treatise on the Putrid Bilious Fever, Commonly Called the Yellow Fever; and Such Other Diseases as Are Indigenous or Endemial, in the West India Islands, or in the Torrid Zone,* 353.

[127] Ibid., 327.

[128] Ibid., 304. My emphasis.

[129] Ibid., 297–8.

and climate. But it was not obvious – despite the West Indies' geographical location within the tropics and its climatic similarity to Africa – that it had always belonged in the latter grouping. Medically speaking, Barbados had, in Hillary's eyes, become part of the Torrid Zone only recently and as a result of human action and human movements.

Conclusion

Although they were bound into a common volume, the two books that made up Hillary's *Observations* spoke to two fairly distinct audiences (one English, one West Indian) and two largely distinct medical traditions. The first, I have suggested, was written under the sign of Hippocrates' *Epidemics I* and *III*, at least as these books were reconceived by members of the Royal Society and other proponents of the new philosophy and mechanical studies of the air. The first book's aim and structure was demonstrably similar to that of an earlier medico-meteorological diary Hillary had produced in England and had appended to his first publication, a Newtonian account of smallpox and its treatment. Although the conceit of many weather diaries was that they detailed the air and diseases in a given location, Hillary's example makes clear that geographical specificity was, in fact, rather insignificant to the global project James Jurin envisioned, which aimed – as so many natural philosophical projects of the time did – to produce universality out of particularity.

It would not do, of course, to overstate the blindness to geographical diversity of works that drew upon *Epidemics*, but a broad pattern may nonetheless be discerned. One may see it most clearly in John Huxham's *Observations on the Air and Epidemical Diseases*, where *Epidemics* was cited on the first page for its description of 'the Constitution of the Air preceding the common Diseases'. Huxham turned to another Hippocratic text – *Airs, Waters, and Places* – to make a point about geographical difference, invoking presumably familiar arguments about the change of diseases across space to defend the mapping between seasonality (thus, temporality) and illness that characterised *Epidemics*.

But if the various Temperatures of the Air in different Climates produces Diseases altogether different, why should not different Tempers of the Air, even in the same Country, produce also different Affections for the Body? And so in Truth it happens, for Instance, in the Spring-Season, especially if dry, north-easterly Winds continue a long Time, inflammatory Fevers, Pleurisies, Peripneumonies, Squinsies most certainly prevail. – In Autumn on the contrary slow and putrid Fevers, Quartans, Cholerae, Dysenteries almost always rage. – Thus in like Manner humid, warm Weather brings on quite different Disorders from such as are found in cold and dry.[130]

---

[130] Orig. Latin is 1739. English trans, 1758, John Huxham, *The Works of John Huxham, M. D. F. R. S. In Two Volumes*, II vols., vol. I (London: W. Bent, 1788), xxvi–vii.

Using *Epidemics*, Hillary could produce a weather diary based on the climate and diseases of Barbados to contribute to universal (read: metropolitan) debates, repeatedly drawing attention to similarities between the West Indies and England. In his *Treatise on the Putrid Bilious Fever*, however, *Airs, Waters, and Places* formed the model for an account of the particularity and peculiarity – the differences – of the West Indian disease environment. The book's intended readers were not metropolitan physicians and natural philosophers collating material for a global project, but West Indian medics interested in the treatment and cure of the local afflictions with which they grappled every day. Huxham, or Boerhaave could be their guides for diseases known in Europe, Hillary's text was concerned with medicine as local knowledge.

Towne, also using *Airs, Waters, and Places* as a guide, had earlier discussed the island's endemial diseases, noting that most were also common in England. In Hillary's book, by contrast, commonalities between the diseases of the West Indies and Europe were ignored or at least underplayed. In the *Treatise* the Barbadian disease environment emerges as a profoundly foreign space. Yellow fever – thoroughly native and utterly novel – served as the most fundamental marker of this foreignness, the product of a distinctly tropical environment. As such, it was also something of an outlier among Barbados' other endemial diseases, a reminder of how complex are the answers as we try to track the emergence of conceptions of the diseases characteristic not of cities or countries, but of vast geographic regions, such as the Torrid and Temperate Zones. While the putrid bilious fever was indigenous, the majority of other endemial diseases were brought to the island via the movement of slaves. Medically speaking, West Indian difference for Hillary was made, not born.

Demography – the spectacular rise in the slave population of the sugar islands – surely had a large role to play in producing Hillary's vision of a distinct disease environment in Barbados. Just as important, however, were mid-century events in which the West Indian islands were only one among many players. It is to these events, and to the role played by military action and military medical genres in the production of difference, that we turn in the next chapter.

Part II

Empire

3   Seasoning Sickness and the Imaginative Geography of the British Empire

The hapless protagonist of Ebeneezer Cook's *The Sot-Weed Factor* (1708) suffered through a series of misadventures after his arrival in colonial Maryland. Battling poultry invaded his hostel room, making sleep impossible. After giving up on his lodgings and fleeing to an orchard, he encountered a rattlesnake; climbing a tree to make his escape, he then spent the evening tormented by 'curst muskitoes'. When, somewhat later, he finally managed a decent night's rest, he awakened to find his stockings, hat, and shoes had been stolen and thrown into a fire (a footnote informs us that this was common practice amongst planters). Most dangerous, perhaps, he soon found himself falling victim to disease: a local affliction known as 'the seasoning'.

> With Cockerouse as I was sitting,
> I felt a Feaver Intermitting:
> A fiery Pulse beat in my Veins,
> From Cold I felt resembling Pains:
> This cursed seasoning I remember
> Lasted from *March* to cold *December*:
> …
> And had my Doctress wanted skill,
> Or Kitchin Physick at her will,
> My Father's Son had lost his Lands,
> And never seen the *Goodwin-Sands*[1]

The idea of *seasoning* was a common one by the 1700s. The term dates back to at least the fifteenth century, when one finds the verb *to season* used in a sense very similar to the most common modern understanding: 'to render (a dish) more palatable by the addition of some savoury ingredient'. The word derives from the Old French *saisonner*, meaning 'to ripen, to render (fruit) palatable by the influence of the seasons'.[2] A second, somewhat different

---

[1] Ebenezer Cooke, *The Sot-Weed Factor, or, a Voyage to Maryland a Satyr: In Which Is Describ'd, the Laws, Government, Courts and Constitutions of the Country, and Also the Buildings, Feasts, Frolicks, Entertainments and Drunken Humours of the Inhabitants of That Part of America: In Burlesque Verse* (London: B. Bragg, 1708).

[2] Oxford English Dictionary Online, accessed 15 Aug. 2014. 'Season, *v*'.

and later English term flows from this original French usage, for one also speaks of seasoned timber, or seasoned metal. The analogous use of the term for people – to be inured to conditions by training and experience – appears already in the early seventeenth century.[3] 'Tis an unseasoned Courtier, Good my Lord', says the Countess of Rossillion to Lord Lafew in *All's Well that Ends Well* (1623), 'Advise him'. Then, as now, soldiers required considerable seasoning to adequately perform their tasks. Baker's *Chronicle* (1665) placed the blame for the Earl of Montross' defeat in battle to his reliance on 'unseason'd Orkney men'.[4]

Cook's usage, however, was rather different to these, for he was alluding to the notion of a 'seasoning sickness', an illness that helped habituate the sufferer to a foreign clime.[5] In 1707, Hans Sloane – then Secretary and later President of the Royal Society – offered the following explanation of 'what is call'd the Seasoning', derived from the time he spent in the West Indies:

that is to say, that every New-Comer before they be accustomed to the Climate and Constitution of the Air in *Jamaica* are to have an acute Disease, which is thought to be

---

[3] Joyce Chaplin has suggested that the term was already in usage in North America in the 1550s, although all the cited examples are from the seventeenth century and afterward. Chaplin, *Subject Matter: Technology, the Body, and Science on the Anglo-American Frontier, 1500–1676*, 151.

[4] Richard Baker, *A Chronicle of the Kings of England: From the Time of the Roman's Government Unto the Death of King James. Containing All Passages of State and Church, with All Other Observations Proper for a Chronicle. Faithfully Collected out of Authors Ancient and Modern; and Digested into a New Method* (London: Nathaniel Ranew and Jonathan Robinson, 1665), 647.

[5] We know a good deal about seasoning and 'acclimatisation' during the nineteenth century. We know a great deal less about the seventeenth and eighteenth centuries, although this situation has changed considerably with the publication of Harrison, *Medicine in an Age of Commerce and Empire: Britain and its Tropical Colonies, 1660–1830*. For early medical histories of the diseases of warm climates in the British Empire, see David Arnold, *Warm Climates and Western Medicine: The Emergence of Tropical Medicine, 1500–1900* (Amsterdam; and Atlanta: Rodopi, 1996); D. Arnold, 'India's Place in the Tropical World, 1770–1930', *Journal of Imperial and Commonwealth History* 26, no. 1 (1998). On Human acclimatisation in Britain, see David N. Livingstone, 'Human Acclimatization: Perspectives on a Contested Field of Inquiry in Science, Medicine, and Geography', *History of Science* 25 (1987); 'Tropical Climate and Moral Hygiene: The Anatomy of a Victorian Debate', *British Journal for the History of Science* 32, no. 1 (1999). For the specific case of Australia, see Anderson, *The Cultivation of Whiteness: Science, Health and Racial Destiny in Australia*. For French botanical and zoological acclimatisation, see Michael A. Osborne, *Nature, the Exotic and the Science of French Colonialism* (Bloomington: Indiana University Press, 1994); 'Acclimatizing the World: A History of the Paradigmatic Colonial Science', *Osiris* 15 (2000). The former contains excellent references to histories of acclimatisation societies around the world. For human acclimatisation in France, see Eric T. Jennings, *Curing the Colonizers: Hydrotherapy, Climatology, and French Colonialism* (Durham, NC: Duke University Press, 2006). For acclimatisation and anthropology in Germany, see Pascal Grosse, *Kolonialismus, Eugenik Und Bürgerliche Gesellschaft in Deutschland 1850–1918* (Frankfurt and New York: Campus, 2000); 'Turning Native? Anthropology, German Colonialism, and the Paradoxes of the "Acclimatization Question", 1885–1914', in *Worldly Provincialism: German Anthropology in the Age of Empire*, eds. H. Glenn Penny and Matti Bunzl (Ann Arbor: University of Michigan Press, 2003).

very dangerous, and that after this is over, their bodies are made more fit to live there, with less hazard than before: and this is not only thought so in that Island, but in *Guinea* and all over the remote Eastern parts of the world.[6]

Seventeenth and eighteenth-century travellers, doctors, soldiers, and sailors all paid a great deal of attention to an illness that seemed to be a disease of *place*. Seasoning affected neither 'natives' nor those who had spent a good deal of time in a specific locale. Only those habituated to one location who ventured to another in which they were strangers fell ill. If they survived their affliction, their bodies were then inured to the novelties of the environments in which they now found themselves.

Of particular interest in Sloane's definition is its geographical reach. The idea of seasoning, it would seem, was a commonplace of parts of the Americas, Africa, and Asia. Just as interesting as the locations included were those left out. Sloane was an English physician writing for a British and European audience that was presumably unfamiliar with the term. His phrasing – '*what is call'd* the Seasoning' – invoked distance. Seasoning was a distemper that plagued English bodies out of place: it made up a discourse of anti-nativity.

I offer in this chapter a history of seasoning in the eighteenth-century British Empire and through this a history of the medical construction of what Edward Said has termed an 'imaginative geography', a conceptual creation of a division of the world.[7] '[E]mpires', Mary Luise Pratt has noted, 'create in the imperial center of power an obsessive need to present and re-present its peripheries and its others continually to itself'.[8] My purpose is to examine the ways in which medicine and medical discourse functioned precisely as part of this far from static re-presentation (and representation) of peripheries to an imperial centre.

The chapter is divided chronologically into two halves. In the first (covering roughly the early seventeenth through the mid-eighteenth centuries) I examine seasoning discourse in its presence throughout the periphery and its relative absence at the centre. In part two I look first at the effect of the wars of the late 1730s and 1740s in bringing seasoning talk to the metropole, before concentrating on the role played by James Lind, author of the most important eighteenth-century medical treatise in English on the diseases of the periphery: *An Essay on Diseases Incidental to Europeans in Hot Climates* (1768). In Lind's work, as we will see, seasoning became a global discourse, as applicable to Britain as elsewhere. Seasoning remained a strangers' affliction, but in the newly and unsettlingly large empire that followed British victories in the Seven Years War, even familiar locations contained pockets of strangeness.

---

[6] Sloane, xcviii.

[7] Said, *Orientalism*.

[8] Mary Louise Pratt, *Imperial Eyes: Travel Writing and Transculturation*, 2nd ed. (London and New York: Routledge, 2008), 4.

3.1   Seasoning on the Periphery

My suspicion is that early military – particularly naval – deployments were the source for the earliest usages of the notion that one needed to endure illness in order to become seasoned to a place. It is in the writings of soldiers and sailors – or at least those discussing war – that I have found the first mention of the term. John Smith, in his accounts of the first European plantation in Virginia, for example, described a battle with local inhabitants in 1608. His company had been drastically reduced due to illness: 'were we but fiue (with our captaine) [that] could stand: [f]or within 2. daies after wee left *Kecoughtan*, the rest … were sick almost to death (vntill they were seasoned to the country)'.[9] In 1640, John Pym addressed parliament and discussed a number of grievances. Among them was King Charles' failure to engage in war with Spain over the West Indies. In New England, Virginia, the Caribbean, and the Bermudas, Pym argued, there were now 'at least sixty thousand able persons of this nation, many of them well armed and their bodies seasoned to that climate' who could prosecute a conflict to the Crown's advantage.[10] After Charles' execution in 1649, Cromwell initiated a far more aggressive foreign policy. A year after the Protector's forces seized Jamaica in 1655, a letter from a ship lying in wait for the Spanish Fleet off the coast of Havannah noted that 'as many of us are left are in good health, being seasoned to the country'.[11]

One may multiply other naval examples of the use of the concept of seasoning in the seventeenth and early eighteenth centuries. Yet, at least within the New World, seasoning would soon also pass into common, civilian parlance. Daniel Denton, in 1670, alluded to the term's popularity, even as he denied its application to New York. The climate there, he argued, 'hath such an affinity with that of England, that it breeds ordinarily no alteration to those who remove thither; that the name of seasoning, which is common to some other Countreys hath never there been known'.[12] Colonists elsewhere had no such reservations in applying the term. 'My sister has had her seasoning …

---

[9] Edward Arber, ed. *Capt. John Smith, of Willoughby by Alford, Lincolnshire; President of Virginia, and Admiral of New England: Works. 1608–1631* (Birmingham: The English Scholars Library, 1884), 117. Smith was fairly complimentary about the climate, however. 'The temperature of the Country doth agree well with *English* constitutions, being once seasoned to the Country'. See ibid., 47, 343.

[10] Charles Kendall Adams, *Representative British Orations* (New York: Putnam, 1884), 82.

[11] Thomas Birch, ed. *A Collection of the State Papers of John Thurloe, Esq; Secretary First to the Council of State and Afterwards to the Two Protectors Oliver and Richard Cromwell* (Burlington: TannerRitchie, 2005), 367.

[12] Daniel Denton, *A Brief Description of New-York, Formerly Called New-Netherlands: With the Places Thereunto Adjoyning: Together with the Manner of Its Scituation, Fertility of the Soyle, Healthfulness of the Climate, and the Commodities Thence Produced: Also Some Directions and Advice to Such as Shall Go Thither … Likewise a Brief Relation of the Customs of the Indians There* (London: John Hancock and William Bradley, 1670), 59.

two or three fits of a feaver and ague', noted William Fitzhugh to a doctor in the Chesapeake in 1687. Two weeks later he wrote similarly to his brother: she has had 'two or three small fits of a feaver and ague, which now has left, and so consequently her seasoning [is] over'.[13] Despite clear differences in climate, seasoning discourse could be found in the North as well as the South. Christopher Merret, surveyor of the port of Boston, published a short 'Account of several Observables in Lincolnshire' in the Philosophical Transactions in 1696 in which he drew attention to 'Agues (here called *Holland Baylies*) [that] are very rife, few strangers escaping without a seasoning'.[14] In his treatise on the *British Empire in America* (1708), John Oldmixon treated the seasoning not as the affliction of a single colony, but of many of them: 'The *Seasoning* here, as in other parts of *America,* is a Fever or Ague, which the Change of Climate and Diet generally throws New Comers into'.[15] By the early years of the eighteenth century, Robert Beverley had already become critical of what he saw as the overuse of the term. His *History of the First Settlement of Virginia*, dedicated a section to the diseases of Virginia and a subsection to 'The Seasoning', yet he dismissively noted that 'The first sickness that any New-Comer happens to have there, he unfairly calls a Seasoning, be it Fever, ague, or any thing else, that his own Folly, or excesses bring upon him'.[16]

Fear of the illness kept the schoolmaster James Kirkwood in Scotland, after apparently being offered a position as professor of Greek and Latin at the College of Jamestown. 'Persons', claimed Kirkwood, had informed his wife that 'it was ten to one of the whole Family should go there alive; and when they are arrived, commonly they are seiz'd on with a Fever, call'd a Seasoning, of which as many die as escape'.[17] One wonders who Kirkwood's informants were, since it was more common to treat the seasoning as one might treat most other fevers: an annoyance that had the potential to become fatal, but was unlikely to. John Norris framed his *Profitable Advice for Rich and Poor* (1712) as a dialogue between James Freeman, a Carolina Planter, and Simon Question, a

---

[13] Darrett B. Rutman and Anita H. Rutman, 'Of Agues and Fevers: Malaria in the Early Chesapeake', *The William and Mary Quarterly* 33, no. 1 (1976): quoted on 43–4.

[14] Christopher Merret, 'An Account of Several Observables in Lincolnshire, Not Taken Notice of in Camden, or Any Other Author', *Philosophical Transactions* 19 (1695–97): 351.

[15] Rutman and Rutman, quoted on 45.

[16] Robert Beverley, *The History and Present State of Virginia, in Four Parts. I. The History of the First Settlement of Virginia, and the Government Thereof, to the Present Time. II. The Natural Productions and Conveniencies of the Country, Suited to Trade and Improvement. III. The Native Indians, Their Religion, Laws, and Customs, in War and Peace. IV. The Present State of the Country, as to the Polity of the Government, and the Improvements of the Land. By a Native and Inhabitant of the Place.*, 1st ed. (London: R. Parker, 1705), 69.

[17] James Kirkwood, *The History of the Twenty Seven Gods of Linlithgow Being an Exact and True Account of a Famous Plea Betwixt the Town-Council of the Said Burgh, and Mr. Kirkwood* (Edinburgh: 1711), 51.

West Country farmer, which included the following exchange, suggesting that the seasoning was unlikely to claim as many victims as Kirkwood had feared:

S. QUESTION: *Have you not some Distempers there peculiar to the Country which is not usual here in* England?

J. FREEMAN: There is, in the Spring of the Year, a Feaver and Ague seizes many that are settled on the lowest Marsh Land, especially when they are new Comers into the Country, which is commonly called a Seasoning to them; after which, if their Habitations is on dry, healthy Land, they are, generally, very healthful, if temperate.[18]

James Oglethorpe pursued a similar theme in 1732, putting the threat of dangerous illness down to intemperance rather than the climate. 'In this country', he wrote, 'as almost in every new Climate, strangers are apt to have a seasoning; an ague, or sort of a Fever, but then 'tis very slight: And for the rest, People very seldom want Health here but by Intemperance (which indeed is too common)'.[19]

In the West Indies, the term was both common enough and geographically specific enough that Edward Phillips, in his *The New World of Words* (1706) defined a plural noun, *seasonings* as 'An Aguish distemper, which strangers are subject to, in the West-Indies, upon their first coming'.[20] Not all, however, were willing to buy the claim that newcomers were disproportionately afflicted by disease. Barbados had its own Denton in the physician Thomas Trapham, who insisted in 1679 that the island possessed fewer diseases than England and that it was those who had become habituated to the warm air who were most likely to be afflicted by distempers caused by cool night time breezes. Trapham granted that the area around the Port of Jamaica and other places near the water were better suited to the 'well inured *Jamaica* Man than any later arrived persons', but for the most part he ascribed the diarrhoeas and fluxes that greeted the stranger to the isle either to new drinks and diet or to 'rejoicing intemperance', rather than any insalubrious quality of his 'Summer Country'.[21]

As one might tell from Sloane's remarks, Trapham was probably in a minority, at least by the last decade of the seventeenth century. For Sloane and his informants, the question was not whether a seasoning sickness existed, but

---

[18] John Norris, *Profitable Advice for Rich and Poor: In a Dialogue, or Discourse between James Freeman, a Carolina Planter, and Simon Question, a West Country Farmer. Containing a Description ... Of South Carolina* (London: J. How, 1712), 28.

[19] J. Edward Oglethorpe, *A New and Accurate Account of the Provinces of South-Carolina and Georgia: With Many Curious and Useful Observations on the Trade, Navigation and Plantations of Great-Britain* (London: J. Worrall, 1732), 24.

[20] Edward Phillips, *The New World of Words: Or, Universal English Dictionary*, 6th ed. (London: J. Phillips, 1706). The word is not to be found in the first edition (1658). However, too much should not be made of this, since no meanings of the word 'season' are to be found in the earliest edition.

[21] Trapham, 23, 3.

rather the specific nature of the disease. Sloane dismissed the idea that jaundice seasoned strangers, on the grounds that it afflicted old hands and often spared newcomers. Instead, he argued that the true seasoning was marked by the eruption of small red boils all over the body. Positing that the pustules were caused by the body's attempt to remove from the blood the 'heterogenous and unaccustom'd Particles it had from the warm Sun', Sloane insisted that the illness was a salutary one, and was not to be checked:

therefore instead of prescribing a Remedy for its Cure I told those who importun'd me, that I thought this Distemper was the greatest advantage they could have, and that this was the effect of the change of Climate, and a proper seasoning, and what might secure them from future sickness by purging the blood from hot and sharp parts, and rather than check it, wish'd them to help the expulsion with a little *Flos Sulphuris*.[22]

What Sloane termed jaundice, however, was likely what later authors described as yellow fever, and it was that disease, more than any other, that became associated with the seasoning in the West Indies. Indeed, as we saw in the last chapter, the fact of seasoning soon became a point of contention in a dispute between Towne and Warren over actiology. Warren's text would be instrumental in disseminating the connection between yellow fever and seasoning and, relatedly, the idea that a bout of the seasoning protected one from later virulent illness. Agues and generic fevers might recur: only a small number of diseases struck only once. As John Lining noted in *A Description of the American Yellow Fever* – a work heavily indebted to Warren's: 'it is a great happiness that our constitutions undergo such alterations in the smallpox, measles, and yellow fever, as for ever afterwards secure us from a second attack of those diseases'.[23] By the early nineteenth century, the yellow fever was literally synonymous, at least in the New World, with the seasoning.[24]

One tends to find the concept more than the language of seasoning in those parts of the periphery with more impermanent British settlement. Harrison has pointed to the existence of seasoning discourse about India in the late seventeenth and early eighteenth centuries, although the examples given seem only to indicate an awareness that European bodies were out of place in warmer climes. Thus Ovington's description from *A Voyage to Suratt in the Year 1689*: the English in India, he claimed, are 'as Exotick Plants brought home to us, not agreeable to the soil'.[25] The Italian Gernelli Caveri, travelling in India around

[22] Sloane, Vol. 1, 25.
[23] John Lining, *A Description of the American Yellow Fever* (Edinburgh: G. Hamilton and J. Balfour, 1756), 7.
[24] George Pinckard and Andrew Dickson White, *Notes On the West Indies, Including Observations Relative to the Creoles and Slaves of the Western Colonies, and the Indians of South America: Interspersed with Remarks Upon the Seasoning Or Yellow Fever of Hot Climates.* 2d ed. (London: Baldwin, Cradock and Joy [etc.], 1816).
[25] Quoted in Harrison, *Climates* 39.

the same time as Ovington, noted a similar, but general, discomfort: 'Generally throughout all Indostan the heat is excessive, except near the mountains. We Europeans fare ill there because of the seasons differing from ours; because their winter begins in June and ends in September'.[26] Sloane's remarks would indicate that a discourse concerning seasoning *sickness* probably existed in the late seventeenth and early eighteenth centuries, yet examples are fairly rare. In 1711, Charles Lockyer wrote of a 'Seasoning Sickness, that we commonly meet, soon after our arrival in *India*', yet it is worth noting his insistence that the cause was diet rather than climate.[27] We find little mention of diseases that particularly strike strangers in Bontius' *Account of the Diseases, Natural History, and Medicines of the East Indies* (1629), but William Dampier's *A New Voyage Round the World* (1699) contains an account of the gold mines of Achin in Sumatra and the miners who are seasoned to the illnesses that arise there:

That at the mines it was so sickly that not the half of those that went thither did ever return again; tho they went thither only to Traffick with the Miners, who live there, being seasoned ... that some there made it their constant imployment to visit the Miners once every year; for after they are once seasoned, and have found the profit of that trade, no thoughts of danger can deter them from it.[28]

If the ideal climate required no seasoning, one might also find climates where habituation seemed virtually impossible. James Houston, physician for the Royal African Company and Chief Surgeon at Cape Coast Castle, mentioned the seasoning as the first disease to strike newcomers, but without the sense that, as Sloane had phrased it, 'after this is over, their bodies are made more fit to live there, with less hazard than before'. 'There is but one other Disease epidemically fatal to your Servants, which they call the *Seasoning*, known to all *Europeans* that come under the *Torrid Zone*, which is nothing but a Fever, caus'd by the change of the Climate'.[29] None were as scathing about

---

[26] Quoted in Harrison, *Climates*, 45.

[27] Charles Lockyer, *An Account of the Trade in India Containing Rules for Good Government in Trade ... With Descriptions of Fort St. George ... Calicut ... To Which Is Added, an Account of the Management of the Dutch in Their Affairs in India.* (London: Samuel Crouch, 1711), 177.

[28] William Dampier, *A New Voyage Round the World: Describing Particularly the Isthmus of America, Several Coasts and Islands in the West Indies, the Isles of Cape Verd, the Passage by Terra Del Fuego, the South Sea Coasts of Chili, Peru and Mexico, the Isle of Guam One of the Ladrones, Mindanao, and Other Philippine and East-India Islands near Cambodia, China, Formosa, Luconia, Celebes, &C., New Holland, Sumatra, Nicobar Isles, the Cape of Good Hope, and Santa Hellena: Their Soil, Rivers, Harbours, Plants, Fruits, Animals, and Inhabitants: Their Customs, Religion, Government, Trade, &C.* (London: James Knapton, 1697–1703), 133. On Dampier's debts to the questions raised in Robert Boyle's 'General Heads for a Natural History of a Countrey', see Malcolmson, 182.

[29] James Houstoun, *Some New and Accurate Observations Geographical, Natural and Historical. Containing a True and Impartial Account of the Situation, Product, and Natural History of the Coast of Guinea* (London: J. Peele, 1725), 56.

the disease environment as Willem Bosman, whose writings we encountered in Chapter 1. As Bosman made clear, not only were newcomers liable to illness in Guinea, even those 'who have long continued here' remained under threat. Only those born to what he referred to as 'the Stench' were immune.

However inured they may have been to their own climate, African bodies suffered just as those of Europeans did in the move to the New World. In an age before the rise of theories of racial fixity, the key questions concerned nativity and habituation. Slaves newly arrived to the Caribbean suffered enormously from the seasoning, a fact commonly described by slavers in economic terms. Some planters in the Antilles, we are informed in Volume V of the *Atlas Geographus* (1717), possessed 20000 pounds worth of slaves 'and many Planters are undone in a time of Mortality for want of Money to renew their Stock, which must be filled up every Year, because a 4th part die in Seasoning'.[30] James Grainger combined economic and moral reasoning in 1764 in what he claimed to be the first medical tract 'purposely written on the method of seasoning new Negroes'. It was not sufficient, Grainger insisted, to care for slaves when they were ill:

they should also be well clothed and regularly fed. Neglecting either of these important precepts is not only inhuman, it is the worst species of prodigality. One Negroe saved in this manner more than pays the additional expences which owners of slaves by this means incur. But, supposing it did not, it ought seriously to be considered by all masters, that they must answer before the Almighty for their conduct towards their Negroes.[31]

'New Negroes', Grainger argued, needed to be gradually accustomed to labour and no new slave could be said to be seasoned before they had been in the West Indies for at least a year. Nor were those newly arrived from Africa the only labourers in peril. Creoles who moved from one island to another also underwent a seasoning. Once seasoned, however, a slave commanded a higher price than a 'salt-water' Negroe. And those born in the region were the most valuable of all, hence the admonition that 'too great care cannot be taken either of Negresses when pregnant, and in the month, or of infants when born'.[32] Seasoning, it becomes clear, was central to the language – economic, moral, and medical – of both settlement and slavery.

While examples certainly exist, one finds comparatively little said about seasoning closer to the British Isles. Where seasoning is mentioned, it tends to be in the context of what, to British authors, were intra-European peripheries.

---

[30] Herman Moll, *Atlas Geographus: Or, a Compleat System of Geography, Ancient and Modern*, vol. V (London: J. Nutt, 1717), 492.

[31] James Grainger, 'An Essay on the More Common West-India Diseases, James Grainger, MD (1764), with Additional Notes by William Wright, MD, FRD (1802)', in *On the Treatment and Management of the More Common West-India Diseases (1750–1802)*, ed. J. Edward Hutson (Kingston, Jamaica: University of the West Indies Press, 2005), 51.

[32] Ibid., 13.

In 1708, for example, John Polus Lecaan – who had been employed as a physician in the service of King William – offered *Advice to the Gentlemen of the Army of her Majesty's Forces in Spain and Portugal*, which advice he proposed would be useful in all hot climates, including 'our Plantations in the West-Indies, &c'.

As in other Countries the Differences of Seasons produce different Effects in our Bodies; for by the more or less Heat the Pores of our Bodies are more or less open, the Air more or less pure, Food more or less spirituous; so without doubt great Difference of Climate, or of Heat and Cold, is very prejudicial to all Strangers, and the cause of numerous Distempers, especially to the *English*, who are very Irregular and Careless in their way of Living.[33]

Were the English instead to adapt their habits to mirror that of locals, such distempers could likely be avoided: 'This way of Living Strangers should observe, especially in the beginning, by which they will season themselves to the Country, and be able to bear the Climate almost as well as the Natives, who are the most abstemious People in the World'.[34]

I have found fairly few examples of the term seasoning applied to an English affliction before mid-century, although each is telling in its own way. Closest to the meanings explored here are comments found in John Graunt's *Natural and Political Observations ... Upon the Bills of Mortality* (1676). Graunt was attempting to explain why London's rate of burials outstripped its number of christenings in the period from 1603 to 1644. The reason he gave was that London's air was, for artificial reasons, particularly harmful. The problem was not intrinsic climate, but the effects of what moderns would call urbanisation. As William Cowper would phrase it: 'God made the country, and men made the town'.[35] London had been *made* a place where visitors from other parts of England required a new habituation.

As for unhealthiness, it may well be supposed, that although seasoned Bodies may, and do live near as long in *London,* as elsewhere, yet new-comers and Children do not: for the *Smoaks, stinks,* and close *Air,* are less healthful than that of the Country; otherwise why do sickly Persons remove into the Country-Air?[36]

London, it would seem, was like a foreign country to those brought up in the purer environs of the English countryside. A quirkier example may be found in Defoe's *Tour Thro' the Whole Island of Great Britain*, where the marital

---

[33] Lecaan, 4.

[34] Ibid., 9.

[35] On similar visions of London in this period, see Roy Porter, 'Cleaning up the Great Wen: Public Health in Eighteenth-Century London', *Medical History. Supplement* 11 (1991).

[36] Quoted in Andrew Wear, 'Health and the Environment in Early Modern England', in *Medicine in Society: Historical Essays*, ed. Andrew Wear (Cambridge: Cambridge University Press, 1992), 130.

habits of the inhabitants of the marshlands of Essex are described. '[A]ll along this Country', Defoe explains, 'it is very frequent to meet with Men that have had from Five or Six, to Fourteen or Fifteen Wives'. The reason had to do with location, the men of the region seeking wives in regions with healthier air. Their brides, brought back, soon fell sick and died, while the men, being 'seasoned to the Place, did pretty well', soon returning to the Uplands to 'fetch another' to replace their unfortunate spouse.[37] But such examples tend to be the exception rather than the rule. While writers in the New World (at least those assuming a local audience) spoke of seasoning with the expectation of being easily understood, those in England often glossed or explained the term, indicating its relative unfamiliarity.[38] This, as we will see, would begin to change after mid-century, in the aftermath of multiple imperial conflicts.

3.2   Seasoning an Empire

The Mid-Century Wars

The Spring of 1738 saw an intensification of the usual hostility between England and Spain over trade and piracy. And just as conflict between the two nations had inspired talk of the need for soldiers seasoned to the West Indian climate a century before, so too it reoccurred now. Parliamentary debates concerned both the question of whether war was advisable and also – should conflict be engaged – whether troops should be raised at home or in the Antilles. In arguing for war, Lord Bathurst rejected the idea that troops be raised from

---

[37] Daniel Defoe, *A Tour Thro' the Whole Island of Great Britain: Divided into Circuits or Journeys. Giving a Particular and Entertaining Account of Whatever Is Curious, and Worth Observation ... By a Gentleman*, 4 vols., vol. I (London: J. Osborn, S. Birt, D. Browne, J. Hodges, A. Millar, J. Whiston, and J. Robinson, 1742), 8–9.

[38] In 1696, for example, Gideon Harvey seemed unaware that the term was not a neologism in the medical context, drawing an analogy with a fired clay pot. 'The suffering of that Distemper [smallpox], I look upon as a seasoning to the demipestiferous Air; for as a new earthen Pot is seasoned, by letting the particles of the Fire gradually enter its pores, whereby they are by little and little widened, and then the Fire entering with a full force and finding no straitness or resistance, passeth through without any injury to the Pot; whereas should it at first be committed to a vigorous Fire, it would soon be crackt by the Fiery particles forcing the pores asunder, and this is called a Seasoning'. Gideon Harvey, *A Treatise of the Small-Pox and Measles: Describing Their Nature, Causes, and Signs, Diagnostick and Prognostick, in a Different Way to What Hath Hitherto Been Known: Together, with the Method of Curing the Said Distempers, and All, or Most, of the Best Remedies: Also, a Particular Discourse of Opium, Diacodium, and Other Sleeping Medicines: With a Reference to a Very Great Case* (London: W. Freeman, 1696), 31–2. Close to a century later, and in the same context as Graunt, Price inserted a parenthetical analogy to aid the reader: 'after that age, the inhabitants consisting chiefly of persons, who (like men *used* to drink) have been *seasoned* to *London*', Richard Price, *Observations on Reversionary Payments; on Schemes for Providing Annuities for Widows, and for Persons in Old Age; on the Method of Calculating the Values of Assurances on Lives; and on the National Debt* (London: T. Cadell, 1771), 266.

the 'few spare hands' working on the West Indian plantations as well as the suggestion that the difference in climates between the two regions would prove an insurmountable obstacle to the deployment of British soldiers and seamen:

It would have been much better to have sent eight or ten thousand of the idle Fellows we have at Home, to some of our most healthful Plantations, in order to have been there ready at a Call; for the Difference of the Climate is so far from being an Argument against, that it is a strong Argument for sending them thither some Months before we have Use for them, that they may have Time to be seasoned to the Climate, and to recover from the Fatigues of a long Voyage, before they are sent upon any Expedition against an Enemy.[39]

By contrast, Lord Hervey was considerably less sanguine about the capacities of men habituated to northern European climes.

[I]f we should strike a blow in the West Indies, it must be struck with the forces that our own settlements furnish. These are the most proper, and our ships will never want abundance of people there, who will be glad to enroll for any expedition of that nature; they are seasoned to the climate, and they know how to deal with the Spaniards. Whereas, if we send forces from this kingdom, one half will probably die in the passage, and the other half will be so sickly and weak when they land, that they can be sent upon no service.[40]

Those agitating in favour of open hostilities soon gained the upper hand. War was declared in October 1739, and British forces scored a first and easy victory at the end of the year in their attack on Porto Bello. The English public responded with enormous enthusiasm (naming the London road for the victory) and – so at least one story goes – singing *Rule Britannia* for the first time in celebration.[41] The country's happy mood would not last, for this would essentially be the last good bit of news for some time. Fired up, English forces decided to attack the much more heavily fortified city of Carthagena. Aiming for their fleet to leave during the summer of 1740, they did not sail until November, by which time scurvy had already broken out on a number of ships. Before they even reached Jamaica, from whence they planned to make the final leg of their journey to Carthagena, their commanding officer, Lord Cathcart, was dead of dysentery. Betrayed by their guides during their assault on the town's fortifications, they were butchered by Spanish troops.[42] But the

---

[39] Ebenezer Timberland, *The History and Proceedings of the House of Lords from the Restoration in 1660 to the Present Time: Containing the Most Healthful Motions, Speeches, Debates, Orders and Resolutions* (London: Printed for Ebenezer Timberland in Ship-Yard, Temple Bar, 1742), vol. 6, 1738–40, 152.

[40] Great Britain. Parliament., *A Collection of the Parliamentary Debates in England, from the Year MDCLXVIII. To the Present Time*, vol. 17 (London: John Torbuck, 1739–42), 450.

[41] Kathleen Wilson, 'Empire, Trade and Popular Politics in Mid-Hanoverian Britain: The Case of Admiral Vernon', *Past and Present* 121 (1988).

[42] J. W. Fortescue, *A History of the British Army*, 2nd ed., vol. II (London: Macmillan, 1910), 55–79.

battle was the least of their worries. It has been estimated that of the 10,000
troops sent to the West Indies, more than 80 per cent died. The Spanish, by contrast, lost only 200–600 men in the defence of Carthegena.[43] And it was from
disease, rather than their wounds, that the vast majority of soldiers and sailors
perished. As Lord Elibank noted in 1740: 'We lost above a 3d of our people as
well officers as soldiers, in 3 weeks that we remained in Carthagena Harbour.
Everybody was taken alike; they call the distemper a bilious fever, it kills in five
days; if the patient lives longer it's only to die of greater agonies of what they
then call Black Vomit'.[44] About 74 per cent of the troops sent to the West Indies
were dead by October, 1742, only 6 per cent of them from their wounds; a large
proportion, probably a majority, died in Jamaica. In July and August, troops
died on the island at the rate of 100 per week. The dramatic difference between
mortality rates on the Carthagenian expedition and most European wars was
not lost on either military or civilian observers. Many would soon note that in
the contemporaneous War of the Austrian Succession, the death rate was about
8 per cent (disease and wounds together); in the Jacobite Uprising a few years
later (1745–6) it was about 2 per cent.[45]

It is hard to overestimate the significance of the mid-century wars on broader
British culture.[46] According to Stephen Conway, around one in fifteen available
men served in the military during the War of the Austrian Succession (1740–8).
One in nine served during the Seven Years War (1756–63), with soldiers and
sailors coming from a wide variety of social backgrounds. The costs as well as
the promises of empire became very tangible to a broad swathe of the population in this period. Kathleen Wilson has pointed to the celebration of Admiral
Vernon, victor of Porto Bello and the face of the opposition to Walpole's
Eurocentrism, as evidence for 'the existence of a vibrant, national extra-
parliamentary political culture'.[47] Vernon was supported by a growing middle
and merchant class and the 'Vernon agitation', Wilson has argued, 'revealed
both the readiness and propensity of urban middling groups in London and
the provinces to engage in a "commercialized" politics, and their capacity for
disciplined political action. Even further, it demonstrates the growing importance of Britain's empire in the nascent political and national consciousness
of ordinary citizens'.[48] Just as important as the changes wrought on military

---

[43] John Robert McNeill, *Mosquito Empires: Ecology and War in the Greater Caribbean, 1620–
    1914* (New York: Cambridge University Press, 2010), 162–3.
[44] Elibank quoted in ibid., 163.
[45] Ibid., 166–8.
[46] Erica Charters, *Disease, War, and the Imperial State: The Welfare of the British Armed Forces
    During the Seven Years War* (Chicago and London: University of Chicago Press, 2014).
[47] Wilson, 'Empire, Trade and Popular Politics in Mid-Hanoverian Britain: The Case of Admiral
    Vernon', 108.
[48] Ibid., 77.

and political culture were those induced in medical attitudes towards the outer reaches of the empire. It was hard for English observers not to suspect that something radically different was happening in the disease environment of the torrid zone.

One of the ways to track this sentiment is by the striking increase in the number of texts published on shipboard diseases and on the diseases of warm climates as they affected soldiers and sailors. Henry Warren's *Treatise on the Malignant Fever of Barbados,* published in 1740, suggested that the King had lost 'upwards of Twenty-Thousand very useful subjects, the much greatest part of whom were Sea-Faring People' to the yellow fever between 1733 and 1739. John Tennent, writing in 1741, described 'that Epidemic Fever so mortal among Northern Foreigners, soon after they arrive in *Jamaica,* and other Parts of the *West-Indies*' and suggested that 'Many Instances prove that Armies suffer as much by marching into hot Climates, from their natural temperate ones, as from a Rencounter with an Enemy; whence appears the Importance of proper Methods, to prevent or cure their mortal epidemic Distempers'.[49] James Lind's *Treatise on Scurvy* was written largely in response to events in the European theatre, in the aftermath of the war of Austrian succession.[50] Charles Bisset's – which treated the West Indian Scurvy – was written while Bisset served in the West Indies during the war with Spain.[51] As J. D. Alsop has argued, 'From 1740, the publications in the medical topography of empire reflected the needs of state and, in particular, the priorities of war'.[52]

The Works of James Lind

Perhaps no works better exemplify Alsop's claim than the medical texts of James Lind. Born in Edinburgh in 1716, Lind began an apprenticeship with a local physician at the age of fifteen. He joined the navy in 1739 as a surgeon's mate and became a full surgeon in 1747, serving in multiple locations throughout the empire, including the Guinea Coast, the West Indies, and Minorca. In 1748 he completed his medical degree at Edinburgh and the following year resigned his military position. The *Treatise on Scurvy* appeared in 1753, with a second edition in 1757, the same year that he published *An Essay on the most Effectual Means of Preserving the Health of Seamen in the*

[49] John Tennent, *A Reprieve from Death: In Two Physical Chapters ... With an Appendix. Dedicated to the Right Honourable Sir Robert Walpole.* (London: Printed for John Clarke, 1741), vi. Cf. Alsop, 35.

[50] Lind, *A Treatise of the Scurvy. In Three Parts. Containing an Inquiry into the Nature, Causes, and Cure of That Disease. Together with a Critical and Chronological View of What Has Been Published on the Subject.*

[51] Charles Bisset, *A Treatise on the Scurvy. Design'd Chiefly for the Use of the British Navy.* (London. R. and J. Dodsley, in Pall-Mall, 1755).

[52] Alsop, 35.

Royal Navy. In 1758 he was appointed Physician-in-charge of the Royal Naval Hospital at Haslar. The second edition of Lind's *Health of Seamen* appeared in 1762. The first edition of the work deemed most important at the time, *An Essay On Diseases Incidental to Europeans in Hot Climates*, was published in 1768. A fifth edition appeared in 1792, two years before Lind's death, with a sixth published posthumously in 1808.[53] For the entirety of the second half of the eighteenth century, Lind was the leading figure in British naval medicine. It is in Lind's writings, I argue, that one may best track radically shifting attitudes towards both medicine and empire. In the early texts, written soon after 1748, Lind maintained differences between Europe and its distant holdings, with his gaze largely on the former. After the end of the Seven Years War, however – which concluded with the dramatic expansion of British imperial holdings – one finds a much more complex attitude toward the familiar and the foreign: an attitude expressed in the language of seasoning.

Today, it may be the *Treatise on Scurvy* that remains most famous, for it was there that Lind offered his description of the first 'controlled trial' of the efficacy of different supposed cures for the maritime disease that had destroyed so many lives, concluding that 'oranges and lemons were the most effectual remedies for this distemper at sea'.[54] For our purposes, however, interest in the text is more limited. As one might expect for a work dedicated to the understanding and cure of a disease whose 'native seat' was to be found 'in the cold northern climates', Lind said little about seasoning. The disease may have been foreign to the ancients, who had lived in warmer, Mediterranean climes and had confined their naval journeys to short coastal voyages, but it was all too familiar to the British.[55] John Pringle's *Observations on the Diseases of the Army* (1752), similarly concerned with afflictions in Northern Europe (particularly the low countries), says nothing about becoming seasoned to the climate. 'By well-seasoned troops are commonly understood', Pringle wrote, 'such as having gone through much fatigue, are therefore supposed best qualified to bear more'.[56] One was to be seasoned, that is, to the service, not to a geographical region.

---

[53] For biographical details, see Louis H. Roddis, *James Lind: Founder of Nautical Medicine* (New York: Henry Schuman, 1950).

[54] Lind, *A Treatise of the Scurvy. In Three Parts. Containing an Inquiry into the Nature, Causes, and Cure of That Disease. Together with a Critical and Chronological View of What Has Been Published on the Subject*, 196.

[55] It had become even more so after the publication of a description of Lord Anson's disastrous circumnavigation of the globe. John Philips, *An Authentic Account of Commodore Anson's Expedition: Containing All That Was Remarkable, Curious and Entertaining, During That Long and Dangerous Voyage: ... Taken from a Private Journal* (London: J. Robinson, 1744). Anson lost half his crew to scurvy in rounding Cape Horn and returned to England with less than 200 of an initial complement of more than 1800 men. Lind dedicated his *Treatise* to Anson.

[56] John Pringle, *Observations on the Diseases of the Army: In Camp and Garrison. In Three Parts. With an Appendix* (London: A. Millar, and D. Wilson; and T. Payne, 1752), 147–8.

Strikingly different was Charles Bisset's *A Treatise on the Scurvy*, published in 1755, two years after Lind's. Bisset, too, was born in Scotland and studied medicine at Edinburgh before joining the service and becoming second surgeon of the military hospital in Jamaica in 1740. He spent five years in the West Indies and America before returning to Britain in 1745 and his book drew heavily on his medical experiences in the New World. Seasoning was central to the published work, which Bisset claimed was only part of a larger tract, concerned with 'the natural constitution of the atmosphere, and the diseases incident to new-comers, seasoned Europeans, and natives of the West Indies'.[57] Bisset paired scurvy with what he termed (combining Warren and Towne's terminology) the 'malignant bilious fever', arguing that one could become seasoned to both. One rarely found scurvy in the West Indies during the winter months, he argued, 'and Negroes, Creols, and seasoned Europeans are not obnoxious to the malignant Bilious Fever, and are seldom much afflicted with the Scurvy'.[58] In the course of a year, Bisset claimed, European bodily fibres gradually became drier, more rigid and more elastic, thus approximating those of 'Creoles and Negroes'. It was this change in the fibres, and concomitant alterations in bodily 'juices' that constituted seasoning. Comparing his analysis to Lind's, Bisset noted that scurvy might strike the European in either hot or cold climes, but in the Torrid Zone it was unseasoned strangers who were most at risk.

It is observed by Dr. Lind, that the principal predisposing cause to the Scurvy, in climates where the winters are cold, is a cold and moist air; and we have shewn, that the chief predisposing cause in the West Indies, consists in an unseasoned constitution to the Torrid Zone, joined with the sultry heat of the hot sun.[59]

Lind would summarise Bisset's main conclusions in the second edition of his *Treatise* and one finds talk of seasoning in Lind's *Essay on ... the Health of Seamen*, also published in 1757. The first edition of *The Health of Seamen*, Lind noted, was published soon after the beginning of what we now term the Seven Years War and what Lind called 'the present war with France'.[60] It was thus largely concerned with the illnesses of sailors, since many more died from disease than from 'shipwreck, capture, famine, fire, or sword'.[61] The second edition was published in 1762 and Lind claimed that he had revised the work so that it could serve not only those on ships, but could also prove useful to those in British colonies and factories.[62]

---

[57] Bisset, 1–2.
[58] Ibid., 10.
[59] Ibid., 41.
[60] James Lind, *An Essay of the Most Effectual Means of Preserving the Health of Seamen in the Royal Navy*, 2nd ed. (London: D. Wilson, 1762), xvii.
[61] Ibid.
[62] Ibid., xviii.

Perhaps because his book was aimed at two rather different audiences – one at sea, one on land – one finds two rather different usages of 'seasoning talk' in Lind's text. Like Pringle and earlier military authors, Lind spoke of the need to use men seasoned to the armed services, particularly the navy. In times of peace, Lind claimed, it was common to find smaller ships of war manned with 'sound and seasoned sailors'.[63] In times of war, however, one often found newer men serving on larger ships, which led to higher incidences of shipboard illnesses, for 'raw sailors and unseasoned marines are often the Occasion of great Sickness in Fleets'.[64] But the only problem was not that one had too many newly raised men and not enough veterans, as was often the complaint in the army. An even more important distinction was that between landmen and those used to a marine life. Larger warships should be made up, Lind urged, of 'seasoned healthy Men from other Ships, and of such Landmen who have been somewhat inured to the Sea'.[65]

Just as the Crown needed men seasoned to the service and to maritime life, it also needed men seasoned to certain climates. It may seem intuitively obvious that one should favour strong young men for a crew, rather than more grizzled, older sailors, but this might well prove to be a mistake. '[M]any hardened veteran Sailors are sometimes to be met with', wrote Lind, 'who enjoy a better State of Health in the *West-Indies* than in *Europe*, having been long seasoned and inured to that Climate, either in the King's, or in the Merchant's service'.[66]

It was fairly rare, in the mid-eighteenth century, to find an author deploying both meanings of seasoning in the same text. Military authors, like Pringle, tended to write of seasoned soldiers; medical writers concerned with the diseases of warm climates tended to emphasise the need to become habituated to a given part of the globe, and often stressed, as we have seen, the promises and perils of a seasoning sickness. Interested in the diseases of both sailors and colonists in Europe as well as the Indies and the Guinea coast, however, Lind was a likely first candidate to bring the two discourses together. That said, in doing so, some of the particularity of the discourse about seasoning in the Torrid Zone dropped away. One became sick because of 'a quick Transition to a new way of life' or because of 'sudden Changes of Climates'.[67] For sailor or settler, the problem was rapid change. Effects were largely the same as well: Lind credited no particular illness with being a seasoning sickness. Indeed, while he acknowledged that yellow fever struck those who had newly arrived to the West Indies, he also argued that the disease was much rarer than earlier authors had claimed.[68] As a result, he could advocate the same prophylactic treatment

[63] Ibid., vii.
[64] Ibid., 9.
[65] Ibid., 10.
[66] Ibid., 11.
[67] Ibid., x.
[68] Ibid., 50.

for the unseasoned. Those unaccustomed to life at sea should be gradually habituated to marine life by first serving on smaller warships and merchant vessels; those travelling to the West Indies from England should leave Britain in the Autumn (when the weather was most like that in the Tropics) and become gradually used to increased temperatures, finally arriving at Jamaica at a relatively healthy time of year.[69] In Pringle's treatment of the diseases of the army, the ideal soldier was one who had avoided illnesses best: 'those troops will be best seasoned to go through the difficulties of a second campaign, whose health has been most preserved in the first'.[70] For Lind, similarly, newcomers became seasoned to a climate by assiduously avoiding what others might see as an evil necessary for eventual habituation:

It has been a received opinion, that the first fever or fit of sickness alters the constitution of the body, so as to season it to a new climate: but I am of opinion, that the sudden changes of climates are greatly the cause of sickness, and that a seasoned constitution in any part of the world is chiefly to be acquired by remaining there for some length of time.[71]

Lind's most extensive account of seasoning came in his most widely cited work, *On Diseases Incidental to Europeans in Hot Climates*. He himself pitched the text as a 'sequel' to his earlier studies. Having formerly been concerned with those aboard ships, he now took up the problem of the health of those arrived at their destination in a foreign land. One might also regard the text as the longest and most detailed meditation on the problem of seasoning published in the eighteenth century. That fact is not obvious from its superficial structure, for in many ways the book fits into an established mode. Emulating Hippocrates' *Airs, Waters, and Places,* a number of works had been written that treated of the diseases of regions far from home. Some – perhaps the larger number – considered the afflictions of a given location. A smaller number imitated Hippocrates more directly, and offered a scholarly appraisal of the diseases endemic or native to all places in the known world.[72] Lind's *Hot Climates* would seem to fit into this latter mould, for it discusses diseases found, successively, in Europe and North America, Africa, the East Indies, and the West Indies. And yet, whereas earlier works had taken as their implicit patient a *native* of a given region of the world, almost two-thirds of Lind's work was explicitly concerned with the diseases that attacked *strangers* to a given climate. That is, Lind's was a work concerned with anti-nativity, with diseases that plagued those who were not seasoned to a climate. And the number of the unseasoned, as he noted, was increasing.

---

[69] Ibid., 9, 48.

[70] Pringle, 150.

[71] Lind, *An Essay on Diseases Incidental to Europeans in Hot Climates: With the Method of Preventing Their Fatal Consequences. To Which Is Added, an Appendix Concerning Intermittent Fevers,* 188.

[72] See, for example, Hoffmann and Ramazzini.

Few persons visit the East or the West Indies for their pleasure, but thousands leave England every year, with the design of settling in some of our colonies. Numbers have lately gone to people those parts of America and the West Indies ceded to us by the last treaty of peace. Regiments are often sent out from England, to relieve others stationed in the most distant parts of the globe; and recruits for those regiments are still more frequently ordered abroad.[73]

The traveller, Lind suggested, was like a plant in foreign soil, requiring care to ensure its survival. And while many soils could be salutary, those that were far beyond Europe and in which Europeans now had particular interests were unhealthy, even possibly fatal.[74] Jamaica's climate was deadly to the point that it strained belief. Lind cited a 'common computation' suggesting that a number equivalent to the entire white population died every five years.[75] In many factories on the Guinea Coast, one-third of Europeans might die in a year.[76] It was on these grounds that Lind used the idea of seasoning not – as abolitionists had and would – against slavery, but in slavery's defence. Europeans, especially those newly arrived, were safest on board ship, away from the unhealthy effluvia of the shore. Of particular danger were uncultivated lands, precisely the kinds of places where unseasoned men were often sent to collect wood. 'If the purchasing of negroes on the coast of Guinea can be justified', he wrote, 'it must be from the absolute necessity of employing them in such services as this. It does not seem consistent with British humanity to assign such employments to a regiment of gallant soldiers, or to a company of brave seamen'.[77] 'British humanity', of course, seemed only to apply to the British and their near neighbours. Lind clearly saw no irony in a defence of enslavement that sought to incite the reader's pity for the poor treatment of others. '[N]othing can be more inhuman', he opined, 'that sending unseasoned Europeans high up from the mouths of the rivers, into an uncultivated country, especially during the rainy season, and where there is no shelter from the pestiferous noctural air'.[78]

One should be clear, however, that the issue at hand was one of nativity and seasoning, rather than race, as we might understand that term from the nineteenth century onwards. The capacity to survive in a dangerous climate was not innate. In Africa, Lind twinned 'natives, and such others as are perfectly seasoned to the country'.[79] In the West Indies he paired 'Negroes and Creoles', both of whom could apparently sleep outside on dewy ground – an act against which he strongly counseled European strangers. That this could

[73] Lind, *An Essay on Diseases Incidental to Europeans in Hot Climates: With the Method of Preventing Their Fatal Consequences. To Which Is Added, an Appendix Concerning Intermittent Fevers*, 2.
[74] Ibid., 2–3.
[75] Ibid., 9.
[76] Ibid., 151.
[77] Ibid., 134.
[78] Ibid., 139.
[79] Ibid., 141.

be done by some without hurt was 'a proof how far the Constitution may be framed and accustomed to bear what otherwise is so highly prejudicial'.[80] This anti-essentialist logic had a political corollary. Native factors could be highly useful for British trade – as they were for the Portuguese – and such utility should be rewarded with all the privileges of British subjecthood. Europeans might, over time, become habituated to the climate of the Guinea coast, and Africans could become naturalised servants of the crown.[81]

Although his status may have added medical legitimacy to such claims, Lind was hardly unusual either for views that defended the slave trade or those that advocated for the promotion of useful 'natives'. Where Lind was unlike many of his contemporaries, however, was in refusing to regard extended regions of the globe as inherently dangerous to Europeans. The concluding summary of his remarks on the diseases that afflicted strangers across the earth pointed to peculiar similarities and differences. Hippocratic and neo-Hippocratic texts on *Airs, Waters, and Places* tended to emphasise differences in native diseases due to location: Lind effaced these differences in his focus on newly arrived foreigners. '[T]he diseases of strangers in different climates', he wrote, 'bear everywhere a great similitude to one another'. Difference could be found elsewhere, however, for no country could be regarded in monolithic terms. Seemingly deadly regions had their 'healthy and pleasant seasons' during which strangers could visit with impunity. And insalubrity was archipelagic:

The most unhealthy spots in the world have in their neighbourhood, and often at no great distance from them, places which afford a secure retreat and protection from diseases and death ... In a word, the diseases most fatal to strangers in every country, seem not only to be confined to particular seasons, but even during those seasons to certain places only.

The corollary, then, was that one could be safe or unsafe almost anywhere, depending on whether one was habituated to a given climate. Seasoning had earlier been a discourse that had divided the world into a (northern) European centre and an extra-European periphery. In Lind's hands, the dichotomy ceased, fundamentally, to be explicable in purely geographic terms. What mattered now was only strangeness and habituation. Hence the fact that Lind's survey of the globe's illnesses began at home, with an account of the diseases that afflicted those unseasoned to England's more dangerous regions. Strangers in this context included not only those born outside the country, but even English soldiers unused to the diseases of places like the Hilsea Barracks in Portsea. But strangeness could, with care, be overcome. Lind counselled newcomers to stay on board ship as much as possible, to arrive at the right time

---

[80] Ibid., note 69.
[81] Ibid., 224–5.

and disembark at the right place, and to avoid diseases until one was inured to the new environment. A merchant, sailor, or factor who did so, Lind claimed, was then worth 'ten newly arrived unseasoned Europeans'. Yet the protections of nativity might also be lost. Lind suggested that 'many persons, dreading what they may again be exposed to suffer from a change of climate, choose rather to spend the remainder of their lives abroad, than to return to their native country'.[82] Imperial power came with a medical price.

Conclusion

In this chapter, I have attempted to trace the changing nature of seasoning discourse across the first two-thirds of the eighteenth century, following the ways in which medical logics shifted along with dramatically new conceptions of the relationships between a British centre and its hinterlands. In the earlier eighteenth century, as we have seen, the foreign and the familiar had possessed fairly fixed referents. The metropole was treated as an unmarked category: one needed to be seasoned only to lands in the periphery. By the late 1760s, in medical discourse, centres and peripheries lived cheek by jowl. England had its sites of foreignness, Jamaica could become so familiar that a Briton could fear returning home. Seasoning discourse changed fundamentally in Lind's hands and across his publications, and did so in ways that mirrored equally fundamental changes in the nature and scope of Britain's imperial holdings. The British Empire was dramatically larger after the victories of the Seven Years War than it had been before. With the rapid growth in size came, according to Linda Colley, an uncertainty about the very question of what it was to be British. Before the war, she has suggested, 'Britain's empire had been small enough and homogeneous enough to seem reasonably compatible with the values that the British, and above all the English, believed they uniquely epitomized'.[83] After 1763 and until at least the American Revolution, however, the British found themselves in a state of 'collective agoraphobia', unsettled by new territories that were 'at once too vast and too alien'.[84] Seasoning would appear to play the role of medical counterpart in this shift in an imperial sense of self. In the first half of the century, seasoning had served to define regions of potentially dangerous climatic difference. Such certainty would seem to have eroded by the time of Lind's publication of *Hot Climates* in 1768. Now difference was temporally specific and spatially archipelagic. England was no haven, the imperial periphery contained multiple sanctuaries, and one might be a stranger anywhere.

[82] Ibid., 146–7.
[83] Colley, *Britons: Forging the Nation, 1707–1837*, 103.
[84] Ibid., 105, 02.

4   Imperial Medicine and the Putrefactive Paradigm, 1720–1800

Introduction

James Lind, younger and less famous cousin to the author of a *Treatise on Scurvy*, with whom he shared a name, spent the first half of the 1760s in service as surgeon on the *Drake* Indiaman. In 1762 he found himself in North-Eastern India. Four years later he visited China and in 1768 he graduated with a medical degree from Edinburgh, with a thesis (translated from the Latin in 1776) on a fever he had observed while in Bengal.[1] Concise and straightforwardly written, with clear invocations of the intellectual resources upon which it was drawing, the dissertation provides a fine exemplar of thinking about the diseases of warm climates in the third quarter of the eighteenth century. The cause of the illness, a 'putrid and remitting marsh fever', was the putrescency of a sufferer's bodily fluids.[2] European seamen arriving at Bengal in the autumn were particularly subject to it. 'They are predisposed to it from the nature of their food, their confinement on board ship, the very great heats they are exposed to during the voyage, and their lying, for hours together, exposed to the night colds'.[3] The heat they endured on their voyage was less than that experienced once they arrived in India, but was still 'too much for a European constitution to bear', for it brought on the body's relaxation and promoted the corruption of its humours. The meat that made up a substantial part of their diet possessed a 'putrescent disposition', which the small amount of wine and spirits allowed them could not sufficiently correct, and the cold night air to which they were exposed when sleeping outdoors checked their perspiration, meaning that the 'excrementitious fluid' produced by the body could not be expelled through the pores.[4]

---

[1] T. C., 'Lind, James, M. D. (1736–1812)', in *Dictionary of National Biography*, ed. Sidney Lee (London: Smith, Elder, and Co., 1893).

[2] James Lind, *A Treatise on the Putrid and Remitting Marsh Fever, Which Raged at Bengal in the Year 1762* (Edinburgh: C. Elliot, 1776).

[3] Ibid., 30.

[4] Ibid., 31–3.

The body in warm climates thus possessed a 'putrid diathesis [tendency]'. In such a state, it was particularly susceptible to the environmental dangers posed by Bengal's swampy and insalubrious terrain. 'This part of the country', Lind wrote with obvious distaste, was 'infected with the putrid parts of dead animals, insects and rotten vegetables. The Ganges, besides, is the common receptacle of all the filth and nastiness of the inhabitants; they never ease nature anywhere else; and are constantly washing themselves and their cloaths in it'. Citing John Pringle, whose *Observations on the Diseases of the Army* had almost instantly become the standard reference for surgeons and physicians throughout Britain's armed forces after its publication in 1752, Lind argued that the 'most powerful' of the remote causes of the fever were 'the effluvia of marshes replete with putrid animal substances'. Rising from swampland and encountering bodies already inclined to internal putrefaction, air containing putrid particles induced a potentially deadly illness, one spread as easily by dead as by living victims. Water from old graves flowed into new ones, infecting grave-diggers and mourners alike. Once the disease was present it could be spread contagiously, although it was far more likely to effect newcomers than natives. Just as one could become habituated to quantities of poison that could kill those unused to the substance, so those who lived in 'countries replete with fenny miasmata' could find the air less dangerous than those newly come to the Calcutta garrison.[5]

Lind's was a fairly straightforward application of medical ideas that had become familiar since mid-century. His critiques were mild, tending to affirm general logics while questioning particulars. Pringle had correctly pointed to the rot of animal substances as the cause of putrid diseases, Lind opined, but his theory lacked specificity. After all, every kind of putrefaction did not have the same effect. Tanners and butchers were not more often afflicted by putrid diseases than others; nor were ship-stewards, 'who spend most of their time amongst the putrid and rancid effluvia' of the places where provisions were kept more at risk than their ship-mates. But such objections did not shake his overall faith. '[W]e are well assured', he claimed, 'by the testimony of Sir John Pringle, and other practical writers, that some putrid fermentations produce noxious vapours, which, united with those marshes, render them pernicious.[6]

Lind's position was orthodox, but it had not been so for long. Both his terminology and his stress on putrefaction as a cause of contagious disease tended to mask the novelty of what had rapidly become a widely accepted medical view. 'Putrid fevers', as a category of illness, dated back to antiquity, although

[5] Ibid., 67, 12–13, 33, 38–9.
[6] Ibid., 33–4.

there was considerable flexibility in the meaning of the term.[7] As the older Lind would note in 1768, 'the antients do not seem to have understood by the term putrid, when applied to a fever, that kind of putrefaction which a dead body naturally undergoes'. He suggested that the term derived from Aristotle's dictum 'Omnia quae putrescunt calidiora siunt', because the fever's distinguishing characteristic was a remarkable and disagreeable heat felt on the patient's skin.[8] This is perhaps too minimalist a definition, for it was common to associate putrid fevers with the corruption of humours (rather than, for example, their imbalance).[9] In the middle ages, putrid fevers were categorised according to which of the four humours was affected.[10] Putrefaction was also, as Andrew Wear has demonstrated, 'a crucial component in most accounts of disease' in the early modern period, providing a rare area of agreement among adherents to the old and new philosophies in the seventeenth century.[11] Surgeons, of course, encountered gangrene and sepsis in their daily work, but rot was, more generally, omnipresent in an age before the massive public health programs of the nineteenth and twentieth centuries. As a result, '[t]he corruption and putrefaction of the humours, of parts of the body and of food in the body were especially potent and widespread images of physical disorder and disease'.[12]

And yet, just as with the word putrid, 'putrescency' and 'putrefaction' were rather imprecise terms until the eighteenth century. Putrefaction was largely synonymous with corruption, and corruption could come in many forms.[13] As

---

[7] On the longer history of the term, I have found very useful Christopher Hamlin, 'What Is Putrid About Putrid Fever?', in *History of Science Society Annual Meeting* (Chicago: 2014). 'Putrescence was a vague concept', writes Harrison, 'but its vagueness accounts for its longevity'. Harrison, *Climates & Constitutions: Health, Race, Environment and British Imperialism in India, 1600–1850*, 38.

[8] Lind, *An Essay on Diseases Incidental to Europeans in Hot Climates: With the Method of Preventing Their Fatal Consequences. To Which Is Added, an Appendix Concerning Intermittent Fevers*, 13.

[9] Christopher Hamlin, *More Than Hot: A Short History of Fever* (Baltimore: Johns Hopkins University Press, 2014), 48.

[10] Faith Wallis, 'Medicine, Theoretical', in *Medieval Science, Technology, and Medicine: An Encyclopedia*, ed. Thomas F. Glick, Stephen Livesy, and Faith Wallis (New York: Routledge, 2005), 339.

[11] A. Wear, *Knowledge and Practice in English Medicine, 1550–1680* (Cambridge: Cambridge University Press, 2000), 136. For its use in explaining the fourteenth century plague, see J Arrizabalaga, 'Facing the Black Death: Perceptions and Reactions of University Medical Practitioners', in *Practical Medicine from Salerno to the Black Death*, ed. Luis Garcia-Ballester et al. (Cambridge: Cambridge University Press, 1994).

[12] Wear, 136. On surgeons and putrefaction, see 255.

[13] The most obvious classical reference was Aristotle's work 'On Generation and Corruption', but one finds little discussion of the material nature of corruption there. More specific detail may be found in 'On Meteorology', where putrefaction is delineated as 'the strictest general opposite of true becoming'. Everything, according to Aristotle, can putrefy, except fire: 'for earth, water and air putrefy, being all of them matter relatively to fire. The definition of putrefaction is: the destruction of the peculiar and natural heat in any moist subject by external heat,

Stephen Bradwell noted in a tract on the plague in 1625: 'For noisome vapours arising from filthy sincks, stincking sewers, channels, gutters, privies, sluttish corners, dunghills and uncast ditches; as also the mists and fogs that commonly arise out of fens, moores, mines and standing lakes; doe greatly corrupt the Aire; and in like manner the lying of dead rotten carrions in channels, ditches and dunghills; cause a *contagious* Aire'.[14] Lind's theory, by contrast, limited the cause of his putrid fever to – in his cousin's words – 'that kind of putrefaction which a dead body naturally undergoes'. This narrower understanding, and the suggestion that 'fens, moores, mines, and standing lakes' were dangerous because they contained 'putrid animal substances' was a very recent development, to be traced directly, in many cases, to the arguments laid out in Pringle's hugely important mid-century text on the diseases of the army. In Pringle's work, in fact, one can find the earliest and clearest articulation of what I term the 'putrefactive paradigm', a set of ideas and practices that dominated understandings of the diseases of warm climates for more than three decades.[15] Encompassing a theory of disease, a method of cure and prevention, and an investigative methodology, the paradigm consisted of five elements. The first was nosological: in the new understanding of mid-century, putrid fevers became a much larger and more significant class of illnesses than they had been before. In earlier taxonomies of disease, putrid fevers made up a smaller subclass of a larger grouping, often determined by the periodicity of the affliction's remittance. Thus, in Boerhaave's *Aphorisms,* the putrid fever is a kind of continual fever, with continual fevers differing from other fevers by the fact that they occur 'without any distinct paroxysms or remissions'.[16] In Pringle's hands, however, putrid fevers encompassed a good deal more: all fevers could be divided into two kinds: inflammatory and putrid, which in turn

---

that is, by the heat of the environment'. Putrefaction was thus an entirely general process, rather than (for example) one specific to living things.

[14] Quoted in Wear, 301.

[15] I use the term here in a rather loose Kuhnian sense. On the one hand, clear continuities to both earlier and later ideas make it clear that there can be no talk of incommensurability or, really, of revolutions. I have, elsewhere, been sceptical of any use of the term 'crisis' except where the word is explicitly used by one's historical actors. On the other hand, it seems clear that many, if not most, writers about the diseases of warm climates from the 1750s to the 1780s shared certain assumptions about cause and cure of fevers and that a good deal of work looked like 'normal science' as Kuhn defined it, involving the extension of the paradigm to encompass new disorders in the field and to discover new antiseptic curatives in the laboratory. Thomas S. Kuhn, 'The Structure of Scientific Revolutions', (Chicago: University of Chicago Press, 1962); Suman Seth, 'Crisis and the Construction of Modern Theoretical Physics', *British Journal for the History of Science* 40, no. 144 (2007). Hamlin also takes Pringle as one of the prime expositors of ideas about putrid diseases. See Hamlin, 114–24.

[16] Herman Boerhaave, *Boerhaave's Aphorisms: Concerning the Knowledge and Cure of Diseases. Translated from the Last Edition Printed in Latin at Leyden, 1715.*, trans. J. Delacoste (London: B. Cowse, and W. Innys, 1725), 168.

corresponded to the characteristic illnesses of the army in barracks and in the field. For John Huxham, whose *Essay on Fevers* appeared in 1750 and was very widely cited thereafter, there were three kinds of fevers, corresponding to different internal bodily conditions. To the two main states of the fluids and solids in illness (either over-elastic and rigid fibres, and very dense, viscid blood or too lax a state of the solids and weak, thin blood), Huxham added a third: 'But, besides these, there is moreover a third State of Blood, *of more dangerous Consequence than either;* I mean a State of it, that more immediately tends to *Dissolution* and *Putrefaction'.*[17] This description brings us to the second element of the paradigm: putrid diseases were characterised by the putrefaction (or tendency to putrefaction) of the bodily solids or fluids – most commonly blood or bile – that they induced. As noted above, this putrescence was a literal decay, not merely a corruption of the humours. The body was understood to be rotting (or having a diathesis to rot) from within. Such putrefaction was taken, thirdly, to have two possible causes. Either conditions (such as heat and/or humidity) promoted a spontaneous decay or else external matter (often described as effluvia and associated particularly with marsh- and swampland) made its way into the body and sponsored putrefactive decay. In the latter case, it was assumed that marshes were themselves sites of putrefaction, moist and muddy ground being a promoter of the rot of vegetable and (especially) animal matter. External putrefaction, taken into the body (most likely through the breath) produced internal putrefaction. The nature of the proposed cure for such afflictions, fourthly, re-affirmed the etiological reasoning of the paradigm. Since the cause of the disease was sepsis within the body, the cure should involve antiseptics taken internally. That substances known to retard putrefaction (such as citrus juices) seemed to work so well against putrid afflictions such as scurvy provided indirect but strong confirmation of the theory's assumptions. Lind explained the efficacy of the Peruvian bark against the putrid fever of Bengal – and the reason that it did not work against other afflictions – on precisely these grounds, deploying Pringle's two-fold taxonomy as he did so.

The bark, when too hastily administered in the fevers of cold climates, is so far from checking them, that it greatly endangers the life of the patient. This is owing to the inflammatory diathesis which accompanies these fevers. But we may give it sooner in fevers of warm climates; for here there is a putrid diathesis, the reverse of the inflammatory, to which the antiseptic virtue of the bark cannot be too soon opposed.[18]

---

[17] Huxham, *An Essay on Fevers, and Their Various Kinds, as Depending on Different Constitutions of the Blood: With Dissertations on Slow Nervous Fevers; on Putrid, Pestilential, Spotted Fevers; on the Small-Pox; and on Pleurisies and Peripneumonies*, 41.

[18] Lind, *A Treatise on the Putrid and Remitting Marsh Fever, Which Raged at Bengal in the Year 1762*, 67–8.

Fifth and finally, evidential support for the paradigm came not only from medical observations and practice, but from experimental analysis in the chemical laboratory. The internal state of the living body was essentially unobservable for the physician. In its place, Pringle made observations on meat and bodily fluids, demonstrating that a variety of substances could function as effective antiseptics and then arguing that such substances could function to the same end within the body. Experimental natural philosophy thus worked in the service of medicine, but it did not do so uncontested. As we shall see, many would find the idea that one might use dead flesh as a model for the workings of the living body a deeply problematic assumption.

This chapter offers a history of the rise and fall of the putrefactive paradigm, extending the analysis offered in the previous three chapters, which have tracked theories concerning the diseases of warm climates from the sixteenth century to the mid-1700s. The main part of the narrative here begins with the publication of John Pringle's *Observations on the Nature and Cure of Hospital and Jayl-Fevers* in 1750 and ends in the late 1790s, after two major texts on the diseases of the West Indies (published by Benjamin Moseley in 1787 and John Hunter in 1788) made it clear that putrefactive theories no longer had the salience they had once possessed. I should make clear from the outset that what is novel about the analysis here is not the observation that putrefaction was central to understandings of the diseases of warm climates around the middle of the eighteenth century. That point was made at least as early as 1837, as H. H. Goodeve offered a Sketch of Medical Progress in the East, which characterised the period under discussion here as one in which 'the fear of putrescency preserved its full sway', with the bark prescribed as an antiseptic to check the body's 'putrid tendency'.[19] In recent scholarship, Mark Harrison has been responsible for detailing the fundamentality of Pringle's putrefactive theory to medicine in the British Empire and particularly in the colonies.[20] 'Putrefaction', Harrison notes, 'loomed large in works issuing from the pens of most East India Company surgeons', and he has tracked the changes in medical therapeutics that accompanied the rise of putrefactive theories, as bleeding declined in favour of the administration of the antiseptic Bark.[21] Although he uses the term more loosely than do I, it is from Harrison that I draw the term the 'putrefactive paradigm'.

---

[19] H. H. Goodeve, 'Sketch of Medical Progress in the East', *The Quarterly Journal of the Calcutta Medical and Physical Society* (1837): 128.
[20] Harrison, *Medicine in an Age of Commerce and Empire: Britain and its Tropical Colonies, 1660–1830*, 64–88.
[21] Ibid., 69. 'The rapid and almost complete abandonment of bloodletting in the East Indies reflected the dominance of putrefactive notions of illness, and in particular, of the bilious theory of fevers', ibid., 127.

What this chapter offers is an intellectual history of the putrefactive paradigm, one that allows a specification of precisely what was novel about it. To understand what distinguished Pringle's ideas from earlier conceptions of putrid diseases or miasmatic theories requires detailing, as I do in Section 4.2, the roots of these ideas. Pringle's debts to his teacher, the famed Leiden professor Herman Boerhaave whom he referred to as his 'master', have long been acknowledged, if rarely spelled out. Just as important, however, were the writings of his effective patron, the physician Richard Mead. As we shall see, despite the fact that Mead has been overshadowed by other eighteenth-century figures, his works on poison and the plague would provide an essential resource for articulating the putrefactive paradigm. In Section 4.3 I explicate Pringle's own arguments before turning, in Section 4.4, to the application of these and similar (if not identical) claims by Huxham and the older Lind to work on scurvy and the diseases of warm climates. Section 4.5 then turns to the critiques of the paradigm that one begins to find in the early 1770s. These would grow across the decade, as former proponents turned against putrefactive theories and, somewhat ironically, as the kinds of laboratory experiments suggested by the paradigm's logics seemed to undercut its claims. The end result would be the rejection of the paradigm's theoretical claims but the retention of many of its practices.

Before turning to a discussion of the roots and fruits of Pringle's ideas, however, one further point should be made. While it is true that putrefactive theories characterised discussions of the diseases of warm climates after mid-century, it is also true that such discussions were not limited to the colonies. Pringle was almost certainly the most important figure in British medicine generally in the two decades after 1750, providing the bridge between the earlier period dominated by Boerhaave's teachings and a later one similarly dominated by William Cullen's. With this in mind, we might re-evaluate the significance and meaning of the characterisation of this period by Charles Creighton in his classic *History of Epidemics in Britain*. For Creighton, the middle third of the eighteenth century could be described, in Sydenhamian terms, as possessing a 'putrid constitution', coinciding 'within the great outburst of putrid or gangrenous sore-throat … and it included an extensive prevalence of fevers which were also called putrid or nervous, and sometimes called miliary'.[22] In that period, medical authors in multiple locations – including Rouen, London, Worcestershire, Ireland, and Barbados – described their attempts to grapple with putrid disorders. For Creighton, the cause of such 'putridity-talk' was the rise and spread of a new disease. 'It was certainly not a mere fashion in medicine',

---

[22] Charles Creighton, *A History of Epidemics in Britain, vol. II. From the Extinction of Plague to the Present Time* (Cambridge: Cambridge University Press, 1894), 120.

he wrote, 'which produced these accounts of a similar fever, for these accounts came from places far apart and were independent of one another'.[23] Even if one accepts the realist logic of such an argument, however, there is no reason to assume that multiple observers were compelled to regard the new affliction as specifically putrid. The disease's *label* might surely be considered a matter of 'fashion' and in accounting for its spread it does not seem unreasonable to point both to Pringle's work and to an inversion of the kinds of spatial logics that have long been assumed to govern the dispersal of scientific and medical ideas. It seems necessary to distinguish between those metropolitan writers concerned with what Fothergill in 1748 termed a 'sore throat attended with ulcers' and what Huxham, almost a decade later called a 'malignant, ulcerous sore throat' and those more broadly concerned with putrid diseases. Most of these latter cited Pringle and Lind quite explicitly, several of them drawing on their experiences in warm climates while doing so. Some, like Pringle himself, sought to study putrid diseases (as he understood them) while acknowledging that they were fairly uncommon afflictions at home. What was quotidian in many of Britain's colonies was seen by many as unusual in Britain itself (at least outside heterotopic spaces like army camps, prisons, and hospitals).[24] One might thus explain part of the spread of putrid theories of disease in Britain as an example of the military-imperial tail wagging the metropolitan dog and a case of the incorporation of empire within a previously more geographic-ally limited orthodox medicine. If the last chapter was concerned with medical articulations of imperial imaginaries, then, this chapter describes the rise of imperial articulations of medical logics, a rise that pre-dated Pringle's work. To provide a background for this aspect of the putrefactive paradigm, then, we turn first to a discussion of the ways in which warm climates were entering the medicine of the British Isles in the early 1700s.

4.1   Tropical Climates in Metropolitan Medicine

By the 1720s and 1730s, the periphery had begun to make its mark on metro-politan medicine. Medicinal products had already profoundly shaped medical practice before then, of course, with tea, coffee, cinchona, and many other substances native to warmer climates being added to traditional *materia medica* in the sixteenth and seventeenth centuries. From the eighteenth cen-tury, however, one finds mention not only of products *from* warm climates, but also of bodies *in* warm climates. Medical meteorological reflections seemed to

---

[23] Ibid., 121–2.
[24] Michel Foucault, 'Of Other Spaces: Utopias and Heterotopias', *Architecture/Mouvement/ Continuité*, no. October (1984).

lead writers almost unerringly to considerations of the climates and illnesses of foreign locations. Arguing that physicians should pay attention to seasonality, Huxham made the case by assuming that his readers would agree that attention to geographical differences mattered: 'What Celsus says of Difference of Places is equally true of Difference of Seasons'.[25] John Arbuthnot's *Essay Concerning the Effects of Air on Human Bodies* (1733) abounded with references to countries between the tropics, helping to make the general case that 'The Effects of Air on Human Bodies are as various as the Diversity of the Weather, Climates, and Countries'.[26] Thus, we are informed that barometers registered less variation in the Tropics, 'The Cold in the Parallel of *London* is much greater in the *West-Indies*', there are hot African winds that can kill elephants, and mountains in Ceylon where one might find snow.[27]

The point may seem obvious: were one interested in the effect of the aerial environment on distempers it would seem to make sense to compare spatially – and hence climatically – distinct areas. Yet, however obvious it might appear, this was not the approach taken fifty or sixty years earlier, when Britain's empire was less developed and had intruded less into the medical imagination. Sydenham's comparisons of epidemic constitutions in the 1660s, for example, were temporal, not spatial. Diseases had a yearly rhythm, corresponding to the seasons, but seasons in different years might lead to different diseases. There is, in fact, something surely telling about the structure of Huxham's argument in his *Observations on the Air and Epidemical Diseases*. Rather than letting the authority of Sydenham (or, indeed, of Hippocrates in his *Epidemics*) make the case for seasonal analyses, Huxham instead relied on classical arguments which proved the importance of geographic difference, and then analogised climates to seasons.[28] Asserting the need for a flexibility of practice, for example, Huxham suggested that 'the Physicians of different Countries abundantly testify by using different Methods, all which however very happily succeed. Is it not necessary therefore to have due Regard to the different Constitutions of the Atmosphere even in the same Country?'[29] Sydenham appeared to assume a readership interested in the diseases of London. Huxham assumed that his audience would accept claims about practice in Britain derived from evidence gleaned around the world. A global sensibility was to inform even the most local treatment.

---

[25] Huxham, *The Works of John Huxham, M. D. F. R. S. In Two Volumes*, I, xxvii.

[26] Arbuthnot, 119.

[27] Ibid., 75, 77, 81, 84.

[28] Not all Huxham's evidence, however, was derived from familiar classical sources. He cited both Boerhaave and the naturalist Joseph d'Acosta, for instance, for their views on the appropriate temperature for respirable air. Huxham, *The Works of John Huxham, M. D. F. R. S. In Two Volumes*, I, v, ix.

[29] Ibid., xxvii.

Huxham was hardly alone in this new global medical sensibility. Indeed, as a Fellow of the Royal Society, he was in good company.[30] The Reverend Stephen Hales, for example, was elected a Fellow in 1718 and was cited by all those working on the effects of airs on health. Of particular interest to many was how improving air might benefit the lives of those expanding Britain's trading empire and colonial holdings. Noxious effluvia were particularly dangerous in confined spaces such as that found on ships. Hence Hales' efforts to invent a ventilating system that could pump unhealthy air out of a ship's hold.[31] Preserving the lives of the sailors who made up 'by far the most numerous and Powerful Fleet in the World' also led Hales to a series of 'philosophical experiments' intended for those undertaking long sea voyages.[32] The question of how to preserve drinking water fresh had bedevilled fleets throughout Europe, as had the problem of producing sweet water from salt. Past failures, however, were not reason enough for Hales to give up the task, for the issue was now more pressing than ever. The numbers of those who plied their trade on the oceans, he wrote, 'have within little more than a Century, greatly increased, by a more enlarged Commerce through the World; so are they like to increase more and more in future Generations; and That especially on the vast *Atlantick Ocean*, in proportion as the *European* Colonies in *America*, may more and more increase in number of Inhabitants'.[33] Herman Boerhaave weighed in on the question of how to improve drinking water for sailors and those in warm climates in his *Elements of Chemistry*, a text one would not necessarily assume had a good deal to do with the torrid zone. He suggested that water that had grown putrid could be rendered wholesome by boiling it and then adding an

---

[30] On the Royal Society as part of 'a nascent British imperial complex' see Mark Govier, 'The Royal Society, Slavery, and the Island of Jamaica, 1660–1700', *Notes and Records of the Royal Society of London* 53 (1999).

[31] Stephen Hales, *A Description of Ventilators: Whereby Great Quantities of Fresh Air May with Ease Be Conveyed into Mines, Goals, Hospitals, Work-Houses and Ships, in Exchange for Their Noxious Air. An Account Also of Their Great Usefulness in Many Other Respects: As in Preserving All Sorts of Grain Dry, Sweet, and Free from Being Destroyed by Weevels, Both in Grainaries and Ships: And in Preserving Many Other Sorts of Goods. As Also in Drying Corn, Malt, Hops, Gun-Powder, &C. And for Many Other Useful Purposes* (London: W. Innys and R. Manby; T. Woodward, 1743).

[32] *Philosophical Experiments Containing Useful, and Necessary Instructions for Such as Undertake Long Voyages at Sea. Shewing How Sea-Water May Be Made Fresh and Wholsome: And How Fresh-Water May Be Preserv'd Sweet* (London: W. Innys and R. Manby; T Woodward, 1739), ii.

[33] Stephen Hales, *Philosophical Experiments: Containing Useful, and Necessary Instructions for Such As Undertake Long Voyages at Sea: Shewing How Sea-Water May Be Made Fresh and Wholsome: and How Fresh Water May Be Preserv'd Sweet. How Biscuit, Corn, &c. May Be Secured from the Weevel, Meggots, and Other Insects. and Flesh Preserv'd in Hot Climates, by Salting Animals Whole. to Which Is Added, an Account of Several Experiments and Observations on Chalybeate or Steel-Waters ... Which Were Read Before the Royal-Society, at Several of Their Meetings* (London: W. Innys and R. Manby [etc.], 1739), 3

acid. 'This is found to be of excellent service under the Equator, and between the Tropics', he noted.[34] Also of excellent service 'both to the *English* and *Dutch*' were jellies made from fruits, which would counteract the diseases suffered by sailors on long journeys, forced to subsist on salted, dried, and smoked provisions.[35]

Increasing commerce led to more cases of disease at sea, but it also brought diseases home. Contagion followed trade routes. Historians are familiar with the involvement of leading Fellows in the battle against contagious disease in the 1720s.[36] The plague appeared across the Channel in 1719, leading to the passage of the Quarantine Act in 1721, designed with the aid of Arbuthnot, Sloane, and Mead. In his *Short Discourse Concerning Pestilential Contagion*, Mead laid the blame for the spread of infectious diseases firmly at the feet of commercial interests. The plague, he claimed, was not indigenous to England, but was 'an *African* Fever, bred in *Aethiopia* or *Aegypt*, and the *Infection* of it carried by Trade into the other Parts of the World'.[37] Severe smallpox epidemics had swept England in 1710, 1714, 1719, and 1721, 1722, and 1723. Jurin produced tables comparing mortality rates with and without inoculation while Sloane advised King George I on a proposed experiment on six condemned prisoners at Newgate before turning to the inoculation of two of the Princess of Wales' children. This was Society medicine in the service of the state and the state extended far beyond the British Isles. According to Larry Stewart, Sloane's interest in smallpox 'was part of a general interest in contagion and especially the relationship between the British trade routes and epidemiology. This interest grew out of a network of communication which Sloane assiduously cultivated through his influence with the South Sea Company and the African Company in particular'.[38] Sloane substantially added to his natural historical collections through his correspondences with agents working for the South Sea Company in the Caribbean.[39] Meanwhile, the Duke of Chandos, elected a Fellow in 1694, played a prominent role in the affairs of the Royal African Company, seeking to leverage his connections with the Royal Society (Sloane among them) to improve the company's financial prospects as profits from the slave trade faltered.[40] Chandos and other members of the Company's

---

[34] Hermann Boerhaave, *Elements of Chemistry: Being the Annual Lectures of Herman Boerhaave, M. D.*, trans. Timothy Dallowe, 2 vols., vol. I (London: J. and J. Pemberton, 1735), 348.

[35] Ibid., II: 18.

[36] Larry Stewart, 'The Edge of Utility: Slaves and Smallpox in the Early Eighteenth Century', *Medical History* 29 (1985).

[37] Mead, *A Short Discourse Concerning Pestilential Contagion and the Methods to Be Used to Prevent It*, 20–21.

[38] Stewart, 60.

[39] On Sloane, see Malcolmson., Delbourgo, 'Slavery in the Cabinet of Curiosities: Hans Sloane's Atlantic World'; *Collecting the World: Hans Sloane and the Origins of the British Museum*.

[40] On the Royal Society's direct financial involvement in the African slave trade, see Govier.

Court of Assistants saw smallpox as one of the reasons for their financial woes. Inoculation, they suggested 'would be of great Advantage to Us, could it be put into practice by saving the Lives of great Numbers of Slaves, among whom the Small Pox is very fatall, especially, when it seizes them on their Voyage'.[41] Where smallpox and other epidemic diseases, then, were often a matter of local importance for metropolitan practitioners in the last third of the seventeenth century, they were increasingly a matter of global significance for their successors in the first third of the eighteenth.

4.2   Towards a New Putrescent Medicine

Boerhaave: Fahrenheit's Dog and the Power of Heat

We have already seen that Boerhaave had an interest in the health of sailors and those living and serving outside Europe. His work would also provide a key resource in articulating a new paradigm for understanding the diseases of warm climates. In the context of a detailed survey of theories of fever, Christopher Hamlin has identified three ways in which 'Boerhaave foreshadowed distinct approaches that would dominate the understanding of fever in the centuries to come'.[42] He focused on the nerves and the nervous system as 'the ulterior locus of explanation'; he recognised toxins as remote causes of illness, even where the precise nature or action of the toxin remained unknown; and he was profoundly interested in the body's temperature and the relationship of this to the environment, drawing regularly on the insights of his friend, Daniel Fahrenheit.[43] One might add a fourth element, which often connected the other three: an interest in putrefaction as a cause of particularly dangerous illnesses and – methodologically – the experimental study of putrefaction as a means of understanding disease.

This last element came to the fore in Boerhaave's published work after 1718, when he took up a chair in chemistry at Leiden (adding to his chairs in botany and medicine).[44] He had offered private lectures on chemistry since

---

[41] Quoted in Stewart, 65.

[42] The language of foreshadowing is useful here. If Boerhaave was not the sole inventor of such approaches (and he was not), he nonetheless synthesised and packaged them for his near-innumerable students. Hamlin, 83–6, quote on 83.

[43] Ibid., 83. 'Of what infinite use therefore are *Fahrenheit's* mercurial thermometers?' he would write: 'How certainly do they point out to us the danger that arises from the Heat in acute Diseases?' Boerhaave, *Elements of Chemistry: Being the Annual Lectures of Herman Boerhaave, M. D.*, II, 245.

[44] On the centrality of chemistry to Boerhaave's medical theory across his career, however, see John C. Powers, *Inventing Chemistry: Herman Boerhaave and the Reform of the Chemical Arts* (Chicago: University of Chicago Press, 2012).

1702, drawing a large paying audience. With the chair came public lectures and access to the university laboratory. An unauthorised edition of the lectures appeared in 1724, spurring Boerhaave to produce an official version, *The Elements of Chemistry*, which was published in two volumes in Latin in 1731 and in English translation in 1735.[45] The first volume examined the theory of chemistry, the second described a series of detailed experiments.[46] Putrefaction was a theme throughout. Boerhaave worked to carefully distinguish putrefaction from fermentation, a distinction that was crucial for his medical analyses. Many of those who had previously combined chemistry and medicine, he claimed, had assumed that fermentative processes governed the body in sickness and health. For example, Jean Baptiste van Helmont (the particular focus of Boerhaave's critique) had explained digestion by suggesting that a series of specific ferments worked with stomach acid to break down and transform food into the nourishment the body required.[47] Van Helmont and his many followers also assumed that the body's humours fermented in illness.[48] On the basis of his experiments, Boerhaave was willing to declare that one could now remove from medicine 'those idle notions of Ferments … introduc'd into it by some Dablers in Chemistry'.[49] At multiple points throughout the body, Boerhaave replaced fermentation with putrefaction.[50]

Boerhaave's logic was chemical. The results of fermentation were acidic, those of putrefaction were alkaline, and Boerhaave's experiments appeared to show that the humours did not tend towards acidity.[51] His object of analysis was urine, which he used as a marker of the body's internal state. Urine, he

---

[45] G. A. Lindeboom, *Herman Boerhaave: The Man and His Work* (London: Methuen, 1968), 109–207.

[46] Boerhaave, *Elements of Chemistry: Being the Annual Lectures of Herman Boerhaave, M. D.*, I; ibid., II.

[47] Boerhaave singled van Helmont out by name. *Elements of Chemistry: Being the Annual Lectures of Herman Boerhaave, M. D.*, II, 115. Other Iatrochemists were also roundly mocked, particularly for Sylvius' acid-alkali theory, in 'Discourse on Chemistry Purging Itself of Its Own Errors', in *Boerhaave's Orations: Translated with Introductions and Notes by E. Kegel-Brinkgreve and A. M. Luyendijk-Elshout*, ed. E. Kegel-Brinkgreve and A. M. Luyendijk-Elshout (Leiden: Brill, 1983). On van Helmont's theory of digestions, see, briefly, Allen G. Debus, *The Chemical Philosophy* (Mineola, NY: Dover, 2002), 368–71. In more detail, see Walter Pagel, 'Van Helmont's Ideas on Gastric Digestion and the Gastric Acid', *Bulletin of the History of Medicine* 30 (1956).

[48] On van Helmont's theory of disease, see 'Van Helmont's Concept of Disease – to Be or Not to Be? The Influence of Paracelsus', *Bulletin of the History of Medicine* XLVI, no. 5 (1972). Van Helmont used the term 'ferment' very generally, deploying it to describe any vital agent that facilitated the transformation of one chemical substance to another. Powers, 85.

[49] Boerhaave, *Elements of Chemistry: Being the Annual Lectures of Herman Boerhaave, M. D.*, II, 132.

[50] Thus, for example, on digestion: 'Of all Operations therfore, both artificial, and natural, Putrefaction best explains the first Action of the Mouth, Stomach, and Intestines', ibid., 202.

[51] For a clear statement of the difference between fermentation and putrefaction, see ibid., 116.

claimed, 'exhibits to us those Humours, that of all are by far the most changed by the powers of our Nature, and indeed too much to be of any farther advantage to the Body'.[52] In a healthy body the humours were neutral – neither acid nor alkaline – a fact that could be determined by noting that healthy, fresh urine was also neutral, regardless of diet. If one allowed urine to sit somewhere warm, however, it rapidly putrefied and became more alcalescent, and from this observation Boerhaave drew conclusions about the body in sickness. For urine contained 'those Salts and Oils which are the nearest to a state of Putrefaction', discharged from the body before injury could result. If diseases caused such 'putrid particles' to be retained, on the other hand, the results could be fatal.[53]

Even the healthy body, then, was constantly *inclined* towards putrefaction. At temperatures lower than that of the living body, after all, humours and dead flesh corrupted very quickly. What prevented the entire frame from being 'dissolved by Putrefaction' (as would certainly otherwise happen in a burning fever) was air, food, drink, and medicine, which could work to resist, retard, and reverse putridity. Those in most danger were those whose bodies were warmest. 'How necessary, therefore, are Water, Acids, arescent Substances, and Saline ones, to those Persons who live in hot Climates, or are daily exercised with hard Labour?'[54] In Boerhaave's hands, the processes most commonly at work in the human body were to be analogised not to those of the kitchen – in the making, for example, of beer or bread – but to those of the charnel house.

One suspects that one of the appeals of an explanation involving putrefaction rather than fermentation, for Boerhaave, was its simplicity and universality. Fermentation often required specific ferments, which were multiplied in complex processes. Putrefaction, however, required only heat and moisture, and all animal and vegetable substances could be made to rot. In terms of etiological understandings of disease, putrefaction also allowed a movement from individual afflictions to those spread through contagion. In Volume I, Boerhaave described an experiment carried out on his behalf by his 'friend and kinsman' Jodocus Provost and 'that industrious Gentleman Mr. Fahrenheit'. Having noticed that the air in rooms where sugar was dried was hot to the point of near-suffocation, Boerhaave asked his colleagues to test the effect of such high heats on an animal.[55] '[T]here is scarce any Experiment to be met with',

---

[52] Ibid., 215.

[53] 'As Urine now acquires these new qualities so easily, so soon, in a moderate degree of Heat, and in a close Vessel, hence we learn, that the human Nature does not generate Vinegars ... and consequently does not act by Fermentation, but causes the same alterations that Putrefaction does, and therefore in its effects, comes nearest to that'. Ibid., 224.

[54] Ibid., 225, 24.

[55] The letter in which Fahrenheit described his results to Boerhaave was undated. In an earlier letter, dated 12 December 1718, Fahrenheit alluded to the request, but noted that 'the people there are unwilling to have such an experiment done in their building, although I still propose

Boerhaave declared, 'that will help us better to understand the effects of this heat of Air upon the Bodies, Humours, and parts of Animals. Nor perhaps, is there any other, that is of greater service in the Art of Chemistry'.[56] The room, it was determined, was heated to 146 degrees. A Sparrow introduced into it perished, struggling and panting, after seven minutes; the cat lasted longer and died drenched in sweat. The most striking result, however, came from observations made as the dog expired. It, too, struggled and panted, but it also salivated continuously, exuding a liquid 'which was perfectly reddish, and stank so intolerably, that no body present was able to bear it'.[57] So noxious was the smell that one of the experimenters fainted and had to be revived. For Boerhaave, the conclusion was straightforward: heat so extreme (almost 50 degrees higher than that measured in the mouth of a child in health) could produce a fatal disease in an instant.

But how surprizingly, must all of the humours of the Body here be changed, as they gave such evident signs of a most fetid putrefaction? Certainly there is not in nature a more abominable stench than this terrible rancid one, more loathsome than that of a dead carcase, which was so soon produced, and exhaled from this Animal which was perfectly well just before?[58]

One should note the stress placed on the putrefaction of the *humours*. Heat had effected an internal alteration: Boerhaave noted that the flesh of the dead animal hung in the stove did not putrefy, but merely dried out. That the body's juices had changed utterly could be seen from the change in the colour and smell of the dog's saliva. And the smell that emanated from the poor canine's frame – another sign of putrefaction within – was dangerous to all around. Heat had induced a state deadly to the dog, but the product of that heat on a living animal was now capable of harming others: that 'abominable stench ... purely by its contagious quality, brought a strong man ... into imminent danger of present death'.[59] John Arbuthnot was only among the very many that would cite this experiment, but his summary of its significance was pithy: 'it is possible for pestilential Distempers to begin from excessive Heats'.[60] In

---

to try it at some time with a small bird'. Peter Van der Star, ed. *Fahrenheit's Letters to Leibniz and Boerhaave* (Leiden: Rodopi, 1983), 73, 181–3.

[56] Boerhaave, *Elements of Chemistry: Being the Annual Lectures of Herman Boerhaave, M. D.*, I, 163.

[57] Ibid.

[58] Ibid., 164.

[59] Ibid.

[60] The entire set of remarks is worth quoting: 'in A Sugar-Baker's Drying Room, where the Air was heated 146, or 54 beyond that of a Human Body, a Sparrow died in two Minutes, a Dog in 28 Minutes; but the most remarkable thing of all was that the Dog voided a red *Saliva*, foetid and putrid. We owe this luciferous experiment to the industrious *Boerhaave*, from which many important Inferences may be drawn; for why may not this putrid *Saliva* of

warm climates, then, one had to be concerned not only about the effect of high ambient temperatures on an individual body, but on the contagion that might spread to many once it was produced.

Mead: Poisons and Putrefaction

That putrefaction could cause pestilence was, of course, hardly a new claim.[61] One might regard Boerhaave's experiment as proving an assumption that had been made since at least the classical age.[62] There was, however, a particular timeliness to his observations, for the connection between putrefaction and pestilence had very recently been re-emphasised, in the work of Richard Mead, one of Boerhaave's oldest friends.[63] Mead, as we have seen, was interested in explaining the origin and cause of the plague that had recently struck Marseille and threatened England. The disease arose in Africa, where 'animal putrefaction' in the warm, humid climate conspired with some 'ill state of the air', peculiar to that part of the world. In northern climates, where one found the first element, but not the second, distempers also arose, which could prove very fatal, but they did not rise to the level of the true plague. 'For such fevers are often bred', he observed, 'where a large Number of People are closely confined together; as in *Gaols, Sieges*, and *Camps*'.[64] In the work by Boerhaave that Pringle borrowed from most explicitly, putrescence *inside* the body could produce contagious disease; in the key works by Mead, putrescence *outside* the body produced potentially fatal contagion.

Mead's explanation of the origin and spread of the plague drew heavily on his earlier work, particularly a series of essays on poisons, first published

the Dog be infectious? Consequently, it is possible for pestilential Distempers to begin from excessive Heats; no Human Creature can live long in an Air hotter than their own Bodies'. Arbuthnot, 49–50. For other citations to the experiment, see, for example, ibid., 159. John Huxham, *Observations on the Air and Epidemical Diseases, Made at Plymouth from the Year MDCCXXVIII [1728] to the End of the Year MDCCXXXVII [1737], to Which Is Added a Short Treatise on the Devonshire Colic*, 2 vols., vol. I (London: J. Coote; J. Staples, 1758), v. de Monchy, 66.

[61] On putrefaction and early modern medicine, see Wear. See the two chapters on plague (275–349) in particular.

[62] Boerhaave noted the antiquity of the connection himself. 'Physicians long ago asserted, that the plague itself is generated among animals, from an Air that has been both very moist and warm, for a considerable time'. Boerhaave, *Elements of Chemistry: Being the Annual Lectures of Herman Boerhaave, M. D.*, I, 282.

[63] Mead and Boerhaave lived together while attending Leiden University. Their friendship lasted through their lives. In 1731, Boerhaave sent three copies of his *Elementa Chemiae* to England: two for Hans Sloane, one for Mead. Lindeboom, *Herman Boerhaave: The Man and His Work*, 182. For details on Mead's life, see Arnold Zuckerman, 'Dr. Richard Mead (1673–1754): A Biographical Study', PhD Thesis (Urbana-Champaign: University of Illinois, 1965).

[64] Mead, *A Short Discourse Concerning Pestilential Contagion and the Methods to Be Used to Prevent It*, 33–4.

in 1702.[65] Explaining how the tiny amount of venom injected into the body by a viper or tarantula could kill so swiftly was no easy task. Mead's theory, like Boerhaave's, was chemical and mechanical. The 'fiery drop' communicated via the spider's bite, like that of other poisonous animals, 'put the nervous liquor into a ferment'. We might say that venom acted as a catalyst, inducing fermentation or effervescence in the fluids that flowed through the nerves. In other cases, such as the poison communicated by the bite of a mad dog, this effervescence allowed the disease to be passed from one animal to another, less like a catalyst and more strictly like the kinds of fermentation commonly found in the kitchen.

Now as we every day observe, that what is thrown out from liquors in a ferment, is capable of inducing the like motion in another liquor of the same kind, when duly mixed with it; so we may very well suppose in the present case, that the saliva, which is itself one of the most fermentative juices in nature … when it comes by means of a wound to be mixed with the nervous liquor in another animal, must necessarily put it into violent agitations, in the nature of a ferment.[66]

Poison, in other words, could be contagious: fermentation inducing fermentation. But what of its original cause? In animals, one might simply assume that venom was produced as part of their nature. But what of poisons that were not characteristic of all of the same kind of animal; poisons, for example, that were incidental to its nature (such as that of the mad dog) or those communicated via the air, rather than animal to animal? After all, the air itself could be dangerous. That found in caves or grottos might be deadly for those who breathed it too long. Other 'venomous exhalations' might produce contagious afflictions, such as those produced from bodies putrefying on a battlefield.

All Authors do agree, one great Cause of Pestilential Distempers, especially in Armies and Camps, to be dead Bodies, lying exposed and rotting in the open Air: the Reason of which is plain from what we have been advancing; for Battles being generally fought in the Summer Time, it is no wonder if the Heat acting upon the unbury'd *Carcasses* and *Fermenting* the Juices, draws forth those above Particles, which in great quantities filling the Atmosphere, when they are inspired and let into the Stomach, do affect It after the manner already described.[67]

One can see here almost precisely the logic behind Mead's theory of the plague, which laid the blame at the feet of putrefactive animal material, breathed in by those who found their humours corrupting in ways both contagious and (often) fatal. One difference existed, however, and it was important.

---

[65] *A Mechanical Account of Poisons: In Several Essays* (London: Printed by J.R. for Ralph South, 1702).

[66] Ibid., 81.

[67] Ibid., 164.

The plague was no ordinary pestilential distemper and Mead insisted that only Africa could be considered its home, however easily the disease might be passed from person to person in other climates. As a result, he made a distinction between the first production of the poison and the means of the communication of the disease to which it gave rise. 'It must indeed be owned', he wrote, 'that some malignant fevers are contagious, and that contagion is a real Poison: but the original Cause of a disease and the Communication of it, are very different things. Of this I have largely discoursed on another occasion'.[68] That other occasion was, of course, his essay on the plague, which was divided into two sections that described, in turn, the origin and then the spread of the disease. To be honest, however, Mead was rather vague on the mechanism by which the plague's first cause was produced.

All that we know, is this, that the Cause of the *Plague*, whatever it be, is of such a Nature, that when taken into the Body, it works such Changes in the Blood and Juices, as to produce this Disease, by suddenly giving some Parts of the Humours such corrosive Qualities, that they excite *Inflammations* and *Gangrenes*, wherever they fall. But we are acquainted too little with the Laws, by which the small Parts of Matter act upon each other, to be able precisely to determine the Qualities requisite to change animal Juices into such acrimonious Humours, or to explain how all the distinguishing Symptoms attending this Disease are produced.[69]

Once produced, the disease spread from person to person by familiar mechanisms. In a later edition of the collected essays on poisons, Mead explicitly drew a comparison between the means of passing along the poison in a dog bite and that in a malignant fever like the plague. Putrefaction produced a poison, which induced a fermentation in the blood, which allowed the communication of the disease through the transfer of ferments from person to person. But putrefaction without did not breed putrefaction within. For that step, one required Pringle and the notion of a 'putrid ferment'.

4.3   John Pringle: The Putrefactive Turn

Given his training, Pringle was perfectly poised to bring Boerhaave's and Mead's logics together. Born in 1707, Pringle began his medical studies at Edinburgh at age 20.[70] After only a year he moved to Holland and in 1730 he

---

68 In the 1702 edition of his essay on poisons, he had briefly flagged this distinction, noting a 'Difference of Contagion from the first Invasion of Malignant Distempers; the Effects of the *One* are the Cause and Beginning of the *Other*'. 'A Mechanical Account of Poisons: In Several Essays (4th Ed.)', in *The Medical Works of Richard Mead* (Dublin: Thomas Ewing, 1767), 106.

69 Mead, *A Short Discourse Concerning Pestilential Contagion and the Methods to Be Used to Prevent It.*, 37–8.

70 The biographical material below is derived from Dorothea Singer, 'Sir John Pringle and His Circle. Part I. Life', *Annals of Science* 6, no. 2 (1949).

completed his dissertation, on senile decay, under Boerhaave in Leiden. In 1734 he was appointed to the faculty at the University of Edinburgh, as Professor of Pneumatics and Moral Philosophy and also received his license to practice from the Royal College.[71] He became a Fellow of the College the following year. In 1742 he published a long essay on a specific remedy for dysentery and the same year became physician to the Earl of Stair, then commanding the British Army fighting against the French in Flanders. In 1745 the Duke of Cumberland promoted him to Physician General and physician to the Royal Hospitals in the low countries and overseas. It was that year that he became a Fellow of the Royal Society (his name likely first put forward by Mead). In 1749 he was appointed physician to the Duke of Cumberland. His most famous publication, *Observations on the Diseases of the Army in Camp and in Garrison,* appeared in 1752, following upon a short work on hospital and jail fevers (1750) and a series of papers which also appeared in 1750, on 'Septic and Antiseptic Substances', for which Pringle was awarded the Copley medal.

All of these last three works were connected. Pringle argued (following Mead) that external putrefaction led to internal putrefaction and (following Boerhaave) that one might cure putrid diseases by the internal application of substances that resisted sepsis. In doing so, he would need to make literal a connection that had been less direct in the past. Pringle first addressed the relationship between putrescence and disease in an epistolary essay, addressed to Mead, on hospital and jail fevers. The latter had broken out 'in such a manner as to alarm the town' as Pringle was revising the notes he had gathered for his work on the diseases of the army.[72] Both distempers were essentially the same, Pringle argued, brought about in situations where men were crowded together in poorly ventilated, dirty spaces, 'or what is the same, wherever there is a collection of putrid animal steams, from dead or even diseased bodies'.[73] Jails were filthy; hospitals filled with the 'effluvia' of wounds and excrement. The distemper also found a home on ships, where men had little space and breathed in the air that rose from bilge water, and in the less salubrious areas of cities. Addressing Mead directly, Pringle summarised:

In general, whenever in the less airy and cleanly parts of large and populous cities, a slow and low fever prevails ... we may conclude it belongs to this class of diseases; whereof the first and most exquisite, is the true plague, which YOU have shewn to arise from a high degree of putrefaction of animal substances in a sultry climate.[74]

---

[71] Pneumatics, or pneumatology, was the study of spirits or spiritual beings. One might thus best regard the position, as Singer notes, as a joint professorship in religion and moral philosophy.

[72] John Pringle, *Observations on the Nature and Cure of Hospital and Jayl-Fevers, in a Letter to Doctor Mead, Physician to His Majesty, &C.* (London: A. Millar and D. Wilson, 1750), 1.

[73] Ibid., 8.

[74] Ibid., 9–10.

Dissections gave a sense of the changes the fever wrought in the body. The putrefactive cause had a putrefactive effect. In life, the body gave off 'putrid sweats' and smelled offensive; in death one could observe the mortification of a part of the body or the production of an abscess in the brain. This 'tendency to putrefaction', Pringle declared, allowed the physician to reduce this disease to a class of other afflictions, which included the malignant smallpox, certain hectic fevers and 'the ardent and bilious fevers of moist and hot countries'. All were caused by putridity, either external or internal to the body. That the body was rendered rotten as a result could be determined from the cures for the affliction. The successful remedies were all, Pringle noted (in one of the earliest uses of the term) 'of the anti-septic kind'.[75]

These arguments were substantially elaborated upon in Pringle's most famous work, *Observations on the Diseases of the Army*, based on material he had gathered between 1742 and 1748, serving the British armed forces in Flanders in the War of the Austrian Succession.[76] The main text was divided into three parts, the first two intended for both officers and physicians, the last more technical and intended for the latter alone. An appendix then reproduced the papers that had gained Pringle the Copley medal, his experiments making clear the range of substances that could be used to retard putrefaction in meat and vegetable matter and hence the substances that could be taken internally to halt and even reverse the putrefactive tendency of the body's humours in illness. Part one supplied a medical meteorological journal of the years spent with the troops in Germany, Flanders, Britain, and Dutch Brabant. Absorbing a lesson from the Italian, Giovanni Lancisi, who had described the illnesses due to the stagnant and filthy waters around Rome in 1717, Pringle declared Zealand to possess the worst air, since it was low and watery and surrounded with 'oozy and slimy beaches'.[77] If the lower reaches of Flanders and the Netherlands produced summer and autumnal diseases of an 'extreme' kind, however, nowhere could be considered safe if it possessed swampy soil. In the summer the heat inclined the humours towards putrescence within, while warmth and moisture encouraged rot in the bodies of animals without.[78]

---

75 Ibid., 30, 31, 32.
76 Such a work was needed, Pringle argued, because no medical writers of the classical age had composed a text on the diseases of the army. Nor had any modern authors: none, at least, that one could trust. Works existed, but they had been written, Pringle sniffed, by those who had never (or hardly ever) been in the service. His *Observations*, then, ostensibly combined the expertise of the physician and the soldier. *Observations on the Diseases of the Army: In Camp and Garrison. In Three Parts. With an Appendix*, iii, v.
77 A translation may be found in Giovanni Maria Lancisi, 'Of Marshes and Their Effluvia', in *The Medical Repository*, ed. Samuel Latham Mitchill and Edward Miller (New York: Collins & Perkins, 1810). Pringle cites Lancisi (the first citation of the main part of the book) on 4.
78 Pringle, *Observations on the Diseases of the Army: In Camp and Garrison. In Three Parts. With an Appendix*, 2, 12, 5.

Having considered diseases peculiar to a given geographical region, Pringle next turned, in Part Two, to diseases peculiar to armed service. These could be divided into two kinds: those due to the weather and those due to infection. In each, putrefaction played a key role. Distempers related to the weather could be further divided according either to whether one considered the state of the season (summer or winter) or the state of the body (inflammatory or bilious diseases). The taxonomic outcome was equivalent, for inflammatory diseases were those of the winter, bilious diseases those of the summer. Seasons in turn corresponded to military sites. In summer, troops were in camp; in winter they were quartered. The long-standing analogy between seasons and climates then allowed a seemingly simple connection to be made between the diseases of the army at particular kinds of locations and those of warm climates at all times. Both could be termed 'bilious', following a tradition dating back to antiquity that had ascribed the cause of distempers such as cholera or dysentery to either an excess of bile or the corruption of that humour. 'In effect', wrote Pringle, 'in all hot countries, and in camps, where men are so much exposed to the sun, the gall, if not more abundant, is at this time more corrupted than usual'. What was true of seasons, then, was true of sites: '[W]e shall find the antient maxim, that held "the summer and autumn to be the most sickly seasons", not only verified with respect to the warmer climates, but also to a camp, where men are so much exposed to heat and moisture, the cause of putrid and contagious diseases'. Warm weather relaxed the body's solids and 'dispos[ed] the humours to putrefaction'.[79] When heat was coupled with moisture and humidity, the body could no longer effectively remove these corrupting humours through perspiration. Putrid diseases resulted.

But high temperatures had another role to play in producing illnesses, for warm, humid weather also promoted putrefaction in the body's surroundings. The 'most fatal, and the least understood' cause of sickness, asserted Pringle, was air 'corrupted by putrefaction'. Breathed in by bodies already inclined to rot, such air could produce deadly results. Proceeding taxonomically again, Pringle divided 'bad air' into four kinds, according to its source: stagnant marshes; human excrement; rotten straw; and crowded spaces, such as hospitals, barracks, and transport ships. Preventing illness in camps then boiled down to removing or controlling sources of dangerous effluvia. Camps should be situated away from swampland, straw should be changed regularly, a 'slight penalty, but strictly inflicted' should be imposed 'upon every man that shall ease himself any where about the camp, but on the privies', and confined spaces should be regularly ventilated, using Hales' invention.[80]

[79] Ibid., 91, 96 7.
[80] Ibid., 103, 24.

As striking as Pringle's obsession with putrefaction in and around the body was the fact that his focus on this single cause of illness led him to dramatically downplay the etiological logics deployed by previous authors of works on military diseases. Most had tended to point to problems in the diet of soldiers and sailors, emphasising their reliance on salted and hard to digest food. Many also adopted a moralistic tone, faulting men in service for their intemperance and lax behaviour, thereby effectively blaming soldiers and seamen for their own afflictions. Pringle would have none of it, on either account. Whoever chose to look at the seasonal periodicity of diseases and the state of the air would be convinced, he claimed 'that neither the abuse of spirits, or of fruit, or of drinking bad water, could have any considerable share in producing them'.[81] To those who would chastise soldiers for their drinking, Pringle was unsympathetic. They seemed not to understand precisely what life in campaigns was like. 'Let us not confound the necessary use of spirits in a camp', he insisted, 'with the vice of indulging them at home; but consider that soldiers are often to struggle with the extreams of hot and cold, with moist and bad air, long marches, wet cloaths and scanty provisions'.[82] That said, if Pringle placed relatively little blame on the average man in service, he also accorded him little agency. In preserving men from sickness, one could not rely on medicine or 'depend upon any thing a soldier shall have in his power to neglect'.[83] The solution was to regulate camp life, with orders that appeared reasonable and that men were compelled to obey. In Pringle's vision of the army, health and hygiene were matters of collective, rather than individual action.

The third part of the text then considered the cause and cure of specific illnesses. Inflammatory afflictions were given comparatively short shrift. Cold-weather distempers were well known and well treated elsewhere. The lion's share of the section (close to 80 per cent) was given over to discussions of putrid diseases: bilious fevers, the dysentery, and the hospital fever. Pringle was clear on the inapplicability of much of his analysis to ordinary, civilian life in Britain.

[W]e are not to confound the ordinary checks given to perspiration in Britain (where the weather is seldom close, moist, and hot for any considerable time) with what happens in other climates, subject to such intemperature, and where the inhabitants having in summer and autumn humours of a more putrescent nature, require a more constant evacuation of what is corrupted.[84]

---

81 Ibid., 111.
82 Ibid., 107.
83 Ibid., ix.
84 Ibid., 216–7. The difference, however, was as much of degree as kind. 'It may be proper to take notice, that we have also fevers of a bilious kind in this island; and that both our remitting and intermitting fevers and dysentery, seem no less the effects of a putrid cause than those of other countries. But I must add, that such is the driness of the soil, and its freedom from marshes,

The Low Countries were dangerous; Hungary, where cold and damp nights followed sultry days, was even more so; but the deadliest parts of the world were 'the marshy countries of the south', where heats were most intense and protracted. Pringle, of course, had not served in the latter, and he turned to literature both classical and modern to make his case. Celsus, Galen, and Livy offered evidence on Italy, Hippocrates on Greece, Prosper Alpinus on Egypt, Bontius on Java, 'an experienced surgeon, who lived some years in that country' on Guinea, and Warren on the West Indies. In all, heat and humidity rendered the body's solids relaxed, disposed the fluids to putrefaction, and encouraged the rot of 'plants, insects, and fishes' in marshland, producing effluvia that would reach blood primed for corruption.[85]

To understand the precise mechanism by which marsh effluvia caused putrid diseases, one needs to turn to Pringle's experiments on septic and antiseptic substances, and to read them as a direct response, correction, and elaboration of Boerhaave's.[86] The first order of business in Pringle's experiments was to demonstrate both that all putrid substances were not alkaline and that alkaline salts did not promote putrefaction. The method was simple, although it cannot have thrilled any neighbours within smelling distance.[87] Most commonly, Pringle took pieces of beef and set them somewhere warm, comparing the state of the flesh alone or in water to that of it combined with another substance. Thus, for example, in Experiment III he compared a phial of lean beef in water and salt of hartshorn (baker's ammonia) to one containing beef, water, and table salt, with a third containing meat and water alone 'to serve by way of index'. All were placed in a lamp-furnace, where the temperature stayed between 94 and 100 degrees Fahrenheit. In less than a day, the contents of the 'index' phial were rank; a few hours later, that containing sea salt was also putrid; but the

---

the constant perflation, and the moderate and interrupted heats of our summers, that, unless in extraordinary hot and close seasons, and in the fenny tracts, these distempers are always gentle, and seldom epidemic'. Ibid., 237.

[85] Ibid., 201–2, 20.

[86] Certainly Pringle noted the relation, commending the man he termed his 'celebrated master' for combining mechanics with chemistry in an understanding of medicine. Pringle also saw himself as continuing in research begun by Bacon and Hoffman. 'Ld. Bacon calls, "the inducing or accelerating putrefaction a subject of very universal inquiry"; and says, "that it is of excellent use to enquire into the means of preventing or staying putrefaction: which makes a great part of physic and surgery"'. Ibid., 367. See Gottlieb Benjamin Bergerus and Friedrich Hoffmann, *Dissertatio Physicomedica Inauguralis de Putredinis Doctrina Amplissimi in Medicina Usus. Praes. F. Hoffmann* (Halle: 1722).

[87] Pringle himself made mention of the distasteful elements of his research. 'Altho' an enquiry into the manner how bodies are resolved by putrefaction, with the means of accelerating or preventing that process, has been reckoned not only curious, but useful; yet we find it little prosecuted in an experimental way: nor is it to be wondered at, considering how offensive such operations are', Pringle, *Observations on the Diseases of the Army: In Camp and Garrison. In Three Parts. With an Appendix*, 367.

phial containing salt of hartshorn (considered in the past a promoter of putrefaction) still smelled sweet.

The range of substances that retarded putrefaction, Pringle discovered, was vast: 'besides salts, fermented spirits, spices, and acids, commonly known to have this property, many resins, astringents and refrigerants are of the number; and even those plants called anti-acids, and supposed hasteners of putrefaction: of which class horse-radish is particularly antiseptic'. Later experiments then turned to the question of whether antiseptics might not only resist, but reverse putrefaction. In the case of the Bark, the answer was an unequivocal yes. The famed specific against certain fevers could not only remove the putrid smell from tainted meat, it could stiffen the fibres rendered lax by rot. Pringle immediately connected these two properties of the Bark, arguing that the substance worked against gangrene and various fevers precisely because such afflictions involved putrefaction. Without marking it, then, Pringle introduced what would prove to be the most controversial element of his analysis, the suggestion that sepsis in dead flesh was identical to – and could cause – rot within a living body. Marsh effluvia, rendered putrid by the rotting animal and vegetable substances within it, were a 'ferment', a term, he quickly clarified (in order to avoid association with the fermentational theories of earlier chemists) he meant only 'to express the assimilating power of all putrid animal substances over the fresh'. Pringle put forward the results of simple experiment to demonstrate the point. A small amount of material taken from the yolk of a putrid egg, when added to water and the yolk of half a fresh egg caused more putrefaction than occurred in the other half, in water alone. This 'putrid fermentation', Pringle asserted, offered a close 'connection' with the action of contagion.[88]

Pringle claimed in the Preface to his *Observations on the Diseases of the Army* that little of the etiological reasoning to be found in the text was properly his. 'The corruption of the humours is hinted at by Hippocrates', he noted, and had been further developed by later authors well into the seventeenth century, before being lost by 'mechanical writers' and then revived by his teacher, Boerhaave.[89] But we should be somewhat wary of accepting his history at face value. Corruption and putrefaction were not necessarily the same thing. His explanation was new – radically so – as one can learn by comparing it to that of one of his own key sources. As we have seen, for Mead, the dead bodies of animals could, in the hot and humid climate of Africa, become 'fit to breed'

[88] Ibid., 379, 68–9, 81–2, 87. Pringle cited Bacon as the first to make the connection between contagion and 'putrid fermentation'. Hoffman, who Pringle cited as another key reference, also pursued the analogy between putrescence and ferments in Bergerus and Hoffmann.

[89] Pringle, *Observations on the Diseases of the Army: In Camp and Garrison. In Three Parts. With an Appendix*, xiii.

plague. The effluvia rising from carcasses could corrupt the humours until they were corrosive enough to damage the body's solids, and the disease could then be spread as ferments hopped from body to body via the air.[90] But Mead's was not an explanation in which putrescence bred putrescence. Literal putrefaction, by contrast – not merely a generalised 'corruption' – was placed at the centre of Pringle's theory of diseases in crowded hospitals, jails, and ships, as well as in warm and humid climes. In the colonies, as we will see, his ideas about sources of sepsis suggested a medical geography, one based on avoiding marshes (and their miasmas) at all costs. On ships, his theory of the effect of putrid disorders on the body's humours suggested a cure: the ingestion of antiseptic substances. Medical men at sea and on land would soon be locked in a battle with rot.

4.4   Putrefaction in the Periphery

Putridity at Sea

Perhaps no single voyage changed medical writing so dramatically as the journey of Lord Anson's fleet. In 1739, tensions were high between Spain and Britain. That year, Vernon would capture Portobello, and the following year George Anson, then Captain of the *Centurion*, was given command of a squadron of six warships and two merchant vessels, with orders to attack and capture the port that serviced Lima and, if possible, the city itself. After losing contact with three of the warships, the remaining ships encountered storms and high seas as they rounded Cape Horn. It was then that scurvy broke out, killing a staggering number of men. In the time since it had left England, the crew of the *Centurion* had been reduced by almost 60 per cent, and that of the *Gloucester* by even more. After eventually completing a circumnavigation of the globe, the squadron returned home in June 1744 to a heroes' welcome. Despite the tremendous loss of life – and the failure to achieve any of their main objectives – the ships had managed some very successful piracy, capturing several smaller ships and one Spanish Galleon. The seized treasure was paraded through the streets of London, Anson's share of the prize money made him a very wealthy man, and in 1751 he was promoted to First Lord of the Admiralty. The official account of the voyage was published in 1748 and was read voraciously, four editions appearing for the same London publishers that year and at least two more in 1749.[91]

---

[90] Mead, *A Short Discourse Concerning Pestilential Contagion and the Methods to Be Used to Prevent It*, 32.

[91] George Anson, *A Voyage Round the World: In the Years MDCCXL, I, II, III, IV. By George Anson ... Compiled from Papers and Other Materials Of ... George Lord Anson, and*

Leading physicians published tracts on the scurvy within only a few years of the squadron's return.[92] In 1747, Huxham described *A Method for Preserving the Health of Seamen in Long Cruises and Voyages*, which he then appended to his 1750 book on fevers.[93] Mead weighed in two years later, with an explanation that should now seem familiar: While a bad diet played a role, for Mead, scurvy was caused by bad air.[94] Mead proposed improving the seamen's food, adding wine vinegar to their provisions, and improving the air by using a ventilator, based on Sutton's design. By far the best known of the scurvy-tracts written in response to the appalling death rates during Anson's voyage was that by James Lind.[95] The book remains famous today, because in it Lind described the results of a trial made to determine which anti-scorbutics worked best. Twelve patients, kept on a common diet, were divided into six pairs. The first was given a quart of cider per day; the second an amount of *elixir vitriol* thrice daily; the third two spoonfuls of vinegar as often as the second; the fourth half a pint of sea water per day; the fifth two oranges and one lemon; and the

Published under His Direction, by Richard Walter ... Illustrated with Forty-Two Copper-Plates (London: John and Paul Knapton, 1748). The book remained enormously popular, in spite of the fact that it had considerable competition from various unofficial accounts of the journey. A fourteenth London edition appeared in 1769.

[92] Kenneth J. Carpenter, *The History of Scurvy and Vitamin C* (Cambridge: Cambridge University Press, 1986).

[93] Huxham, *An Essay on Fevers, and Their Various Kinds, as Depending on Different Constitutions of the Blood: With Dissertations on Slow Nervous Fevers; on Putrid, Pestilential, Spotted Fevers; on the Small-Pox; and on Pleurisies and Peripneumonies*, 259–65. Much like Pringle, Huxham combined his Boerhaavian training with readings of Mead to offer an account of putrid fevers as a class unto themselves (see Introduction). Huxham analogised the cause of this dissolution to the action of poisons, citing Mead, and paid particular attention to the putrefaction of the Bile: 'truly putrid Bile is little less pernicious than an actual Poison', he wrote. Ibid., 41, 114. Huxham argued that the cause of the scurvy was 'bad Provisions, bad Water, bad Beer &c', coupled with a moist, salty aerial atmosphere and foul air between decks. This led to a putrefaction of the blood, which – since in Huxham's view, putrefaction was alcalescent – could be corrected using acidic substances, like apple cider. Huxham prescribed at least a pint per day, in addition to the daily allowances of beer and water. Ibid., 259, 60–1.

[94] Moisture weakened the air's spring; it was full of 'foul particles' breathed out by men crowded together, some of whom were no doubt diseased; filthy bilge-water stagnated and gave off effluvia; and salts were inhaled, some of which may have originated from animals putrefying in the water. When the latter made their way into the blood, they could, 'in the nature of a ferment, corrupt its whole mass'. Richard Mead, 'Discourse on the Scurvy', in *An Historical Account of a New Method for Extracting the Foul Air out of Ships, &C with the Description and Draught of the Machines, by Which It Is Performed: In Two Letters to a Friend, by Samuel Sutton, the Inventor*, ed. Samuel Sutton (London: J. Brindley, 1749), 102. Mead also related the comments made to him by Admiral Charles Wagner, who had supplied his men with oranges and lemons daily. The men ate them and added the juice to their beer. 'It was also their constant diversion to pelt one another with the rinds; so that the deck was always strewed and wet with the fragrant liquor. The happy effect was, that he brought his sailors home in good health'. Ibid., 112.

[95] Lind, *A Treatise of the Scurvy. In Three Parts. Containing an Inquiry into the Nature, Causes, and Cure of That Disease. Together with a Critical and Chronological View of What Has Been Published on the Subject*. The text was dedicated to Anson.

sixth medicine recommended by a hospital surgeon. The citrus fruit won hands down, with one of the two previously scorbutic patients ready for duty only six days later, and the other well enough after some time to serve as nurse for the rest.[96] Cider – recommended by Huxham – did second best.

Nowadays, we regard the scurvy as a disease brought on by a vitamin deficiency. Oranges and lemons provide the requisite Vitamin C. Lind, of course, had no conception of such an explanation. *The principal and main predisposing cause* of the disease 'is a manifest and obvious quality of the air, *viz.* its *moisture*', he wrote, systematically rejecting previous theories that pointed to the harmful effects of sea salt in the diet, the absence of fresh vegetables, or bad and vitiated air. Running sores and stinking gums clearly indicated rot within the body, but Lind rejected both Mead and Pringle's suggestions for the origins of putridity. Putrefaction required no unusual explanation, Lind argued, because it was the body's natural action to tend towards a putrescent state: 'the scorbutic putrefaction … is purely the natural effect of animal heat and motion caused by the action of the body'. Heat and motion produced two effects. The body's fluids tended to degenerate and become corrupted because of their constant mutual actions on each other; the body's solids tended to be abraded by the motion of the fluids, parts of them washed into the channels along which the fluids flowed. An animal body, Lind claimed was 'of all substances, the most liable to corruption and putrefaction'.[97] In a healthy body, the worst of the putrescent particles were removed either by urination or perspiration (particularly insensible perspiration), and the material lost from the solids was replaced by food that had been transformed into a nutritious chyle. Problems arose when insensible perspiration was impeded (when the weather was cold – particularly when it was also damp – and when men failed to exercise sufficiently), and when poor food made the production of useful chyle difficult.

Diet thus mattered, but the key question had less to do with 'freshness' and more to do with the ability of the body to use food to replace what had been lost. The fluids given off in perspiration were the thinnest and the most 'subtilised', thus those most able to pass through miniscule pores. The body also required a thin liquor to repair the abraded solids, since it had to pass through the 'most minute canals' to reach the sites of wear. The staples of sea-life, however – salty, dried food and unleavened bread – were notoriously difficult to break down. Green vegetables worked in their stead because they contained less oil than animal matter and because they were less solidly held together in the first place. 'There is no other particular virtue', Lind noted, 'in which they all agree'. Green vegetables shared with ripe fruits a

---

[96] Ibid., 192 3.
[97] Ibid., 107, 277, 73.

'fermentative quality'. From the fact that such substances seemed valuable remedies for the scurvy, Lind concluded that a fermentative operation, and foods that promoted it, was necessary for digestion and for preventing 'scorbutic corruption'. Vegetables also produced a chyle that tended towards the acidic, which could 'correct the continual putrescent tendency of the animal humours'.[98] Yet Lind was clear on the fact that acidity was not to be taken as the sole reason that oranges and lemons worked so well. Putrid bodies were not always alkaline and alcalescent vegetables, like the famed 'Scurvy-grass' or cresses, worked against the scurvy, the water they contained diluting and thinning the chyle; their viscid parts dulling the acrimony due to putrefaction; and the salts within them acting as a fine antiseptic. Nonetheless, he acknowledged, alcalescent plants did not seem as efficacious as acidic fruits. The ideal solution, Lind advised, was to use a mixture of different ingredients, each of which possessed one or more anti-scorbutic virtue to a high degree and which, when combined, produced a 'vegetable, saponaceous, fermentable acid'. Precisely such an acid was to be found 'in a certain degree' in oranges, which made them very effective as a means of preventing and remedying scurvy, even if they were not to be understood as, in our contemporary language, a magic bullet against the disease.[99]

Putridity on (Warm) Land

The Preface to the third edition of Pringle's *Diseases of the Army* (1761) contains a line not found in the first or second, or in any that followed. 'In reasoning upon the nature of the bilious fevers, the hospital-fever, and the dysentery, I have so much recourse to the *septic principle,* that the Reader may imagine I have considered it as a more universal cause than I really think it; for except in these distempers, and in a few more ... I have hitherto referred no other disorder to that origin'.[100] Pringle had, in fact, been clear about the limitations of his analysis. He had focused on bilious diseases because they were less well treated in the medical literature, since Britons were far more likely to be afflicted by cold weather, inflammatory distempers. Putrid diseases were the illnesses of elsewhere, although some of the elsewheres – hospitals and jails – could be found in the heart of the metropole. If the 'septic principle' was of limited applicability in Britain, however, it would soon become ubiquitous – whether precisely in Pringle's terms or not – in the colonies, where

---

[98] Ibid., 290, 301, 8, 3. Green vegetables could thus produce the ideal chyle, one that could 'dilute and sweeten the acrimonious animal juices, to correct the putrescent tendency of the humours, and to repair the decay of the body'. Ibid., 296.

[99] Ibid., 306, 10.

[100] Quoted in Dorothea Singer, 'Sir John Pringle and His Circle, II', *Annals of Science* 6, no. 3 (1950): 245.

warmth and humidity seemed to make the centrality of rot to medical discourse seem almost natural. For perhaps a quarter of a century after 1750, distempers in the warm climates of the British Empire became putrefactive. Putrescence, one might say, was in the tropical air.

The change wrought in theories of medicine in warm climates around mid-century might be seen by returning to examples from Chapter 2. What Towne called an 'ardent bilious fever' in 1726, what Warren named a 'malignant' one in 1740, what Dale Ingram referred to merely as the 'yellow fever' in 1755, Hillary termed a *putrid* bilious fever' in 1759.[101] There was no talk of putridity or rot in Towne's text at all. Warren, as we saw earlier, modelled his account after Mead's, and presented his fever as a contagious one, brought from the East. But he said little of its original (possibly putrefactive) cause. He followed Mead in arguing that contagious distempers acted like poisons on the body, the particles making them up mixing with the body's fluids and changing them 'into their own Likeness and Nature, and these again infect others in a sort of proliferous Manner, until the whole Mass becomes contaminated'.[102] Like the bites of venomous animals, gangrene could be a result of infection by the contagious poison and Warren described a possible 'gangrenous *Diathesis* of the sanguineous Mass' and labelled the third stage of the distemper the 'Gangrenous State'.[103] Necrotic decay thus seemed to play a role in Warren's theory, but he did not label the fever putrid, nor turn to chemistry as a means of healing. Ingram offered an alternative explanation, which pointed to external putrefaction as a cause of the fever and suggesting that it was 'brought on by a poison, that is, a *poisonous state of the air*' but denied that it was contagious and said little about the internal putrefaction of the body's fluids.[104]

---

[101] Putrefaction played no central explanatory role in Cleghorn's account of the Diseases of Minorca (1751) or in the debate between Williams and Bennet (1750). George Cleghorn, *Observations on the Epidemical Diseases in Minorca. From the Year 1744 to 1749* (London: Printed for D. Wilson, 1751). Williams and Bennet.

[102] Warren, 21.

[103] Ibid., 12, 16.

[104] Dale Ingram, *An Historical Account of the Several Plagues That Have Appeared in the World since the Year 1346. With an Enquiry into the Present Prevailing Opinion, That the Plague Is a Contagious Distemper ... In Which the Absurdity of Such Notions Is Exposed ... To Which Are Added a Particular Account of the Yellow Fever ... Also Observations on Dr Mackenzie's Letters; ... And an Abstract of Capt. Isaac Clemens's Voyage in the Sloop Fawey* (London: R. Baldwin and J. Clark, 1755), 133. The book received a scathing commentary in *The Monthly Review*, which described it as 'this worse than worthless piece'. Anonymous, 'Review of Dale Ingram, "A Historical Account of Several Plagues That Have Appeared in the World since the Year 1346"', *The Monthly Review* (1755): 139. The anonymous author of a 1776 tract on West Indian diseases offered yet another take on the yellow fever's aetiology. It was caused by either excessive heats, which induced putrefaction of the body's juices, or through the action of putrid effluvia, but it was not contagious. All those who shared the same air might become ill, but they did not infect one another. *Practical Remarks on West India Diseases* (London: F. Newbery; F. Blyth, 1776), 72–3.

By contrast, the 'septic principle' was front and centre in Hillary's explanation at the end of the 1750s.

From an attentive Consideration of all the Symptoms which attend this Disease, and a strict Examination of the putrid State, and dissolved gangrenescent Condition in which we find the Blood of those who labour under it; as well as the half putrefied and mortified State in which the Body is found immediately after their Death ... it evidently appears from all the Symptoms which attend it, as well as from their putrid Effects, that a bilious putrefying Diathesis, is actually introduced into the Blood and all the circulating Fluids of the Body.[105]

To effect a cure, one needed first to slow the excessively rapid motion of the fluids and to reduce the fever, second to remove as much of the putrid bile and other humours as possible, and third, to use 'suitable Antiscepticks' to 'put a Stop to the putrescent Disposition of the Fluids, and prevent the Gangrenes from coming on'.[106] Such antiseptics included the Peruvian bark (although it could be hard for a patient to stomach) or a julep made from serpent's root.[107] Hillary rejected so-called alkaline antiseptics, however. He did not mention Pringle by name, but there would seem to be little doubt whom he had in mind when he critiqued experiments 'made on Pieces of dead Flesh, or dead stagnating animal Fluids'. Trials made on the living, he asserted, had made it clear that alkaline salts and spirits brought on putrescence, rather than hindering it. On this point, as on many others, Hillary followed Huxham.[108]

By the early 1760s, one can see the emergence of a new orthodoxy, one that paired internal and external putrefaction and located both, in their most extreme forms, outside Northern Europe. '[A]lmost all Diseases in hot Climates', wrote Lind in his essay on the *Health of Seamen*, 'are thought to be of a putrid Nature'. Citing Pringle's 'excellent Observations' with enthusiasm, Lind also noted the dangers of marshy effluvia: 'The Fens, even in different Counties of *England*, are known to be very dangerous to the Health of those who live near them, and still more so to Strangers; but the woody and marshy lands in

---

[105] Hillary, *Observations on the Changes of the Air and the Concomitant Epidemical Diseases, in the Island of Barbados. To Which Is Added a Treatise on the Putrid Bilious Fever, Commonly Called the Yellow Fever; and Such Other Diseases as Are Indigenous or Endemial, in the West India Islands, or in the Torrid Zone*, 163.

[106] Ibid., 164.

[107] Hillary's treatments were subsequently used throughout the empire. Richard Huck, physician to the general hospital at Havaan noted that many of the medical men he met with recommended Hillary's work on the yellow fever as 'the best upon that distemper'. Quoted in Charters, 60.

[108] See Chapter 2. On Huxham's theory of putrid fevers, see above. Although they differed somewhat on how to cure such afflictions, Pringle was very enthusiastic about Huxham's text, noting that it appeared immediately after his short essay on jail and hospital fevers. Pringle, *Observations on the Diseases of the Army: In Camp and Garrison. In Three Parts. With an Appendix*, xii.

hot Countries are exceedingly more pernicious to the Health of *Europeans*'.[109]
Solomon de Monchy drew heavily on 'Mead, Pringle, Huxham, Lind, Watson,
Bisset, Hillary' in his prize-winning essay in answer to a question on the usual
causes of illnesses among seamen in journeys to the West Indies. We should
thus not be surprised to find putridity given a starring role in his explanations.
The putrid fever, malignant fever, and the scurvy, he claimed, all flowed from
the same cause: putrefaction. Pairing the ship and the colony, he argued that
the source of the putrefaction was 'fetid vapours', found equally in ships'
holds and the 'marshy coasts of the West Indies'. 'This retained putrescent
vapour, or matter', he wrote, 'acting like yeast on the juices ... dangerous,
putrid diseases must necessarily be the result in hot countries'.[110] It is difficult
to date the 'Account of the True Bilious, or Yellow Fever', written by John
Hume, who had served as Surgeon at the Naval Hospital at New Greenwich
in Jamaica between 1739 and 1749, since it was only published after his death
in 1777.[111] My suspicion, however, is that it was composed in the 1760s or
early 1770s, since Hume describes as common the position that Hillary had
first advocated in 1759: 'All practitioners in the West-Indies now agree', he
stated, 'that the principal intentions in the cure of this fever must be, to correct
the too-great tendency of the blood to putrefaction, and to carry off the putrid
bile as expeditiously and safely as possible'.[112] In writing to Donald Monro
in 1773, John Quier – who had practiced almost six years in Jamaica – was
almost certainly right to suspect that Monro would find it surprising to be told
that his correspondent had not 'met with a single case of what might properly
be called an acute putrid disease, except the small-pox'. Of diseases arising
from the corruption of fluids, particularly the bile, there were plenty, but of
'real putrefaction', none. Quier was well aware of his exceptionality, however.
Among the endemial diseases of warm countries, he observed, those disorders
which 'arise from, or are accompanied with putrefaction', were held to be the
most common.[113] Andrew Wilson, Fellow of the Royal College of Physicians in
Edinburgh was critical of the label, but nonetheless noted in 1780 'that tendency
to putridity which so remarkably stigmatizes the diseases of hot climates'.[114]

---

[109] Lind, 25, 66, 64.
[110] de Monchy, 67, 88.
[111] The dates for Hume's tenure as surgeon are those given in Donald Monro et al., *Letters and Essays on the Small-Pox and Inoculation, the Measles, the Dry Belly-Ache, the Yellow, and Remitting, an Intermitting Fevers of the West Indies* (London: J. Murray, 1778), 195–6. Chakrabarti notes, however, that Hume resigned his position in 1746. Chakrabarti, 69. The editor of the volume in which Hume's essay appeared noted that a copy of the original text was made 'some years before his death'. Monro et al., xv.
[112] Monro et al., 197–249, 10.
[113] Letter sent from Jamaica, dated 23 March 1773. Ibid., 151.
[114] Andrew Wilson, *Rational Advice to the Military, When Exposed to the Inclemency of Hot Climates and Seasons* (London: W. Richardson, 1780), 33.

The importance of Pringle to medicine in the armed forces may be seen by the fact that two of the most well-cited texts of the mid-1760s function as essential paraphrases of his main arguments.[115] Richard Brocklesby published his *Oeconomical and Medical Observations* in 1764, having succeeded Pringle as Surgeon-General of the British Army in 1758. Brocklesby referred to Pringle as 'my most philosophical and ingenious immediate predecessor', but noted that Pringle's 'Verulamian' style may have been off-putting for officers reading his text. Hence this 'more popular treatise', describing 'the tender frame of man ... whose body is every instant pervious to all the minute seeds of putrefaction and dissolution'.[116] Donald Monro published his *Account of the Diseases Which were most Frequent in the British Military Hospitals in Germany* the same year. There he noted that, after time, diseases in warm climates 'tend to the putrid kind, and must be treated as such'. To effect a cure, the diet had to be made up of vegetable antiseptics, which could correct the tendency of the blood to putrefy.[117]

By the late 1760s, as can be seen from the text by the younger Lind, one finds Pringle's septic principle being applied to explain diseases in India. In 1773, John Clark, who had previously served as surgeon on the Talbot Indiaman also pointed to noxious exhalations from marshy ground as the cause of many illnesses in the East Indies. All the dangerous diseases of warm climates, he

---

[115] Erica Charters makes a more general argument for the crucial importance of the work of Pringle and Lind to medical practice during the Seven Years' War in Charters.

[116] Richard Brocklesby, *Oeconomical and Medical Observations, in Two Parts. From the Year 1758 to the Year 1763, Inclusive* (London: T. Becket, and P. A. De Hondt, 1764), 27, 167. The cause of decay within the body was decay without: 'Heat and moisture conspire to resolve the dead bodies of reptile and other animals, and the dying parts of vegetables; and the waters, the earth, and the air we breathe, abound with volatile putrescent effluvia, which are at this season scattered around in great abundance, as is fatally experienced by those who are obliged to live in marshy warm countries, near stagnant waters, or on lands annually laid under water by the inundations of great rivers, &c'. Ibid., 167.

[117] Donald Monro, *An Account of the Diseases Which Were Most Frequent in the British Military Hospitals in Germany, from January 1761 to the Return of the Troops to England in March 1763. To Which Is Added, an Essay on the Means of Preserving the Health of Soldiers, and Conducting Military Hospitals* (London: A. Millar, D. Wilson, and T. Durham, 1764), 239. A second and much revised edition appeared in 1780. In it, Monro drew heavily on the work of those in the West Indies, particularly John Hume. *Observations on the Means of Preserving the Health of Soldiers and of Conducting Military Hospitals. And on the Diseases Incident to Soldiers in the Time of Service, and on the Same Diseases as They Have Appeared in London. In Two Volumes. By Donald Monro, M.D*, 2nd ed. (London: J. Murray; and G. Robinson, 1780). 1764 also saw the original Latin publication of Lewis Rouppe, *Observations on Diseases Incidental to Seamen*, Translated from the Latin Edition [1764], Printed at Leyden ed. (London: T. Carnan and F. Newbery, 1772), 81., which continues the theme. Rouppe cited some of his key sources on 82: 'With respect to the effect which such a foul air must produce in the body, consult the histories of epidemical disorders published by *Hoffman, Huxham,* and *Pringle*, as well as *de Monchy*'.

claimed, 'depend upon a putrescent disposition in the fluids'.[118] The same year Edward Ives, whose thoughts on the diseases of Europeans in the East Indies had already appeared in print in Lind's book on Scurvy (and whose book was well known enough to end up on the desk of Immanuel Kant), described a practice in India about which there was 'nothing uncommon' and where 'antiseptic medicines' were regularly administered.[119] A decade later Stephen Mathews noted the 'pernicious' effect of the Indian climate on European constitutions, suggesting that the constant heat produced a relaxation of the body and a sluggish motion of the fluids, leading to obstructions and putrescency. In such a state, the body was particularly vulnerable to 'septic miasmata' with a putrefaction of the fluids a potentially deadly result.[120]

Tracking the spread of putrefactive theories of disease in the British Isles is a task rendered complex by the existence of two distinct (at least initially) conceptions of putrid disorders around 1750: one building upon John Fothergill's 1748 report on the deadly spread of cases of a sore throat attended with ulcers and the other drawing upon the work of figures such as Pringle, Lind, and Huxham on putrid disorders.[121] The disease described by Fothergill killed rapidly, after producing, among other symptoms, a 'Disposition to Putrefaction' of the body in general, and the back of the throat leading to the pharynx in particular. Fothergill ascribed the cause of this disposition to a 'putrid *Virus*, or *Miasma sui generis*', passed contagiously via the breath from person to person.[122] In 1755, Claude-Nicolas Le Cat, Professor of Anatomy and Chirurgery at Rouen, described a number of 'malignant fevers' that raged in the previous few years. Le Cat did not use the term 'putrid' to describe any of

---

[118] John Clark, *Observations on the Diseases in Long Voyages to Hot Countries, and Particularly on Those Which Prevail in the East Indies*. (London: Printed for D. Wilson and G. Nicol, 1773), 149.

[119] Edward Ives, *A Voyage from England to India, in the Year MDCCLIV: And an Historical Narrative of the Operations of the Squadron and Army in India, Under ... Watson And ... Clive ... Also, a Journey from Persia to England, by an Unusual Route. With an Appendix, Containing an Account of the Diseases Prevalent in Admiral Watson's Squadron: A Description of Most of the Trees, Shrubs, and Plants, of India ... Illustrated with a Chart, Maps, and Other Copper-Plates* (London: Edward and Charles Dilly, 1773), 444.

[120] Stephen Mathews, *Observations on Hepatic Diseases Incidental to Europeans in the East-Indies* (London: T. Cadell, 1783), 7, 19.

[121] Almost all of the texts cited by Creighton fall into one of these two camps. The exceptions are those that are too short or too vague for one to determine what, precisely, is meant by a 'putrid disease'. For example, the few lines penned in Latin by 'S' in the *Gentleman's Magazine* in 1755 or the multiple mentions of putrid fevers (with little, if any, discussion of their causes) in Thomas Short, *A Comparative History of the Increase and Decrease of Mankind in England, and Several Countries Abroad ... To Which Is Added, a Syllabus of the General States of Health, Air, Seasons, and Food for the Last Three Hundred Years: And Also a Meteorological Discourse* (London: W. Nicoll, 1767).

[122] John Fothergill, *An Account of the Sore Throat Attended with Ulcers; a Disease Which Hath of Late Years Appeared in This City, and the Parts Adjacent* (London: C. Davis, 1747), 60, 61.

these, but he did make mention of a number of 'gangrenous sore throats'.[123] Two years later, Huxham offered his own account of the disease, citing Fothergill as the first to provide an accurate depiction of it in England.[124]

If these three cases – drawn from Creighton's analysis – point to a metropolitan origin for part of the talk of putrid diseases in Britain at mid-century, many of the other examples Creighton used point towards imperial and colonial resources for this discourse. James Johnstone appears to have been the first to construct a lineage of authors writing about the malignant sore throat that included Fothergill, Le Cat, and Huxham. His work of 1758 was also one of the first (together with Huxham's) to link these studies of a singular disease with a more general discourse concerning putrid afflictions.[125] James Sims drew upon the experiences gained in his practice in Tyrone, Ireland in the mid-1760s and early-1770s in writing his *Observations on Epidemic Disorders*. But his remarks on nervous and malignant fevers in that volume are all offered in dialogue with the writings of Huxham and Pringle.[126] Creighton cited Charles Bisset's *Essay on the Medical Constitution of Great Britain* (1762), but did so without noting that Bisset came to his understanding of putrid disorders during time served as second surgeon to the hospital at Jamaica, beginning in 1740. This experience was reflected in his *Treatise on the Scurvy* (1755), a text which drew heavily on Lind's *Treatise* on the same topic, as well as Pringle's *Diseases of the Army*.[127] Citing Hillary's book on the diseases of the West Indies, Creighton suggested that 'Perhaps the most surprising testimony to the existence of an "epidemic constitution" of slow, continued, nervous fever comes from the Island of Barbados'.[128] Certainly, if one imagines the spread of a specific disease agent, it may be surprising to find it in Barbados as well as Rouen, England, and Ireland. However, if one imagines that what is spreading is a way of understanding disease, and that it spread via imperial networks,

---

[123] Mons. Le Cat, 'An Account of Those Malignant Fevers, That Raged at Rouen, at the End of the Year 1753, and the Beginning of 1754', *Philosophical Transactions* 49 (1755–6).

[124] John Huxham, *A Dissertation on the Malignant, Ulcerous Sore-Throat* (London: J. Hinton, 1757). That said, Fothergill's and Huxham's accounts of the disease – and the role played by putrefaction – were quite different. The former located the specific site of putrefaction (or a disposition to putrefaction) in the throat. For Huxham, however, in keeping with his earlier work on fevers, putrescence was located in the blood.

[125] James Johnstone, *An Historical Dissertation Concerning the Malignant Epidemical Fever of 1756* (London: W. Johnstone, 1758), 7. Johnstone makes explicit reference to Pringle's work on antiseptics on 57.

[126] James Sims, *Observations on Epidemic Disorders, with Remarks on Nervous and Malignant Fevers* (London: J. Johnson; G. Robinson, 1773).

[127] Bisset; *An Essay on the Medical Constitution of Great Britain, to Which Are Added Observations on the Weather, and the Diseases Which Appeared in the Period Included Betwixt the First of January 1758, and the Summer Solstice in 1760*. (London: A. Millar and D. Wilson, 1762). Bisset dedicated the *Medical Constitution* to Pringle.

[128] Creighton, II. *From the Extinction of Plague to the Present Time*, 127.

carried with particularly urgency after the outbreak of the Seven Years War, and travelling not from centre to periphery, but in all directions, the surprise tends to evaporate.[129]

4.5   The End of the Putrefactive Paradigm

Scurvy as Anomaly and the Problem of Method

Putrefactive theories of disease had become standards in texts produced in and about warm climates by the last quarter of the eighteenth century. The idea that marshes produced putrid effluvia that induced decay in the human frame provided a rationale for the placement of residences and soldiers' quarters and pointed towards at least some elements of a regimen of both prevention and treatment by means of the ingestion of antiseptics. In terms of practical medicine, then, views broadly similar to Pringle's had gained a great deal of traction, particularly – and unsurprisingly – within the military. No doubt, part of the appeal was the fact that the new set of explanations in fact recapitulated many older ideas, such as the dangers of marshlands and rotting corpses, and the value of curatives such as fresh produce and the Peruvian bark. Many of these notions would remain, even after the putrefactive paradigm was replaced, the Bark, for example, now employed for its properties as a nervous tonic, rather than an antiseptic.

In 1768, when the younger Lind published his Latin dissertation on the putrid fever of Bengal, the paradigm was orthodoxy. By the time the text was translated into English in 1776, a growing chorus of criticisms could be heard. Some of these criticisms – one suspects they were among the most damaging – came from earlier proponents of putrefactive theories and involved what had been one of the paradigm's earliest extensions and successes. Scurvy had become, after Lind's tract on the subject appeared in 1753, the quintessential putrid disease. With other illnesses one had to hazard guesses about the putrid inner state of the body. In the case of scurvy, the classic symptoms – rotting, stinking gums, running sores, wounds that could not heal or that freshly opened again – seemed obviously to point to decay within. Lind, as we have seen, called into question the classical pedigree of contemporary understandings of 'putrid' fevers in his 1768 text on *Diseases Incidental to Europeans in Hot*

---

[129] As Erica Charters has noted, the circulation between metropole and imperial periphery began before the publication of Lind's and Pringle's works. Both men 'relied on the network of British military medicine in order to empirically inform their theories of disease and treatment. As a result, the first-hand experience of even lowly military surgeons was solicited and assiduously collected, meaning that military medical men in the colonies were considered experts, providing reliable observations and informed medical judgments'. Charters, 35.

Climates. In the third edition of his book on Scurvy, however, he would go much further.[130] In the book's *Postscript*, Lind asked a fundamental question about the blood taken from scorbutic patients: did this substance in fact tend to corruption more than the blood of those in health? 'This is the opinion of most authors', he noted, 'and what I had formerly adopted from them, as the foundation of my reasoning on the theory of this disease'.[131] Now, however, he was not so sure. Blood taken from many different patients suffering from the disease seemed to possess few common traits other than an insipidity to the taste. It corrupted no more quickly than the blood of the healthy and could induce corruption in other substances no more readily.[132] The rottenness of the gums and their smell, Lind argued, was not to be taken as a sign of internal putrefaction, but proceeded 'solely from the corrupt state of the gums. For in their dead bodies, I never perceived any unusual marks of putrefaction'. On the other hand, he acknowledged, other physicians had observed clear signs of putrefaction in the bowels of scorbutics after death and one could note the tenderness and laxity of the body's fibres in dissections, which might indicate that the body was 'inclined to corruption'. Certainly, too, the gums were putrid, as, oftentimes, were scorbutic ulcers.[133] The jury was out, but Lind was doubtful enough to suggest that the terminology being used was too vague to be of service and had, in fact, misled those who had followed the logics implied by it in recommending specific treatments:

The term *putrid*, respecting animal and vegetable substances, is not indeed, in my opinion, sufficiently defined and restricted, so as to serve as a solid basis or foundation for explaining the symptoms of the scurvy. The idea of the scurvy proceeding from animal putrefaction, may, and hath misled physicians to propose and administer medicines for it, altogether ineffectual.[134]

Lind was not alone in his apostasy. In the early 1770s, Francis Milman was on the cusp of an illustrious establishment career. In 1776 he received his M. D. from Oxford; two years later he was elected Fellow of the College of Surgeons in London. In 1806 he would become physician to the King. In 1772

---

[130] James Lind, *A Treatise on the Scurvy. In Three Parts. Containing an Inquiry into the Nature, Causes, and Cure, of That Disease. Together with a Critical and Chronological View of What Has Been Published on the Subject*, 3rd ed. (London: S. Crowder, D. Wilson and G. Nicholls, T. Cadell, T. Becket and Co. G. Pearch, and W. Woodfall, 1772). Carpenter, 69–74; Charters, 34.

[131] Lind, *A Treatise on the Scurvy. In Three Parts. Containing an Inquiry into the Nature, Causes, and Cure, of That Disease. Together with a Critical and Chronological View of What Has Been Published on the Subject*, 511.

[132] On this point, Lind deployed Pringle's methods, steeping thin slices of mutton in the blood's serum and comparing the rate of its decay to that of blood drawn from the healthy. Ibid., 513.

[133] Ibid., 513, 14.

[134] Ibid., 514–5. Cited in Charters, 34.

he published a curious account of two cases of scurvy, not at sea (where the cold, moist air or salted provisions might be invoked as contributing factors), but on land. The case involved two old women who had survived for months on bread and tea alone. 'They pleaded, that the small pittance, allowed them by the parish, would not enable them to procure any better nourishment, during the winter season'.[135] As explanation, Milman invoked a 'gradually accumulated putrefaction', brought on by lack of food.[136] A decade later, however, Milman exchanged the old orthodoxy for a newer one, marking the change explicitly. 'In a paper which I had many years since the honour of transmitting to the College', he wrote, 'I adopted Sir J. Pringle's idea of a gradually accumulated putrefaction; but a reference to those who have examined the actual state of the blood in the scurvy, has taught me the groundlessness of such a notion'. Drawing on Lind and others, Milman now lambasted those who argued that putrid diseases were caused by the putridity of the blood and mocked those who sought recourse in antiseptics. With so many having been discovered in recent years, 'It must surely strike every unprejudiced mind with surprize, that … the idea of a putrid disease should still be matter of so much alarm'.[137] Putridity, he argued, was not the cause of illness, but its effect. It was not that marsh miasma, for example, was not dangerous, or that exposure to noxious effluvia could not lead to a 'disposition to putridity'. It was rather that the direct impact of such effluvia was on the body's solids, not its fluids. Milman's was a nervous theory, which supposed that poison induced debility in the body's vital power.

I have no objection to suppose that these noxious contagious matters, which we will for the present call putrid matters, make their way into the circulation. But the question is, whether, having thus got admittance into the vital stream, they there act as ferments, and assimilate the blood to their own corrupt natures, or whether they produce their mischief by an action on the vital power, without affecting the sensible qualities of that fluid.[138]

Milman's answer – at least in 1782 – was clearly the second of the two options.

---

[135] Francis Milman, 'An Account of Two Instances of the True Scurvy, Seemingly Occasioned by the Want of Due Nourishment; Being an Extract of a Letter Addressed to Dr. Baker, by Francis Milman', *Medical Transactions, Published by the College of Physicians in London* 2 (1772): 476.

[136] Ibid., 477 Milman differed from standard accounts by arguing that the body required not antiseptic substances, but merely sufficient food. 'It is not then the antiseptic nature of the food taken in, which preserves our fluids from putrefaction, but the constant change of them, by which those parts, which are corrupting, and which, if retained would not fail to produce morbid effects, are expelled'. Ibid., 478, 79–80.

[137] *An Enquiry into the Source from Whence the Symptoms of the Scurvy and of Putrid Fevers Arise* (London: J. Dodsley, 1782), Note on 108, 211.

[138] Ibid., 134.

The critiques that both Lind and Milman levelled at putrefactive theories were not merely empirical, having to do with the question of whether the body and its fluids were really in a state of decay. They were also at once epistemological and ontological. Was dead flesh enough like the living body that experiments done on the former could reliably inform practice on the latter? I noted above that Hillary had little time for Pringle's assertion that alkaline substances could be used to treat putrefaction, whatever their abilities to retard the decay of beef may have been. And already, in the first edition of his text on his text on *Scurvy*, Lind offered similar objections to Pringle's method, although, like Hillary, he did not name his antagonist. Noting that salted and dried meat and fish did not putrefy in the air nearly as quickly as fresh flesh did, Lind suggested that one might conclude that salt meat was less likely to produce scorbutic putridity. Yet such a conclusion would be an obvious error:

This only proves how little we can learn of the effects of food and medicines in the body, by experiments made out of it. In a deep scurvy, there is the highest degree of putrefaction which a living animal can well subsist under: yet if we were so lucky as to find out the most powerful antiseptic in nature, it is not probable the scurvy could thereby be cured; although the body, after death, might be preserved by it as long as an *Aegyptian* mummy. On the contrary, the most putrid scurvies are daily cured by what quickly becomes putrescent out of the body, *viz.* broth made of coleworts and cabbage. However contradictory to some modern theories these facts may be, the truth of them is undeniable.[139]

There were clearly limits to the analogy between the dead and living body, however fruitful that analogy might be at times. Huxham was generally sympathetic to Pringle's approach, but he, too, observed that while volatile, alkaline salts might work to 'retard the Putrefaction of the Flesh of animals, and even in some Measure of the Blood, out of the Body ... yet mixed with the Blood, whilst actually under the Power of Circulation and the *Vis* Vitae, they certainly hasten its Dissolution, and consequent Putrefaction'.[140] Characteristically, Milman put the point even more bluntly: 'Many things', he wrote, 'which in the furnace or elaboratory of the chymist resist putrefaction powerfully, have no such action in the animal machine'.[141] He continued in a similarly vitalist vein a few pages later: 'The means of preserving dead substances from putrefaction, are no way applicable to the living moving fibre, a law peculiar to itself'.[142] In 1787, Benjamin Moseley denied that bile had any 'septical properties ... as

---

[139] Lind, *A Treatise of the Scurvy. In Three Parts. Containing an Inquiry into the Nature, Causes, and Cure of That Disease. Together with a Critical and Chronological View of What Has Been Published on the Subject*, note, 295–6.

[140] Huxham, *A Dissertation on the Malignant, Ulcerous Sore-Throat*, 54–5.

[141] Milman, *An Enquiry into the Source from Whence the Symptoms of the Scurvy and of Putrid Fevers Arise*, 225.

[142] Ibid., 228.

has been suggested from fallacious experiments, unconnected with life'.[143] By the 1770s, however, Pringle's theories were coming under fire even from those who agreed with his methods completely.

Problems in Pneumatic Medicine

Pringle was not, of course, alone in arguing for an analogy between what had happened in his experiments and what afflicted the body in sickness. Boerhaave's work provided a robust model for such studies, as had Robert Boyle's experiments on blood in the seventeenth century. Others quickly followed Pringle's lead, with some drawing upon the new pneumatic chemistry to do so. In 1754, Joseph Black had announced the discovery of a new kind of air, different from common atmospheric air. The air released when a given salt (magnesia alba) was heated or treated with acid had peculiar properties, being denser than common air, unable to support respiration or a flame, and turning lime water milky when bubbled through it. Black used the term 'fixed air', used by Hales to describe the air given off by various substances when they were decomposed by heat. In 1764, the surgeon David Macbride published a series of *Experimental Essays*, which he claimed to have designed as a sequel to the work of Hales, Black, and Pringle. In Macbride's account, dead bodies became putrid by losing fixed air. Replace the air artificially, and one could retard or even reverse putrefaction. In 1773, Pringle cited MacBride and others as the sources for Joseph Priestley's idea that water impregnated with antiseptic fixed air might work as a means for combating scurvy on long sea voyages.[144]

The next year, Priestley found himself defending Pringle's theories against a somewhat unlikely antagonist. In two books, one written in 1768, the other in 1771, the surgeon (and then doctor) William Alexander[145] proceeded to dismantle most of the central claims of the putrefactive paradigm, doing so by using Pringle's own tools.[146] In his first book, Alexander made it clear that

[143] Moseley, *A Treatise on Tropical Diseases; And on the Climate of the West-Indies*, 126.

[144] John Pringle, *A Discourse on the Different Kinds of Air, Delivered at the Anniversary Meeting of the Royal Society, November 30, 1773* (London: Royal Society, 1774), 15–16.

[145] Helping to make the point that putrid diseases were seen as afflictions more properly belonging to sites beyond the ken of the average metropolitan practitioner, Alexander noted that he had not personally encountered many cases of such distempers, though he had seen a number of putrid malignant fevers among French soldiers during the Seven Years War. William Alexander, *Experimental Essays on the Following Subjects: I. On the External Application of Antiseptics in Putrid Diseases. Ii. On the Doses and Effects of Medicines. Iii. On Diuretics and Sudorifics* (London: Edward and Charles Dilly, 1768), ii–iii, 6.

[146] In fact, Alexander made it a point to defend the use of experiments on dead flesh as a means of understanding the living body, while noting that 'it has been much litigated whether putrefaction be the same in the living and the dead animal'. It had been shown, he claimed, that a

he was in good company among those who found preposterous Boerhaave's suggestion – on the basis of his experiment on the dog in the sugar-baker's stove – that high heats alone could cause putrefaction within the living animal.[147] Putrid distempers required 'putrid particles' in the air, either due to 'putrid miasmata' or 'septic particles' flying from the breath of the diseased.[148] Alexander also advocated a change in treatment. Tests made on both dead rats and live patients made it clear that the best way to administer antiseptics was externally, by bathing or washing the patient in the substance. By this means, a much greater quantity of antiseptic could be introduced than would be possible were the treatment swallowed; the antiseptic would enter immediately into the blood, rather than travelling via the stomach; the stomach could not alter the substance by its action; and there was no danger of the patient's stomach rejecting (and ejecting) the cure.[149] The last point seemed to particularly recommend this method to the anonymous author of some *Practical Remarks on West India Diseases*. When vomiting was incessant in the yellow fever, the practitioner recommended a warm bath in which vinegar and nitre had been added, which by their 'antiseptic virtue' could resist the body's putrefaction.[150]

Alexander dedicated his second book to Pringle – as Priestley noted with some justifiable incredulity – even as it threatened Pringle's single most original argument: the claim that marsh miasmata caused putrid illnesses. Wherever else they may have disagreed, most previous medical writers (including Alexander only a few years earlier) seem to have found unproblematic the suggestion that effluvia arising from putrefying matter encouraged putrefaction in dead flesh. When he tested this supposition, however, Alexander found it wanting. Dangling pieces of meat above 'necessary houses' and swamps, he determined that such pieces lasted longer without putrefying than those kept in common air. Marshy vapours and the airs from human excrement (such

---

putrefying dead animal could communicate a putrid disease to a living one, which suggested that living and dead putrefaction were 'pretty nearly allied to each other'. This 'alliance' worked in both directions, since the breath of a diseased person could make meat rot faster than the breath of a healthy one. He also observed that the best modern physicians treated putrid disorders with substances proven to be antiseptic when applied to dead flesh. William Alexander, *An Experimental Enquiry Concerning the Causes Which Have Generally Been Said to Produce Putrid Diseases* (London: T. Becket and P. A. de Hondt, and T. Cadell, 1771), 47–8.

[147] Alexander cited a Dr Shebbeare who 'exclaims bitterly against Boerhaave, for inferring from an experiment he made, that a very great degree of heat is the cause of animal putrefaction', and noted that he had been told that a dissertation entitled *De Colore* had recently been published in Germany 'which asserts the same thing, and intirely overturns the Boerhaavian doctrine, of heat being the cause of putrefaction'. Alexander, 50–1.

[148] Ibid., 55–7.

[149] Ibid., 75.

[150] Anonymous, *Practical Remarks on West India Diseases*, 77.

as those in privies in camps) not only failed to encourage rot, they actively hindered it.[151]

The conclusion to be drawn from this experimental result seemed obvious and inescapable: however dangerous marshes might be, they could not be blamed for putrid diseases, for neither marsh water, nor the effluvia rising from it promoted putrefaction. Precisely the connection that Pringle had made central to the arguments of *Diseases of the Army* did not hold. Alexander went on, however, to make a second and even more radical claim. That he was aware of how radical it was may be seen from his hedging:

I do not mean here to plead the innocence of marsh miasmata, or to assume that marshes are salutary, because I have found the water of them to be antiseptic. I am not ignorant that almost all of the authors who have treated on this subject, and especially Lancisis, have agreed that it was hurtful, and adduced many instances of cities and armies having been attacked with putrid malignant diseases when exposed to it.[152]

Yet Alexander argued precisely not only that the noxious qualities of marshes might be 'a little doubtful', but that military observers may, in fact, have been systematically mistaken in associating swampy ground with illness. After all, it seemed likely that those in the army only paid attention to their marshy surroundings when sickness began to rage. Quizzed on the point, 'several military gentlemen' remembered that they had camped near putatively dangerous grounds with no ill effects, while suffering outbreaks of illnesses when nowhere near a marsh. In civilian life, it did not seem credible that boggy terrain proved uniquely deadly when those employed to drain such land did not seem adversely affected by their occupation. Perhaps, Alexander suggested, the problem was not putridity, but moisture alone. Humidity reduced perspiration, which could lead to many illnesses. Yet that explanation suggested that marsh water was no more dangerous than the water of the purest, clearest lake on a warm day. '[A]lmost all the authors who have treated on this subject' had indeed argued for the insalubrity of the putrid effluvia of marshes: Alexander was disagreeing with them all.[153]

In his 'Letter from the Rev. Dr. Priestley to Sir John Pringle', published in the *Philosophical* Transactions, Priestley could find little to dispute in Alexander's findings, but he firmly rejected the author's conclusions. 'I was particularly surprised, to meet with such an opinion as this', Priestley remarked to Pringle, making the stakes of the dispute clear, 'in a book inscribed to yourself, who have so clearly explained the great mischief of such a situation, in

---

[151] Alexander, 41.
[152] Ibid., 77–8.
[153] Ibid., 65, 80, 78.

your excellent treatise on the diseases of the army'.[154] Priestley offered his own explanation for the seemingly antiseptic properties of marsh air, relying on an unstated analogy with the role accorded common air in the phlogistic theory of combustion. Just as the flame of a candle burning under a glass would eventually die out because the phlogiston being released could no longer be absorbed by the saturated air, Priestley argued that putrid marsh air was already saturated, could absorb no more putrid effluvia from rotting substances, and hence worked to preserve them from further putrefactive processes. This did not mean, however, that such putrid effluvia were not enormously harmful when breathed into the lungs. That air remained 'very unfit for respiration'.[155]

Priestley portrayed Alexander as frankly irresponsible for suggesting that it might be safe to sleep, camp, or live near swampy terrain. He was not alone in this. In 1781, Thomas Dancer, who had served as physician for the expedition against Fort San Juan that had left Jamaica in 1780, made his objections clear. 'Alexander is of opinion', he declared, 'that marsh miasmata are not putrescent, but antiseptic; and he infers, therefore they are not hurtful: but the conclusion is both against reason and fact'.[156] Alexander Wilson, a physician trained by William Cullen, acknowledged in 1780 that it was hard to reconcile the antiseptic properties of marshes with 'their known effects in bringing on a putrescent tendency on living bodies', but proffered an explanation that echoed Priestley's nonetheless.[157] Marsh air, he argued, citing Priestley on the point, contained an 'overabundance' of phlogiston. In such air, lungs could not emit their own phlogiston-laden air, so that putrid diseases arose less because of what was taken *in* to the lungs and more because of what could not be expelled.

Although many of those with allegiances to Pringle and his ideas did not walk through it, Alexander's results opened a door towards the destruction of the putrefactive paradigm. Indeed, in saving Pringle's recommendations, Priestley had sacrificed the former's theoretical assumptions. In the seventh edition of *Diseases of the Army*, which appeared in 1775, even Pringle himself drew back from his earlier claims. He was careful, he noted, 'to avoid all denominations of fevers, communicating either no clear idea of their nature,

---

[154] J. Priestley, 'On the Noxious Quality of the Effluvia of Putrid Marshes. A Letter from the Rev. Dr. Priestley to Sir John Pringle', *Philosophical Transactions* 64 (1774): 91; Christopher Lawrence, 'Priestley in Tahiti: The Medical Interests of a Dissenting Chemist', in *Science, Medicine, and Dissent: Joseph Priestley*, ed. C. J. Lawrence and R. Anderson (London: Wellcome Trust/Science Museum, 1987).

[155] Priestley, 92.

[156] Thomas Dancer, *A Brief History of the Late Expedition against Fort San Juan, So Far as It Relates to the Diseases of the Troops; Together with Some Observations on Climate, Infection, and Contagion* (Kingston: D. Douglass & W. Aikman, 1781), 34.

[157] Alexander Wilson, *Some Observations Relative to the Influence of Climate on Vegetable and Animal Bodies* (London: T. Cadell, 1780), 154.

or a false one. The terms therefore of *nervous, bilious, putrid,* and *malignant,* applied so commonly to fevers, will either not occur at all, or be so defined as to occasion no ambiguity'.[158] To say that the air that arose from stagnant ponds was dangerous was not to say that it induced putrid diseases. And both Priestley and Wilson's explanations rested – either implicitly or explicitly – on a denial of the similarity between results on the living human body and those found in the laboratory based on dead flesh. More hostile readers, like Milman, cited Alexander's work with more enthusiasm, invoking it to critique the value of antiseptic treatments. Clearly, without following Alexander fully, one could hold on to a view that held marsh miasmas to be potentially deadly – a position that could not be countered with impunity – while rejecting the underlying logic of putrefactive explanations. External putridity did not lead directly to internal rot.

A New Paradigm

Of course, paradigms do not fall merely because they are criticised. One needs an alternative mode of explanation. Such alternatives were, particularly in the 1780s, both many and various. For some, a resource was the work of William Cullen, the Edinburgh professor who was, for the second half of the eighteenth century what Boerhaave had been for the first.[159] Indeed, one may note that most of the main proponents of the putrefactive paradigm (such as Huxham, Hillary and Pringle himself) were all students of Boerhaave's, Pringle being among the last to work with the Leiden professor.[160] A number of those most critical of the paradigm tended to be students of Cullen, who so denied the utility of the category of 'putrid fever', that he did not include it in his nosology.[161] He noted that both ancients and moderns ('who are in general much disposed to follow the former') had distinguished between putrid and non-putrid fevers,

---

[158] John Pringle, *Observations on the Diseases of the Army,* 7th ed. (London: W. Strahan, J. and F. Rivington, W. Johnston, T. Payne, T. Longman, Wilson and Nicoll, T. Durham, and T. Cadell, 1775), xv.

[159] For brief and elegant summaries of Cullen's ideas, see Lester S. King, *The Medical World of the Eighteenth Century* (Chicago: University of Chicago Press, 1958), 139–43; W. F. Bynum, 'Cullen and the Study of Fevers in Britain, 1760–1820', *Medical History (Supplement)* 1 (1981). See also A. Doig et al., eds., *William Cullen and the Eighteenth Century Medical World: A Bicentenary Exhibition and Symposium Arranged by the Royal College of Physicians of Edinburgh in 1990* (Edinburgh: Edinburgh University Press, 1993).

[160] Huxham began his medical degree at Leiden under Boerhaave in 1715. Due to financial reasons, he was forced to complete the degree at Rheims. R. M. McConaghey, 'John Huxham', *Medical History* 13, no. 3 (1969): 280.

[161] Dale C. Smith, 'Medical Science, Medical Practice, and the Emerging Concept of Typhus in Mid-Eighteenth-Century Britain', *Medical History (Supplement)* 1 (1981): 132.

but Cullen could not see the utility of the distinction.[162] It was not, he made clear, that he denied that putrescency was possible. In the 1784 edition of his *First Lines of the Practice of Physic* (but not in the first, 1777 edition) he alluded to the debates discussed above. 'I have no doubt', he wrote, 'how much soever it has been disputed by some ingenious men, that a putrescency of the fluids, to a certain degree, does really take place in many cases of fever'.[163] The problem, however, was that such putrescency attended many different kinds of fevers, and to varying different degrees. Putrefaction might be present, but it was not characteristic and hence was not usefully diagnostic. Putrescency was an effect and not a cause of fever, he argued (presumably this was the source of Milman's similar claims). Hence, the expulsion of putrid fluids could not effect a cure.

Where putrefaction retained an important role in Cullen's work was in his discussion of the remote causes of epidemic fevers. These Cullen limited to two: contagions and miasmata.[164] Contagions were effluvia deriving from the bodies of people in illness; miasmata derived from non-human substances. Each had similar causes and effects: 'They arise from a putrescent matter; their production is favoured, and their power increased, by circumstances which favour putrefaction, and they often prove putrefactive ferments with respect to the animal fluids'.[165] They caused fevers, however, not by the induction of putrefaction, but by the fact that putrid matter was a powerful sedative. In Cullen's scheme, this sedative power, when applied to the nervous system, diminished the brain's energy and induced debility. The body then reacted in such a way as to obviate these negative effects, entering a cold state as a means of stimulating the increased action of the heart and larger arteries (experienced as a fever), which would in turn raise the energy levels of the brain. Fevers, then, 'do not arise from changes in the state of the fluids', but rather 'chiefly depend upon changes in the state of the moving powers of the animal'.[166] Internal putridity

---

[162] William Cullen, 'First Lines of the Practice of Physic (1784)', in *The Works of William Cullen*, ed. John Thomson (Edinburgh and London: William Blackwood; T. & G. Underwood, 1827), 526.

[163] Ibid. Compare *First Lines of the Practice of Physic. For the Use of Students in the University of Edinburgh*, vol. 1 (London and Edinburgh: J. Murray; William Creech, 1777), 63. The mid-1780s seems to have been the high point for this debate. Another author noted in 1785 that '[t]he influence of putrid effluvia on the human system, has of late been the subject of much controversy'. M. de Lassone, 'Histoire de divers Accidens graves, occasionnés par les miasmes d'animaux en putrefaction, et de la nouvelle methode de traitment qui a été employé avec succés dans cette circonstance', *Medical Commentaries* 9 (1785).

[164] In discussing marsh effluvia or miasmata, Cullen drew heavily on 'Dr Lind's ingenious work on the preservation of health of Europeans in warm climates'. Cullen, 'First Lines of the Practice of Physic (1784)', 506. The quoted lines are from Cullen's notes on the manuscript for his text, added by Thomson.

[165] Ibid., 546.

[166] Ibid., 506.

might accompany a fever, but the seat of the illness was in the nervous system, not in the blood or bile.

One finds a related, although not identical, argument in the work of Benjamin Moseley, who studied medicine in London, Paris, and Leiden before establishing a practice in Jamaica in 1768. There he was appointed surgeon-general, returning to England after roughly a dozen years. He received his M. D. in 1784 and in 1787 published *A Treatise on Tropical Diseases; And on the Climate of the West-Indies*, a work that was the first to use the term 'tropical diseases' and that self-consciously set itself the task of supplanting Towne's and Hillary's works as the standard references on the illnesses of the West Indies. 'Worthy of imitation as the laudable efforts of Towne, and respectable as Hillary's accuracy is describing what he had actually seen, were, much improvement in the treatment of diseases has since their time taken place in that part of the world'.[167] There was no more reason, Moseley added, 'why all progress should stop with Towne and Hillary, than that it should have ceased with Hippocrates'.[168] The *Treatise* largely succeeded in its aims. A second edition appeared in 1789 under a slightly altered title, a German translation in 1790, and a fourth edition in 1803. One finds it cited throughout the literature on the diseases of warm climates at the end of the eighteenth and the beginning of the nineteenth centuries.

Hillary had declared the yellow fever to be a putrid distemper. Moseley rejected the general applicability of the category to the diseases of the West Indies.

Much has been said by writers concerning putrid fevers, and the tendency of all fevers to putrefaction, in hot climates. But such opinions are not founded on practice, however much they may seem to agree with theory. The great endemic there is the *Nervous Remittent Fever*, which is unattended with any putrid symptoms, and which has its seat in the nervous system; or, as I have often thought, in the brain itself.[169]

He was particularly scathing about those who took the antiseptic properties of wine, punch, and spirits as an excuse for revelry, arguing that this faulty prophylactic practice had resulted in the 'death of thousands'.[170] As can be

---

[167] Moseley, *A Treatise on Tropical Diseases; And on the Climate of the West-Indies*, 382.

[168] Ibid., 383.

[169] Ibid. That said, elsewhere Moseley seemed to use the term unproblematically, suggesting that it was perhaps the totalising element of putrefactive explanations to which he was opposed, rather than their specific deployment: 'Stagnant waters and swamps load the air with pernicious vapours, that are productive of obstinate intermittent fevers, diseases of the liver, and putrid diseases'. Or, later in the text, where he accepted Pringle's terminology as well: 'Dysenteries, as well as other disorders, in hot climates, in Autumn, have more of the putrid, than of the inflammatory diathesis' Ibid., 36, 196.

[170] Ibid., 48.

seen, Moseley subscribed to something like Cullen's nervous theory of disease, although he regarded tropical heat as the cause of the body's debility, rather than miasmatic effluvia. Indeed, in Moseley's explanation, marshes were not at fault at all in producing the characteristic diseases of the climate. Nor was heat alone a problem. Moseley followed a long tradition in noting that he had experienced equally warm temperatures in Europe (in Naples, Rome and Montpellier).[171] As long as heat and humidity promoted perspiration, in fact, climatic conditions carried their own remedy with them. 'The mischief they produce is, that they dispose the body to the slightest impressions from cold', for even a slight change in the temperature was experienced as considerable by the debilitated tropical body. Drawing on a sub-element in Cullen's theorising, Moseley declared that it was this experience of sudden cooling that inspired the onset of fever.[172] '[H]owever paradoxical it may appear', he wrote, 'cold is the cause of almost all the diseases in hot climates, to which climate alone is accessory'.[173]

John Hunter was just as critical of putrefactive theories as Moseley, but he found less inspiration in Cullen, despite having been a student at Edinburgh from 1770 to 1775. After completing his thesis, Hunter was admitted as a licentiate to the Royal College of Physicians in 1777 and was then appointed physician to the army.[174] He served as Superintendent of the military hospitals in Jamaica from the beginning of 1781 to May 1783, after which he returned to London and began private practice. His *Observations on the Diseases of the Army in Jamaica* appeared in 1788.[175] Like Moseley's, Hunter's text became a standard reference for medical men in the West Indies and throughout the Tropics. Among its most oft-cited sections was that which supplied a long disquisition on Jamaica's remitting fevers, of which the most severe was probably the disease known as the yellow fever or black vomit. Previous authors, Hunter noted in a very fine summary of the logics of the putrefactive paradigm, had

---

[171] Ibid., 41–2.

[172] Although Cullen regarded human and marsh effluvia as the main cause of fevers, he also looked at other causes, cold included. In doing so, he stressed the historicity, so to speak, of the bodily experience of temperature, just as Moseley would: 'The *relative* power of cold with respect to the living human body, is that power by which it produces a sensation of cold in it; and with respect to this, it is agreeable to the general principle of sensation, that the sensation produced is not in proportion to the absolute force of impression, but according as the new impression is stronger or weaker than that which had been applied immediately before'. Cullen, 'First Lines of the Practice of Physic (1784)', 547.

[173] Moseley, *A Treatise on Tropical Diseases; And on the Climate of the West-Indies*, 47.

[174] It may well be this thesis – an early contribution to race-science – that remains Hunter's most famous work today. John Hunter, *Disputatio Inauguralis, Quaedam De Hominum Varietatibus, Et Harum Causis, Exponens* (Edinburgh: Balfour and Smellie, 1775).

[175] Hunter, *Observations on the Diseases of the Army in Jamaica; and on the Best Means of Preserving the Health of Europeans, in That Climate.*

laid blame for the distemper at the feet of a corrupted bile or a putrid state of the blood.

Next to the opinion that the fever proceeds from bile, none is more prevalent than that it is of a putrid nature; and that the whole mass of humours are running violently into putrefaction. If it be asked what is meant by the term *putrefaction*, it will doubtless be answered, that species of fermentation or change, which dead animal matter in a certain degree of heat and moisture, joined to an admission of air, spontaneously undergoes. That such is the acceptation of the term cannot be doubted, when it is observed that in reasoning on this subject, whatever is found to check putrefaction out of the body, is supposed to have the same effect taken internally, and is therefore recommended in diseases believed to be putrid; and whatever promotes putrefaction out of the body, is supposed to be noxious, and is therefore avoided.[176]

Hunter, however, found little to support in this account. It was true, he acknowledged, that putrefaction led to the dissolution of flesh and fluids and was often accompanied by a noxious smell and that, in fevers, the blood was sometimes found to be in a dissolved state and the patient's body emitted an 'extremely disagreeable' odour.[177] But there the similarity ended. In dead bodies the skin turned a greenish colour: no such change was observed in the living. The phenomena might be saved by arguing that putrefaction proceeded differently in the living and the dead, but then one could no longer make inferences (as Pringle had) from one to the other. In any case, Hunter argued, 'the opinion of the putrid nature of the disease is founded on a vague analogy, which will not stand the test of experiment, or observation'.[178] The dissolution of the blood was often observed in scorbutic cases, but (here he cited Lind) such blood did not putrefy any faster than the blood of anyone else. 'If the dissolved state of the blood in scurvy do not depend on putrefaction', he stated, making clear the once-paradigmatic stature of scurvy as a putrid disease, 'there is little reason to suppose, that in fevers it is owing to that cause'.[179]

What, then, was the cause? Hunter rejected several of Cullen's arguments, seeing no evidence that the fever arose as a reaction to a 'cold fit' and denying that symptoms all flowed from an 'affection of the brain and nervous system'.[180] He did, however, cite Cullen in support of the notion that marshy effluvia produced the illness by acting as a poison on the human frame, and Priestley for the fact that part of the air breathed in by the lungs made its way to the blood and hence might carry the poison with it.[181] Precisely how

176   Ibid., 172–3.
177   Ibid., 173.
178   Ibid., 175.
179   Ibid., 175–6.
180   Ibid., 179, 82–3.
181   Ibid., 184, 85.

such a poison produced a fever, Hunter professed not to know: 'Our ignorance of the animal economy absolutely precludes us, from giving any adequate answer to this question'. The operation of other poisons on the body provided an analogy, however. The symptoms of poisoning could be much like those of a febrile disease: vomiting, convulsions, a dissolution of the blood (in the case of the viper's bite), jaundice, weakness, fainting, and even death. Yet, however apt the analogy might be, it could only be of limited utility: no one properly understood how any other poisons, even the most common, actually worked. At the beginning of the eighteenth century, Mead had drawn on iatrochemical theories of ferments to explain the action of poisons and had then transferred that explanation to his theory of the plague. Almost at the end of the century, in an ironic twist, Hunter turned to more recent work on poisons, but eschewed any explanations for their action, seeming similarly agnostic about the cause of what had once been known as putrid fevers. Common ground, of course, remained across the paradigmatic divide, but it was marshy, perilous, and to be avoided as much as possible.

Conclusion

For Creighton, Britain's 'putrid constitution' ended around 1765, at roughly the time that the industrial revolution can be said to have begun. Christopher Hamlin has suggested that putrid theories reigned until the mid-1770s, at which point nervous theories of fever began to supplant them.[182] Looking at the colonies, Harrison has argued that it is from the 1790s that one begins to see the emergence of a new orthodoxy about the diseases of warm climates, one rooted in Cullenian notions of nervous debility.[183] Certainly one sees Cullen's mark very clearly in the work of William Lempriere, although even here the differences from Cullen's schema are as striking as the similarities. Lempriere served as 'Apothecary to his Majesty's Forces' and published his *Practical Observations on the Diseases of the Army in Jamaica* in 1799, there laying out a step-wise process by which the newly arrived to a warm climate could be afflicted by a 'tropical continued fever'. Those coming from cold climates arrived with tense fibres and a plethoric habit, but their bodies soon began to undergo a relaxation, with the energy of nervous systems declining somewhat. Initially, this loss of energy was counterbalanced by the stimulus provided by the high environmental heat, so that the blood tended to circulate with its usual force. Were this state now changed by the dimunition of the capacity

[182] Hamlin, 'What Is Putrid About Putrid Fever?'.
[183] Harrison, *Medicine in an Age of Commerce and Empire: Britain and its Tropical Colonies, 1660–1830*, 85.

of the voluntary muscles (due to fatigue, excessive heat, or intemperance, for example), the action of the involuntary muscles would increase to make up the balance. Blood would then be forced from the arteries into the veins, with a 'plethoric state of the venous system' as a necessary result. 'Look at the newly-arrived European after common exercise', Lempriere suggested, 'and see how his countenance is flushed, mark the turgescence of his veins, and take the whole of his countenance into your consideration, and you will find it to denote a very unequal circulation. Observe with what facility the robust and the athletic are fatigued, it will prove to you in what degree the voluntary nervous energy is impaired'.[184] And it was now, while a considerable venous plethora existed, that marsh miasmas had their most dire effect on the body, acting as a 'poison, or stimulus, or spasm-forming cause',[185] producing an even greater plethora in the veins and – even worse – congestions within the liver and the brain, where pressure could build to the point of fatality. Marsh miasmata is dangerous here, as in Cullen's *First Lines*, but the effluvia would appear to be a stimulant, rather than a sedative. And it is the heat of the climate that induces a nervous debility in the bodies described by Lempriere, not the poison of putre-factive matter.

For others writing in the 1790s, it seems harder to locate an end of the putre-factive paradigm. In 1793, Thomas Dickson Reide was still dividing fevers into three types: inflammatory, putrid, and those that were both.[186] In offering *Medical Advice to the Inhabitants of Warm Climates*, Robert Thomas seems simply to have ignored the notion that nervous and putrefactive theories might be opposed to one another, discussing nervous fevers and putrid fevers in succession.[187] John Bell denied that the climate – whether it acted on the nerves or the fluids – was much to blame for the suffering of soldiers: the real problem was the soldiers themselves and their near-constant intemperance.[188] It may not be wrong, however, to regard cases like these as hold-outs, for the trend would seem to be clear. Apart from anything else, one might compare the social status

---

[184] William Lempriere, *Practical Observations on the Diseases of the Army in Jamaica, as They Occurred between the Years 1792 and 1797*, 2 vols. (London: T. N. Longham and O. Rees, 1799), 95.

[185] Ibid., 97.

[186] Thomas Dickson Reide, *A View of the Diseases of the Army in Great Britain, America, the West Indies, and on Board of King's Ships and Transports, from the Beginning of the Late War to the Present Time* (London: J. Johnson, 1793), 39.

[187] Robert Thomas, *Medical Advice to the Inhabitants of Warm Climates, on the Domestic Treatment of All the Diseases Incidental Therein: With a Few Useful Hints to New Settlers, for the Preservation of Health, and the Prevention of Sickness* (London: J. Strahan and W. Richardson, 1790).

[188] John Bell, *An Inquiry into the Causes Which Produce, and the Means of Preventing Diseases among British Officers, Soldiers, and Others in the West Indies* (London: J. Murray, 1791).

of critics of the putrefactive paradigm in the late 1780s and 1790s with those who still made use of it. Hunter, Moseley, and Lempriere all held fairly prestigious positions within the British armed forces, while Reide, Thomas, and Bell did not.

As it held sway for roughly four decades after mid-century, the effect of the putrefactive paradigm in shaping attitudes towards the diseases of warm climates was profound. This was not, I think – although the connection seems tempting – because the paradigm aided in making the diseases of the tropics seem distinctive, the heat and humidity of the region encouraging the kinds of rot upon which the theories of putridity were built. For, in many ways, the putrefactive paradigm made it obvious that putrid diseases were not merely products of warm weather. Scurvy, which became the emblematic putrid disease after Lind's work, had long been associated with cold European winters. The putrefactive paradigm, in fact, paired the characteristic diseases of warm climates with the most distinctive disease of shipboard life, suggesting that we might best see the entire theoretical schema as one that encompassed the British Empire outside the metropole: the colonies it held and the fleets that allowed it to rule the waves. The putrefactive paradigm was imperial medicine.

We should also not ignore the significance of the paradigm within the medicine of the British Isles. What Boerhaave's *Aphorisms* had been for almost four decades after their first publication in 1709, and what Cullen's *First Lines of the Practice of Physic* was for several decades after 1777, Pringle's *Observations of the Diseases of the Army* was for the intervening period: a common and standard reference for medical men both civilian and military, both in Britain and throughout the empire. And in dividing fevers into two kinds, the inflammatory and the putrid, the first associated with the diseases of Pringle's home and the second with armies in camp and with warm climates, Pringle made a rather remarkable point. To understand fevers in general, one needed to understand them as they appeared throughout the Empire. It became the physician who wished to master his craft to understand not merely the afflictions of London, but also those of army, navy, and colonial life. There was what we might call an openness to empire about Pringle's vision, one that recalls Lind's archipelagic imaginary of the last chapter and seems characteristic of the period immediately after the victories of the Seven Years War.

That said, the putrefactive paradigm would indeed be partially responsible for later constructions of the diseases of warm climates as distinctive and requiring not a broad and imperial medicine, but one that could grapple with the specific pathologies of the tropics. For, precisely by associating putridity not solely with climate but with locations (jails, hospitals, ships, and warm countries),

Pringle weakened the analogy that had shaped earlier understandings of the illnesses of India, Africa, and the Americas. No longer could one simply associate the diseases of Britain's summer with those of warm climates, for they might as easily come in the cold and damp (as with scurvy) or at any season (as with jail and hospital fevers). The diseases of warm climates may have been seen by practitioners in the tropics as near-universally putrid, but all putrid diseases were not those of warm climates.

The climate/season analogy had, for a long time, worked against the idea that there was something truly distinctive about the diseases of warm countries. In troubling it, the putrefactive paradigm offered in its stead an even larger similitude, one that saw the empire as a whole as the space for British medicine. With the replacement of putrefactive theories by those that located the seat of disease in the nerves, authors like Moseley articulated a different vision of empire, one that saw the colonies as strikingly distinct from – and decidedly subordinate to – the metropole. Colley has noted the irony in conceptions of empire in the second half of the eighteenth century. The victories of the Seven Years War induced a kind of collective angst and thoughtful reflections about the relationship between the British Isles and the large swathe of the Earth that they now commanded. After the loss of the American colonies, however, one finds a counter-intuitive confidence about the imperial mission. 'Instead of being sated with conquests, alarmed at their own presumptuous grandeur as they had been after 1763, the British could now unite in feeling hard done by. Their backs were once more well and truly to the wall, filling many of them with grim relish and renewed strength'.[189] Where 'some leading Britons', she notes, 'had been embarrassed by the weight of empire, even questioning its morality', by the 1780s such scruples had evaporated and London passed a series of reforms (the India Act in 1784, the Canada Act in 1791) aimed at strengthening control of its remaining holdings.[190] In medicine, one finds a similar transition. In the work of Pringle and Lind there is a sense, medically speaking, that we are all in this together. From the 1780s, the colonies increasingly became portrayed as dangerous foreign zones, to be mastered, rather than incorporated. The introduction to Moseley's text addressed the book to those 'impelled by necessity, or induced by interest, to visit the torrid zone' thereby leaving behind 'the delightful climates of the earth … for such as no care, or art, can ever make agreeable'.[191] Later, he simple declared England's climate to be 'the best on the habitable globe – For by what comparison is a climate to be estimated, which produces such a race of people as the English, and in

---

[189] Colley, *Britons: Forging the Nation, 1707–1837*, 146.
[190] Ibid., 147.
[191] Moseley, *A Treatise on Tropical Diseases; And on the Climate of the West-Indies*, 1–2.

which almost every species of animal arrives to their utmost perfection?'.[192] If others were less jingoistic, by 1800 they nonetheless portrayed the relationship between Britain and its tropical holdings as an oppositional one.[193] Among the categories that helped frame this opposition was race and it is to this different kind of difference as formulated in medical discourse that we now turn.

[192] Ibid., 44–5.
[193] Harrison, ' "The Tender Frame of Man": Disease, Climate and Racial Difference in India and the West Indies, 1760–1860'.

Part III

Race

5   Race-Medicine in the Colonies, 1679–1750

Introduction

In 1735, the former naval surgeon John Atkins penned what must be considered one of the more striking understatements of his age. In *A Voyage to Guinea, Brasil, and the West-Indies*, he described the differences between the physical appearance of the inhabitants of Guinea and that of 'the rest of Mankind'. These differences were so profound, he claimed, that 'tho' it be a little Heterodox, I am persuaded the black and white Race have, *ab origine*, sprung from different-coloured first parents'.[1] To suggest that Adam was not the original father of all humankind was, of course, considerably more than a little heterodox. This position, known as polygenism, was very uncommon in the eighteenth century. Yet Atkins was unusual even in his polygenism, for – unlike most polygenists of whom I am aware prior to the middle of the century – he spent very little time in relating his heterodoxy to Biblical views and he proffered his most detailed remarks within a medical text, as opposed to one concerned with theology, natural philosophy, or history.

The fact that Atkins espoused polygenism in the same volume in which he described diseases peculiar to native Africans led one of the few scholars to have considered his texts in any detail to suggest that one might therein find 'connections between concepts of race and concepts of disease'.[2] That Atkins gave up on his polygenism in a later edition of his best known work without significantly changing his etiological understanding leads me to the opposite conclusion. By the 1730s, I suggest, environmentalist understandings of human physical difference were beginning to change. Environmentalist

---

[1] John Atkins, *A Voyage to Guinea, Brasil, and the West-Indies; in His Majesty's Ships, the Swallow and Weymouth* (London: Caesar Ward and Richard Chandler, 1735), 39.

[2] Norris Saakwa-Mante, 'Western Medicine and Racial Constitutions: Surgeon John Atkins Theory of Polygenism and Sleepy Distemper in the 1730s', in *Race, Science, and Medicine, 1700–1960*, eds. Waltraud Ernst and Bernard Harris (London and New York: Routledge, 1999), 34. See also Curtin, *The Image of Africa: British Ideas and Action, 1780–1850*, 41, 83; Jennifer L. Morgan, '"Some Could Suckle over Their Shoulder": Male Travelers, Female Bodies, and the Gendering of Racial Ideology, 1500–1770', *The William and Mary Quarterly* 54 (1997).

understandings of disease, however, particularly with regard to the diseases of warm climates, were not. Atkins provides us with a fine example of a trend that would continue for the majority of the century: the widening gap between 'race-science' with its anatomical focus and what I am here terming 'race-medicine', with its emphasis on racial physiology and pathology.

This chapter and Chapter 7, divided chronologically, are dedicated to a history of race-medicine across the eighteenth century. Section 5.1 in this chapter provides an overview of the main arguments concerning the origins of racial difference from the discovery of the New World to the mid-1700s. Section 5.2 draws on literature that has insisted on reading discourses concerning race together with those concerning gender and sexuality, offering an analysis of the relationships connecting women's diseases, climate, race, and locality. Section 5.3 concentrates on the role played (or not) by racial thinking in medical texts from the late seventeenth century to roughly 1750. Section 5.4 is then dedicated to a close reading of Atkins' several publications from 1729 to 1742, situating his claims in the intellectual contexts previously described. As we shall see, Atkins may best be understood as being pulled in two opposite directions, as the doors to an increasingly anti-climatic racial thinking began to open, while the medicine of warm climates became increasingly Hippocratic and environmentalist.[3]

Before proceeding, however, some comments about terminology. Race-medicine is a neologism: like 'race-science', the term after which it is modelled, it was not an actors' category.[4] One does not find those who called themselves 'race-physicians' or 'race-surgeons', any more than one found, in the nineteenth century, scientists who called themselves 'race-biologists'. Both terms are, moreover, particularly fraught when applied to the eighteenth century, when the word race was only beginning to acquire the meanings we associate with it today. Indeed, those who study race have tended to divide themselves, according to the question of whether it is legitimate to use the term prior to (roughly) 1750 or not. Those who offer an expansivist definition note that observations concerning traits we now regard as quintessentially racialised (skin colour, for example, or hair type) have been made in almost every culture through history, and that one can find xenophobic remarks made against outsiders, who were at least partly distinguished by appearance, in works from the classical age onwards.[5] Those who offer a more restrictive

---

[3] On growing critiques of the climate theory in Britain in the seventeenth century, see Malcolmson.

[4] Stepan.

[5] See, for example, Thomas Gossett, *Race: The History of an Idea in America* (Oxford: Oxford University Press, 1997). The first edition of the text appeared in 1963. Gossett acknowledged that one finds very few examples of statements about the importance of racial differences before the eighteenth century. Nonetheless, he argued that one can find 'racism' and 'race-prejudice' in cultures at least 5,000 years old. Ibid., 3–4. As his title suggest, Benjamin Isaac finds the

reading argue, by contrast, that observations about physical difference carried little weight compared to observations about social or cultural differences. Physical differences made little difference. The real issue was whether one spoke Greek, for example, or (later) whether one was a Christian or pagan, not skin colour or the presence or absence of facial hair. Nancy Stepan, who coined the term, restricted her study of 'race-science' to the years from 1800–1960, a period in which, as Hannah Augstein has lucidly noted, one may identify three rather novel and agreed upon tenets undergirding the science of race: first, that mankind could be divided into 'races', the characteristics of which were fixed (or essentially fixed);[6] second, that all human races did not possess the same intellectual and moral qualities; and third, that intellect and character were determined (at least in large part) by physical characteristics – a position we can term racial determinism.[7] Clearly, nineteenth-century race theory did not closely resemble earlier claims about race, so that the debate over when a historian might begin a history of race comes to resemble that over the history of sexuality. One might identify forms of behaviour that we would regard as 'homosexual' in the classical era (just as we may identify statements that sound 'racist'), but these behaviours (and these statements) did not carry the meanings that we associate with them today. In particular, before a period we might roughly call the 'modern' age, neither sexuality nor race was seen as an essential category.[8]

---

case that racism has always existed less compelling, but locates its origin in the classical age. Benjamin H. Isaac, *The Invention of Racism in Classical Antiquity* (Princeton: Princeton University Press, 2004). One finds the middle ages posited as the origin for the concept in several of the essays in Miriam Eliav-Feldon, Benjamin H. Isaac, and Joseph Ziegler, eds., *The Origin of Racism in the West* (Cambridge: Cambridge University Press, 2009). Francisco Bethencourt, *Racisms: From the Crusades to the Twentieth Century* (Princeton: Princeton University Press, 2013). George Mosse is perhaps the most famous proponent of the view that, as he phrased it: 'Eighteenth-century Europe was the cradle of modern racism'. George L. Mosse, *Toward the Final Solution: A History of European Racism* (New York: H. Fertig, 1978). For a good overview of the literature that has seen racism as part of the 'dark side of the Enlightenment', see Colin Kidd, *The Forging of Races: Race and Scripture in the Protestant Atlantic World, 1600–2000* (Cambridge: Cambridge University Press, 2006), 79–120. See also Justin E. H. Smith, *Nature, Human Nature, and Human Difference: Race in Early Modern Philosophy* (Princeton: Princeton University Press, 2015).

6 Nicholas Hudson makes an important addition to this criterion, by noting that the number of races in the late eighteenth and early nineteenth century are small, with concomitant populations within them then very large. Where once observers noted considerable differences between the inhabitants of a given region (such as the Americas), such differences were subordinated to a larger similitude imposed by the logic of race. Hudson.

7 Stepan; Hannah Franziska Augstein, *Race: The Origins of an Idea, 1760–1850* (Bristol: Thoemmes Press, 1996), x.

8 Michel Foucault, *The History of Sexuality*, 3 vols., vol. I (London: Allen Lane, 1978). Arnold I. Davidson, *The Emergence of Sexuality: Historical Epistemology and the Formation of Concepts* (Cambridge, MA: Harvard University Press, 2001). One of the central loci for this debate concerned the so-called 'Boswell thesis' about attitudes toward homosexuality in early Christianity. John Boswell, *Christianity, Social Tolerance, and Homosexuality: Gay*

My sympathies tend to lie with those offering more restrictive understandings of the terms involved, but there is no need to take understandings of race in the period in which race science became 'normal science' as entirely definitional of the concept. For the eighteenth century, I would suggest, the question should be rather broader: when did race become understood not as an effect, but as itself a cause?[9] A comparison between classical and nineteenth-century examples should make the distinction clear. In Hippocratic thought, physical differences were caused by climate and diet – by the 'Airs, Waters, and Places' in which people lived. Also produced by such environmental causes were forms of government, styles of behaviour, and systems of culture. 'Race' in other words did not cause differences in intellect or morality; it was itself an effect of environmental differences. In the nineteenth century, however, race became, as Robert Knox would infamously phrase it, 'destiny'.[10] Physical differences – understood racially – were taken to be the *cause* of mental differences. Africans had smaller brains, it was argued, and hence lower intellects.[11]

In attempting to identify when race moved from effect to cause, one should note that the debate between polygenists and monogenists may at times be something of a red herring. Darwinian monogenists happily used race as a causal mechanism and polygenism did not necessarily accord physical difference an explanatory role. As we shall see, some adopted the doctrine of special creations as a way of dealing with theological concerns that had little to do with questions of racialised difference, while other early polygenists took such differences as *explanandum*, without then turning to the question of whether they could then be used as *explanans*. It should also be noted that causal explanations in medicine differed from those in natural history or natural philosophy, not least because the questions being asked were different. Thus, while it might be suggested that race science was already, in many ways, race-medicine, since so many of those who have been identified as early prominent race-scientists were trained in medicine, anatomy, or surgery, my target here is rather different. The question is simple: when does one begin to find arguments that related racialised physical differences to the presence (or inclination) to

People in Western Europe from the Beginning of the Christian Era to the Fourteenth Century (Chicago: University of Chicago Press, 1980). For contemporary re-examinations, see Mathew Kuefler, ed. *The Boswell Thesis: Essays on Christianity, Social Tolerance, and Homosexuality* (Chicago: University of Chicago Press, 2006).

[9] I am using the word 'cause' here in its contemporary sense. For excellent discussions of causes in eighteenth-century medicine, see Christopher Hamlin, 'Predisposing Causes and Public Health in Early Nineteenth-Century Medical Thought', *Social History of Medicine* 5 (1992). Margaret DeLacy, 'The Conceptualization of Influenza in Eighteenth-Century Britain: Specificity and Contagion', *Bulletin of the History of Medicine* 67 (1993); 'Nosology, Mortality, and Disease Theory in the Eighteenth Century', *Journal of the History of Medicine* 54 (1999).

[10] Robert Knox, *The Races of Men: A Fragment* (London: H. Renshaw, 1850).

[11] See, e.g. Stephen Jay Gould, *The Mismeasure of Man* (New York: Norton, 1981).

particular diseases in ways that saw them not as sharing a common cause (the environment, for example), but rather in ways that saw race as the *cause* of the affliction? The answer, at least in this chapter, is also fairly simple: with some few possible exceptions, not until at least after the mid-eighteenth century, even as race began to acquire a (limited) causal role in other realms.

Having laid out my question and hinted at my answer, let me lay out what I see as the stakes behind this study. My intention is to offer a contribution towards and correction of much of the work done on the intellectual history of naturalistic understandings of race.[12] The seminal work on the subject was Stepan's *The Idea of Race in Science: Great Britain, 1800–1960*. In retrospect, it seems easy to situate it at the centre of two complementary trends in early science studies. One sought to demonstrate the social, cultural, and political roots of seemingly 'objective' ideas in contemporary science. This brings to mind a number of studies of Darwinian thought, the Forman thesis, and an array of works within feminist history and philosophy of science. The other trend sought to problematise demarcation criteria, pointing out the difficulties in differentiating, methodologically, between 'good' science and so-called pseudo-science. This was the province of some early work in the sociology of scientific knowledge (on 'spoon-bending', and parapsychology, for example) and also work by historians on subjects such as magic, alchemy, phrenology, and eugenics. Science that was judged 'cranky' and objectionable by today's standards was clearly not always regarded as such. Stepan's book combined both of these arguments. On the one hand, she asserted: 'The scientists who gave scientific racism its credibility and respectability were often first-rate scientists struggling to understand what appeared to them to be deeply puzzling problems of biology and human society. To dismiss their work as merely "pseudoscientific" would mean missing an opportunity to explore something important about the nature of scientific inquiry itself'.[13] However troubling it may appear today, race science was good science done by scientists of excellent repute. On the other hand, even the casual reader could not help but notice that Stepan placed Darwin at the centre of her work on 'dubious', culturally-ridden science. 'Good science' (by then-contemporary standards) had produced ideas about racial fixity and racial limits; discourses about fixity and inequality had helped shape 'good science' (by standards that we continue to accept).

It is also in retrospect that we can identify some of the problems induced by the historiographical (and political) aims of Stepan's study. *The Idea of Race in*

---

[12] For my fruitless attempt to introduce the term 'the new intellectual history', see Suman Seth, 'The History of Physics after the Cultural Turn', *Historical Studies in the Natural Sciences* 41 (2011).

[13] Stepan, xvi.

Science joined a growing body of scholarship interested in challenging current norms and ideals and hence tended to emphasise the roots of those elements in the past. Stepan's was a study, for example, of race *science* (largely, biology and ethnology), not of race-medicine, in spite of the fact that many early 'race-scientists' were trained as doctors. James Cowles Prichard, for example, was a Bristol physician; Robert Knox an anatomist who left Edinburgh several years after his involvement in the Burke and Hare body-snatching scandal. The medical grounding of much race science is particularly clear if one looks (as Stepan would in her next monograph) beyond the European metropole.[14] The majority of those with scientific training in the colonies were medical men.

The metropolitan focus of *The Idea of Race in Science* was, of course, a conscious choice. The 'best' men of science were likely to be found in European capitals. Yet this meant that the study of race in science often concentrated on places with little contact between different 'races'. These 'races' were often represented by skulls and skeletons (immutable mobiles if ever such existed). We know too little about the ways in which daily contact between 'races' shaped taxonomic understanding. Beyond questions of 'collecting', our histories of the practices of race science often seem to avoid discussions of slavery and colonialism as quotidian experience.[15]

Finally, Stepan was most interested in race science as 'normal science' during the period in which biology came of age as a discipline in its own right. If seemingly misguided, the questions of race science are demonstrably part of the heritage of 'modern science'. The methods are naturalistic; physical features are assumed to provide adequate guides to mental characteristics. Yet the origins of race science lie (at least) in the eighteenth century and race as a category of analysis has grown dramatically in importance in our genomic age.[16]

My aim in this work is to re-locate race along three axes: discipline, geography, period. This chapter and Chapter 7 offer a history of eighteenth-century ideas about medicine and race largely drawn from texts either written (or drawing upon experiences) in places far beyond European metropoles. Of course, I am hardly the first to suggest that such relocations are necessary, although this book may be unique in arguing that all three should be considered simultaneously. Arguments rejecting the privileging of nineteenth-century understandings of race have already been noted. The eighteenth century has been paid particular attention by Roxanne Wheeler, Colin Kidd and Andrew

---

[14] Nancy Stepan, *The Hour of Eugenics: Race, Gender, and Nation in Latin America* (Ithaca: Cornell University Press, 1991).

[15] See, however, James Delbourgo, 'The Newtonian Slave Body. Racial Enlightenment in the Atlantic World', *Atlantic Studies* 9 (2012).

[16] Suman Seth, ed., 'Focus: Re-Locating Race'. *Isis* 105, no 4 (2014): 759–814.

Curran.[17] The last few decades have also seen compelling arguments made by students of race in the Spanish and Portuguese empires that have convincingly problematised the normalisation of racial views in Northern and Western Europe.[18] The relationship between medicine and race has continued, however, to be under-considered, with Warwick Anderson's study of nineteenth-century Australian medical attitudes towards 'whiteness' remaining a conspicuous exception.[19] At times, the absence can seem striking, as in Wheeler's excellent *The Complexion of Race*, where particular attention is paid to what is termed the 'humoral body', precisely because this body and its relationship to climate 'have been strangely omitted in recent eighteenth-century studies'.[20] Despite tracing the classical roots of such thinking to the works of (among others) Plato, Hippocrates, and Galen (the two latter of whom were, of course, physicians) and despite acknowledging that this was also the occupation of many of those working within a 'humoural' tradition in the eighteenth century, Wheeler nonetheless associates the mode of thought with natural history rather than medicine.[21] Although it would not do to over-emphasise the distinction between medicine and natural history (the two fields shared clear and obvious connections), collapsing one onto the other is equally problematic and speaks more to a persistent failure of communication between the history of science and the history of medicine than it does to the historical facts on the ground. Nor is the point simply a matter of boundary work. Insofar, I would argue, as we are interested in the ways that naturalistic understandings of race did *work* – not just intellectual work, but social and political work – then I think we have been looking in the wrong places. The right place – the place that we can see race in action – is medicine in the colonies.[22]

---

[17] Wheeler. Kidd, 79–120. Curran.

[18] The literature is vast. As a starting point, see Thomas E. Skidmore, *Black into White: Race and Nationality in Brazilian Thought* (New York: Oxford University Press, 1974); Francisco Bethencourt and A. J. Pearce, eds., *Racism and Ethnic Relations in the Portuguese Speaking World* (New York: Oxford University Press, 2012). Richard Graham, ed. *The Idea of Race in Latin America, 1870–1940* (Austin: University of Texas Press, 1990). Jorge Cañizares-Esguerra, 'New Worlds, New Stars: Patriotic Astrology and the Invention of Indian and Creole Bodies in Colonial Spanish America, 1600–1650', *American Historical Review* 104 (1999). In 2011, the *Hispanic American Historical Review* dedicated a special issue (Volume 91, number 3) to examining the significance of Stepan's work on science and medicine in Latin America. Warwick Anderson has very recently surveyed material on 'Racial Conceptions in the Global South' in *Isis* 105 (2014): 782–92.

[19] Anderson, *The Cultivation of Whiteness: Science, Health and Racial Destiny in Australia*. See also Stephen Snelders, 'Leprosy and Slavery in Suriname: Godfried Schilling and the Framing of a Racial Pathology in the Eighteenth Century', *Social History of Medicine* 26 (2013).

[20] Wheeler, 28.

[21] Ibid., 22, 28.

[22] This fact would suggest that scholars may need to reconsider several criteria by which we judge the significance or import of given texts. Some of these texts (Atkins', for example) went through multiple editions, providing some indication of their popularity. Many did not.

5.1   Race: The Terms of the Debate in the Early Enlightenment

By the mid-eighteenth century, the question of the origin of human physical differences had become a familiar one within European philosophy. The
orthodox view was known as monogenism and posited a single act of creation
for all humankind. At some point in the past, humanity had looked similar: if
Biblical narratives were taken literally, the resemblance was a familial one.
Human groups had spread from a common centre through different climatic
zones until their physical and intellectual features displayed the myriad diversity of the human species today.[23] This environmentalist explanation had roots
going back to antiquity, where even the differences between the inhabitants
of nearby city-states were explained by describing their various 'airs, waters,
and places'. But challenges to what might be termed naïve monogenism were
already to be found by the late seventeenth century. In 1665 the anatomist,
Marcello Malpighi, had seemed to identify the difference between black and
white skin by finding, in an African subject, a layer of skin that contained a
dark mucus or fluid.[24] Andrew Curran has termed this 'the most important skin-
related discovery of the early-modern era'.[25] In 1684, the traveller François
Bernier put forward 'A New Division of the Earth According to the Different
Species or Races of Men'. While willing to acknowledge that a myriad of
differences distinguished the nations of men, Bernier insisted that larger

Many (particularly with regard to their views on race) were not cited in subsequent writings.
Understanding their 'reception', then, is difficult and, beyond their published works, the historical record concerning a number of the authors I examine is fairly meagre. On the other
hand, by reading their published material, it becomes clear that many, if not most, of those that
I discuss had substantial medical interactions with populations both 'white' and 'black', free
and enslaved. It seems obvious that medical views on race – on the putative difference, if any,
between the afflictions of 'whites' and 'blacks' – could *make* a difference in both diagnosis and
treatment. By studying these authors, then, we can get a sense of the immediate effect of racial
ideas on the bodies of those who were the subject of discourse concerning race.

[23] It was apparently common, by the seventeenth century, to argue that black skin was a mark of
the curse laid on the descendants of Noah's son, Ham. John Josselyn, in his *Account of Two
Voyages to New England* (1674) noted that: 'It is the opinion of many men, that the blackness of
the *Negroes* proceeded from the curse upon *Cham's* posterity'. Quoted in Winthrop D. Jordan,
White over Black: American Attitudes toward the Negro, 1550–1812 (Chapel Hill: University
of North Carolina Press, 1968), 245. This, however, was a fairly late development. One finds
very little evidence that suggests that Ham or his children were seen as black or were unam-
biguously associated with Africa until around the Renaissance. On the changing understanding
of the curse, see Benjamin Braude, 'The Sons of Noah and the Construction of Ethnic and
Geographical Identities in the Medieval and Early Modern Periods', *The William and Mary
Quarterly* 54, no. 1 (1997).

[24] On Malpighi, see Domenico Bertoloni Meli, ed. *Marcello Malpighi: Anatomist and Physician*
(Firenze: Leo. S. Olschki, 1997). On studies of human skin colour in the early modern period
more generally, see Renato G. Mazzolini, 'Skin Color and the Origin of Physical Anthropology
(1640–1850)', in *Reproduction, Race, and Gender in Philosophy and the Early Life Sciences*,
ed. Susanne Lettow (New York: SUNY Press, 2014); Malcolmson.

[25] Curran, 121.

similarities grouped them into only four or five races, 'whose difference is so remarkable that it may be properly made use of as the foundation for a new division of the earth'. In some, skin colour was a relatively insignificant feature, to be explained by the 'accident' of their location in sunny climes. For others, however, skin colour seemed a more profound mark. The slave trade had produced data that appeared to trouble environmentalism, for new climates seemed to have but little effect on some races. '[I]f a black African pair be transported to a cold country', wrote Bernier, 'their children are just as black, and so are all their descendants ... The cause must be sought for in the peculiar texture of their bodies, or in the seed, or in the blood'.[26] Winthrop Jordan has suggested that some kind of 'fluid theory' was the most common explanation to be found in the early eighteenth century and one finds versions of it in the work of Alexis Littré in 1702 and Pierre Barrère in 1741, with each connecting the black layer to increased levels of black bile in African bodies.[27]

Not all were so impressed, however. The Virginian physician John Mitchell deployed Newtonian optics in arguing that Negro skin was only somewhat thicker than that of whites, so that differences existed 'only in the Degree of one and the same Colour'.[28] The Comte de Buffon did not deny the facts involved in the fluid theory, but he did question their significance. '[I]f one asserts that it is the blackness of the blood or the bile that gives this colour to the skin', he noted logically, 'then instead of asking why the *nègres* have black skin, one will ask why they have black bile or black blood; this is thus to dismiss the question, rather than resolving it'.[29] Buffon's environmentalist arguments, as laid out in 'On the Varieties in the Human Species', published in 1749, played down any notion of intrinsic differences, but they also tried to nuance earlier climatic claims. Most previous commentators had assumed that there was a reasonable correlation between latitude and complexion. Warmer climates produced people of darker skin and those from diverse nations in common latitudinal regions should look reasonably similar. It was becoming clear, however, that

---

[26] François Bernier, 'A New Division of the Earth', in *The Idea of Race*, ed. Robert Bernasconi and Tommy L. Lott (Indianapolis: Hackett, 2000), 2. Siep Stuurman, 'François Bernier and the Invention of Racial Classification', *History Workshop Journal* 50 (2000). Malcolmson suggests that it may have been the publication of Bernier's essay that inspired debates over the origin of human skin colour in the Royal Society in the 1690s. Malcolmson, 69–70.

[27] Jordan, 246; Curran, 121–2; Pierre Barrère, *Dissertation sur la Cause physique de la couleur des nègres, de la qualité de leurs cheveux, et de la dégénération de l'un et de l'autre* (Paris: Pierre-Guillaume Simon, 1741). On responses to Barrère's theories, see Sean Quinlan, 'Colonial Bodies, Hygiene, and Abolitionist Politics in Eighteenth-Century France', *History Workshop Journal* 42 (1996): 112.

[28] Mitchell quoted in Jordan, 247; John Mitchell, 'An Essay Upon the Causes of the Different Colours of People in Different Climates', *Philosophical Transaction* 43 (1744–45); Delbourgo, 'The Newtonian Slave Body: Racial Enlightenment in the Atlantic World'.

[29] Buffon quoted in Curran, 124.

neither of these assumptions properly held. If darker skin was produced by the action of the sun, why were peoples in the tropics and the polar zones both swarthy, while those in temperate climes were pale? According to Buffon, it was because one needed to take into account the effect not only of heat, but also of moisture. Both very cold and very hot environments, he argued, could produce a darkening of the skin because both were also dry.[30] Moreover, physical features could be altered indirectly by the climate. Different regions of the earth, for example, contained characteristically different flora and fauna. Humans who moved into such regions gradually developed different manners of living, ate different diets, and suffered from different diseases, all of which changed their physiognomy and intellectual characteristics in permanent, heritable ways.[31]

Buffon's explanations re-affirmed the brotherhood of man. Humans might come in different varieties, but – since crossings between different human groups produced fertile offspring – we were all one species.[32] Not all varieties were equal, however. The original human type was white, in Buffon's formulation, and all deviation from this original was to be understood as a form and sign of degeneracy. The animals of the New World were, for example, degenerate versions of those in the Old. Why else was there nothing to compare to the lion or elephant? So too were the human inhabitants and if one wished to restore them to their first and higher state they must be removed and transplanted. Given time, French food and a temperate climate could reverse their decline.[33]

Buffon's hierarchical monogenism provided the orthodox naturalistic position for the rest of the century. Much more unorthodox was polygenism, which held that different races had been made in separate acts of creation. This was an old heresy, given much greater weight after the European discovery of the Americas. Monogenetic theories that sought to explain how people had travelled from the Old World to the New abounded. One finds them still in the nineteenth century, as scholars argued, for example, that Native Americans might be descended from 'descendants of the Welsh emigrants of Prince Madog'.[34] Some few iconoclasts, however, found such notions impossible. Paracelsus

---

[30] Georges Louis Leclerc Buffon, 'Of the Varieties in the Human Species', in *Barr's Buffon. Buffon's Natural History Containing a Theory of the Earth, a General History of Man, of the Brute Creation, and of Vegetables, Minerals &C. &C.* (London: H. D. Symonds, 1807), 349.

[31] Ibid., 270.

[32] Phillip R. Sloan, 'Buffon, German Biology, and the Historical Interpretation of Biological Species', *The British Journal for the History of Science* 12, no. 2 (1979).

[33] Phillip R. Sloan, 'The Idea of Racial Degeneracy in Buffon's *Histoire Naturelle*', *Studies in Eighteenth-Century Culture* 3 (1973).

[34] D. W. Nash, 'The Welsh Indians: To the Editor of the Cambrian Journal', *The Cambrian Journal* (1860).

declared in 1520 that 'these people are from a different Adam', while Giordano Bruno – soon to be burned at the stake for related views – claimed that Adam was only one of three Patriarchs.[35] The first sustained polygenetic work, Isaac La Peyrère's *Prae-Adamitae* (*Men Before Adam*) appeared in 1655 to wide condemnation. In February of the following year he was jailed; in June he agreed to repent, apologise to the Pope, and convert from Calvinism to Catholicism.

In La Peyrère's account, the Bible was a description of history and destiny that applied only to the Jews. To them alone had the word of God been revealed. This meant that one need not consider the history of other peoples, for they were not part of the divine plan. Nor did one need any longer to worry about how to square the narrative of creation or the story of the Deluge with new discoveries of men in far-flung locations. Ancient pagans had not derived from the same stock as the chosen people; inhabitants of the New World had not descended from the sons of Noah. On the other hand, as Popkin has noted, La Peyrère was a universal humanist. If only Jews were the subject of a divine history, their Messianic salvation would include all others, pre- and post-Adamic alike.[36]

La Peyrère was a believer. Many of those who would follow in his polygenetic footsteps, however, would see the doctrine of separate creations as a means of mocking – rather than salvaging – Biblical exposition.[37] Thus, one finds 'L. P'. (presumably a nod to La Peyrère) offering a defence of rationalism in the face of biblical literalism in 1695. The work combined two essays, the first of which ridiculed the notion that the Noachic flood, if it had occurred, had spanned the globe. Why drown the earth and all its innocent creations, L. P. asked, when most of the world was uninhabited? Why destroy all on account of 'a few Wanton and Luxurious *Asiaticks*, who might have been drown'd by a *Topical Flood*, or by a particular Deluge, without involving all the Bowels of the whole Mass, and the remote Creatures upon the face of

[35] Quoted in David N. Livingstone, *Adam's Ancestors: Race, Religion, and the Politics of Human Origins* (Baltimore: Johns Hopkins University Press, 2008), 23. On Pre-Adamism before the seventeenth century, see Richard H. Popkin, *Isaac La Peyrère (1596–1676): His Life, Work, and Influence* (Leiden: Brill, 1987), 26–41; Livingstone, *Adam's Ancestors: Race, Religion, and the Politics of Human Origins*, 1–25. On whether it is entirely correct to call Paracelsus a polygenist (on the grounds that he did not necessarily treat non-Adamic peoples as fully human), see Popkin, 34.

[36] Popkin, 69–79.

[37] As Colin Kidd has argued: 'The subversion of scripture was not in most cases a strategy designed consciously to provide new polygenetic supports for white domination of non-European peoples; rather Enlightened critics used the fact of racial diversity as a weapon to undermine the authority of scripture'. Colin Kidd, 'Ethnicity in the British Atlantic World, 1688–1830', in *A New Imperial History: Culture, Identity, and Modernity in Britain and the Empire, 1660–1840*, ed. Kathleen Wilson (Cambridge: Cambridge University Press, 2004), 263.

the Earth, in the Ruin'?[38] The second essay then heaped scorn on the idea that the world had been populated from a single spot, with animals and men travelling vast distances across many different climes to reach the locations in which they were now found. '[H]ow the Animals, that cannot endure the extremity of Cold', he scoffed, 'should climb over inaccessible Mountains or Ice and Snow for many Thousands of Miles together, is hardly explicable to any thinking man'.[39] Nor could one imagine that they had been carried by men. Why would one do this with dangerous creatures and leave behind so many 'mild and useful ones'?[40] The logics that applied to animals would seem to apply to men, as well. In any case, however, there was reason beyond this to doubt that all men were related. As others had, L. P. noted the problems with climatic explanations for differences in skin colour between whites and blacks. One found different coloured people in similar climates; whites did not seem to darken appreciably in warm countries, blacks did not lighten in cooler ones. He declared of Negroes, then, that 'their Colour and Wool are Innate, or Seminal from their first beginning, and seems to be a Specifick Character, which neither the Sun, nor any curse from *Cham* could imprint upon them'.[41] Arguments derived from '*Eastern* Rubbish, or Rabbinical Weeds' could supply no reasonable answer to the questions raised by natural history.[42]

The tone in which Atkins expressed his musings about the several origins of mankind – matter-of-fact, if somewhat apologetic – would be the exception among polygenists in the first half of the eighteenth century. One might, indeed, say that the doctrine of special creations was a sarcastic position in this period. It was nowhere more so than in the writings of Voltaire, who turned La Peyrère's philosemitism on its head. Europeans, in Voltaire's view, had preceded Jews on the Earth. The Jewish patriarch was merely a pale imitation of the original, and Jews would remain a race apart, however long they lived in Western lands.[43] Writing of blacks in *The Philosophy of History,* Voltaire noted that it had now become common practice for the 'curious traveler' passing through Leiden to make a stop to view the *reticulum mucosum* (now known as the Malpighian layer) of a dissected negro.[44] This membrane, he added, is itself black and 'communicates to negroes that inherent blackness, which they do not lose'. The philosopher declared that 'none but the blind' could make of whites, negroes, Albinoes, Hottentots, Laplanders, the Chinese, and

[38] L. P., *Two Essays Sent in a Letter from Oxford to a Nobleman in London.* (London: R. Baldwin, 1695), 14.

[39] Ibid., 20.

[40] Ibid., 22.

[41] Ibid., 27.

[42] Ibid., 23.

[43] Popkin, 133–4.

[44] Voltaire, *The Philosophy of History* (London: I. Allcock, 1766), 6.

Americans anything but distinct races, and if one were to ask about the origins of such races, the answer was equally obvious: 'the same providence which placed men in Norway, planted some also in America and under the Antarctic circle, in the same manner as it planted trees and made grass to grow there'.[45] David Hume concurred in 1753, arguing that all races other than whites were inferior, and that the differences among such races were innate, nature having made an 'original distinction betwixt these breeds of men'. His tone might be captured by reproducing his comments on a counter-example to his claim that no negro had or would ever distinguish themselves through their intelligence. There were those in Jamaica, he noted, who spoke of one as a man of considerable learning. Hume dismissed the thought: "tis likely', he wrote, 'he is admired for very slender accomplishments like a parrot, who speaks a few words plainly'.[46] Heterodox and uncommon, polygenism had nonetheless become a viable philosophical position by the mid-eighteenth century, even if one might regard it – in the main – as a view more reactive and antagonistic than deeply held in its own right.[47]

5.2   Gender, Medicine, and Climate

If the Bible appeared to license a unitary view of human races, it offered a binary conception of human sexes, with Eve produced in a special and derivative creation. Depending on what kinds of elements medical men discussed, this binary was more or less stark. Although scholars have identified cases

---

[45] Ibid., 6, 9. Material on the races of men first appeared in 1734.

[46] The remarks appeared originally in a footnote to the 1753 edition of a work published originally in 1748. David Hume, 'Of National Characters', in *Hume: Essays, Moral, Political, and Literary*, ed. E. F. Miller (Indianapolis: Liberty Fund, 1987), 197–215, footnote on 8. For a discussion of variant readings see 629–30. On the relation of this footnote to the remainder of the essay see Kidd, *The Forging of Races: Race and Scripture in the Protestant Atlantic World, 1600–2000*, 93–4.

[47] As Popkin has noted, one finds a number of thinkers whose views would seem to lead them almost inexorably to polygenism, but who were orthodox enough to draw back from the precipice. Popkin, 132. To offer merely one concrete example, one finds in Ovington's account of his voyage to Suratt and other locations in 1689 a discussion of the difference in skin colour of various peoples. Ovington rejected the idea that climate alone could produce such variation, arguing that diet was of crucial importance. An Indian of very dark colour who was taken into the English service, he claimed, had become noticeably paler by 'tasting wine and eating flesh'. J. Ovington, 'A Voyage to Suratt in the Year 1689', in *India in the Seventeenth Century: Being an Account of the Two Voyages to India by Ovington and Thevenot. To Which Is Added the Indian Travels of Careri*, ed. J. P. Guha (New Delhi: Associated Publishing House, 1976), 219. Differences between peoples, then, were not essential. Ovington, however, was scathing about the people he called 'Hotantots', whom he claimed to be 'the very reverse of human kind'. Were there a middle position 'between a rational animal and a beast', he asserted, 'the Hotantot lays the fairest claim to that species'. Ibid., 218. Yet Ovington remained silent on the question of the cause or origin of this bestial nature.

where even this boundary was blurred, the sources I have examined associated specifically reproductive elements solely with women.[48] The key questions for many physicians and surgeons writing about pregnancy, childbirth, menstruation, and menopause were about the ways in which such processes varied with the climate.[49] On other medical issues, concerning distempers that afflicted both sexes, differences were perceived as a matter of degree and not kind. Effeminate men, like women, were less liable to a fatal bout of yellow fever in climates that favoured the relatively emasculated. The relationships between sex and race were similarly complex, depending on the afflictions involved. As we shall see, one area where sex and race became particularly mutually imbricated concerned the putative threat posed by Afro-Caribbean women accused of prostitution and the spread of venereal disease.

Many of the observations found in medical texts concerning the diseases of warm climates are perhaps best understood as cultural tropes, rather than material aimed at diagnosis or treatment, with numerous authors, for example, discussing the relative ease of childbirth in foreign climes. This was a claim of considerable antiquity, with parts of Hippocrates' *Airs, Waters, and Places* dedicated to the difficulties attending parturition according to location, diet, and environment.[50] At the beginning of the sixteenth century, Amerigo Vespucci made sure that a claim about the Old World was also part of the understanding of the New. The women he observed in his voyage were 'very fruiteful, and refuse no laboure al the whyle they are with childe. They travayle in maner without payne, so that the nexte day they are cherefull and able to walk'.[51] As part of his *Travels*, published in 1687, Jean de Thevenot claimed of Indian women that they 'are easily delivered of their children' and, in common

---

[48] See Thomas Laqueur, *Making Sex: Body and Gender from the Greeks to Freud* (Cambridge, MA: Harvard University Press, 1990); Barbara Duden, *The Woman beneath the Skin: A Doctor's Patients in Eighteenth-Century Germany* (Cambridge, MA: Harvard University Press, 1991).

[49] All doctors did not take up the question of specifically female complaints in any detail. Neither Towne nor Hillary listed any specifically female illnesses among those they deemed characteristic of the West Indian climate. Thomas, in 1790, was one of the few to include a section on 'Women's diseases'. Towne. Hillary, *Observations on the Changes of the Air and the Concomitant Epidemical Diseases, in the Island of Barbados. To Which Is Added a Treatise on the Putrid Bilious Fever, Commonly Called the Yellow Fever; and Such Other Diseases as Are Indigenous or Endemial, in the West India Islands, or in the Torrid Zone*. Thomas. Those primarily treating soldiers and sailors made up a class of practitioners with understandably little dealing with female patients. For concrete descriptions of cases involving women – and hence more material useful for a history of *practice*, see for example, Sloane. On whom, Churchill. Of the twenty-four cases discussed by James Hendy, ten involved women and one a female child of eleven years. James Hendy, *A Treatise on the Glandular Disease of Barbadoes: Proving It to Be Seated in the Lymphatic System* (London: C. Dilly, 1784).

[50] Hippocrates, 'Airs, Waters, and Places'.

[51] Quoted in Jennifer L. Morgan, *Laboring Women: Reproduction and Gender in New World Slavery* (Philadelphia: University of Pennsylvania Press, 2004), 17.

with women all over the Indies, could 'walk about' the day after giving birth.[52]
By the early eighteenth century, the topic was standard enough that Friedrich
Hoffman, in his neo-Hippocratic survey of *Endemial Diseases*, considered it a
common axis upon which to compare the various peoples of the world:

In *Aethiopia* the Women are blessed with peculiarly easy and happy Labours, and are
generally delivered on their Knees ... *Borlaeus* ... mentions the like Hardiness and
Strength in the *Brasilian* Women, who, as he informs us, 'do not keep themselves up for
five or six Weeks after Labour, like the *European* Women, but set about their ordinary
Business next Day after their Delivery, though their Bodies, however firm and healthy,
are yet very small'. I have often heard and read that in *Batavia*, the women immediately
after their Delivery go into running Water, and wash both themselves and their Children,
without any Danger to either.[53]

Less painful childbirth might seem to have been a positive characteristic, but
it was not necessarily taken to be so. Since the agony of parturition was part
of the punishment inflicted upon Eve, the suggestion that some women were
spared could carry with it a whiff of polygenism. Edward Long, who espoused
polygenist beliefs, and who – as we will see in the next chapter – would raise
the status of Orangutans to that of men in order to lower the status of Africans
to those of beasts, was characteristically offensive and distasteful in discussing
African women, who 'are delivered with little or no labour; they have therefore
no more occasion for midwives, than the female Oran-Outang, or any other
wild animal. A woman brings forth her child in a quarter of an hour, goes the
same day to the sea, and washes herself'.[54] Consistent with Long's belief that
the transportation of Africans to the West Indies improved them, he also argued
that 'Child-birth is not as easy here as in Afric'.[55] Increased pain in parturition,
in other words, could be read as civilisational improvement. And, of course, in
less abstract terms, asserting that Afro-Caribbean women could labour even in
the last months of pregnancy and return to work within days afterward served
to license a gruelling slave regime.[56] Benjamin Moseley declared that 'hot
climates', in general 'are indeed very favourable to gestation and parturition',
that difficult labours were uncommon, and that the lying in period was short.
'Indians and Negroes', he claimed, 'sometimes make it an affair of a few days,
and sometimes of a few hours only, and then pursue their occupation'.[57] That

[52] Jean de Thevenot, 'The Third Part of the Travels of Mr. De Thevenot, Containing the Relation
of Indostan, the New Moguls and of Other People and Countries of the Indies', in *India in the
Seventeenth Century: Being an Account of the Two Voyages to India by Ovington and Thevenot.
To Which Is Added the Indian Travels of Careri*, ed. J. P. Guha (New Delhi: Associated
Publishing House, 1976 [1687]), 80, 143.

[53] Hoffmann and Ramazzini, 30.

[54] Edward Long, *The History of Jamaica*, 3 vols., vol. II (London: T. Lowndes, 1774), 380.

[55] Ibid., 436.

[56] Bush; Dunn, 'Sugar Production and Slave Women in Jamaica'.

[57] Moseley, *A Treatise on Tropical Diseases; And on the Climate of the West-Indies*, 61.

said, as we shall see in Chapter 7, abolitionists would focus upon the appalling treatment of pregnant and nursing women in propaganda that successfully turned public opinion against slave owners. One wonders whether this might have been an impetus behind the Jamaican doctor, John Quier's correction of Donald Monro's comments on this point.[58] Monro had read a letter from Quier on inoculation to the Royal College of Physicians in London in 1771 and had inserted a note concerning the propriety of inoculating pregnant women. Since the women involved were African, Monro insisted, one need not worry too much: 'Negro women and others of hardy constitutions', he opined, 'who are much exposed to the open air, often bear children, and go about their daily labour in a day or two afterwards, and undergo many other things without the least inconvenience, which would be in danger of destroying those of delicate habits, who have been educated in European luxury'.[59] Perhaps aware that such comments could be regarded as callousness, Quier rejected them in a second letter. '[W]hatever hardiness negroes may possess', he noted, 'I do not find that the females enjoy that immunity from the evils of child-bearing, at least in this country, that you seem to imagine'. As a result, Quier claimed, such women were 'carefully nursed for a fortnight; and excused from all kinds of labour', sometimes not emerging from her house for a month.[60] Whatever the truth of this claim – and there were many who suggested that slave women received no such careful nursing – its timing is worth noting. In 1773, a year after the Somerset case appeared to outlaw slavery on English soil, the plight of slaves was a matter of newly-urgent public discussion. Quier may well have seen the value in not adding fuel to the fire with talk of the physiological differences that putatively justified the comparative neglect of enslaved mothers.[61]

As common as the trope that related warm climates and easy parturition was one that pointed, within the same regions, to sexual precocity and a concomitantly early decline. 'Girls soon arrive at Maturity', wrote George Cleghorn in his *Observations on the Endemical Diseases in Minorca* (1751), 'and soon grow old'. The menses usually appeared before fourteen, frequently as early as eleven, and could sometimes 'return twice a month'.[62] No others reported a

---

[58] Cf. Schiebinger, 'Human Experimentation in the Eighteenth Century: Natural Boundaries and Valid Testing', 402–4. Schiebinger associates comments concerning the hardiness of Negroes with Quier and then suggests that he 'backtracked' on these in a subsequent letter. Quier, however, refers to '[t]he note, you have inserted concerning gravid women' in his letter of 28 March 1773 to Monro. The letters are reproduced in Monro et al., 1–104, the quotation is to be found on 54. See also Schiebinger, *Secret Cures of Slaves: People, Plants, and Medicine in the Eighteenth-Century Atlantic World*, 104–9.

[59] Monro et al., 12.

[60] Ibid., 55.

[61] I discuss the Somerset case in detail in the next chapter.

[62] Cleghorn, 53.

fortnightly period, but it was not uncommon to report that those living in warm climates might enter puberty at ten or eleven when, as Thomas observed, it seldom appeared before fifteen in colder regions.[63] Long imagined a speeding up of existence in general for creole white women in Jamaica, who 'attain earlier to maturity, and sooner decline' than their northern counterparts, and who were not unseldom mothers at twelve. 'They console themselves, however, that they can enjoy more of real existence here in one hour, than the fair inhabitants of the frozen, foggy regions do in two'.[64] Such a positive spin on precocity and early senescence was not granted to mulatto women, who arrived at puberty quickly, but then declined dramatically after the age of twenty-five 'till at length they grow horribly ugly'.[65] By 1787, Moseley seemed to be aware of how familiar observations of this kind were, for he both confirmed the fact of early menstruation, while rejecting the applicability of the wilder tales that filled travel narratives. 'Though females do arrive at early maturity in hot climates, there are none of those wonderful instances of early pregnancy in the West-Indies, that travellers speak of, and such as are said to have happened in other parts of the world'.[66]

Perhaps more interesting than the repetition of this familiar refrain concerning menstruation were observations about the benefits it conferred on women with regard to susceptibility to diseases otherwise unconnected to reproduction.[67] A sizeable portion of the authors who wrote about certain kinds of fevers (usually including the yellow fever) noted a peculiarity about those most badly afflicted by it. The disease laid low the strongest and most robust of men. In his *Description of the American Yellow Fever*, John Lining observed that while the disease was almost always fatal to 'valetudinarians', and often deadly to the intemperate, and those not habituated to the climate, it also seemed to particularly afflict 'those of an athletic and full habit'.[68] Lewis Rouppe, in a tract in the diseases of sailors, similarly pointed to 'young robust men' as those likely to die the soonest from bilious fevers, as did John Hume who noted that 'strong muscular men' were most liable to the 'true bilious, or yellow fever' while 'those of a lax habit are least liable to it, and most likely to recover'.[69] A 'lax

---

[63] Thomas, 279.

[64] Long, II, 285.

[65] Ibid., 335.

[66] Moseley, *A Treatise on Tropical Diseases; And on the Climate of the West-Indies*, 60.

[67] This was not, in general, uncommon. It had been believed since antiquity that some diseases – often precisely those that could be aided or cured through venesection – were less likely to afflict women, who lost blood naturally on a monthly basis.

[68] John Lining, *A Description of the American Yellow Fever, Which Prevailed at Charleston, in South Carolina, in the Year 1748* (Philadelphia: Thomas Dobson, 1799), 25–6.

[69] Rouppe, 413–4; John Hume, 'An Account of the True Bilious, or Yellow Fever; and of the Remitting Fevers of the West Indies', in *Letters and Essays on the Small-Pox and Inoculation,*

habit' could be acquired in many ways, from dissolution to simple aging, but it was also an effect of heat or humidity. Moisture and warmth could cause the strings of a well-tuned instrument to sag; so, too, could the tense and rigid fibres of a strong male body. The body best suited to the tropics, then, was the diametric opposite of that which was the perfect symbol of British manliness at home. As a reviewer of Charles Bisset's *Essay on the Medical Constitution of Great Britain* (1762) phrased it in rejecting the author's (unusual) assertion that northern Europeans were *less* likely to suffer from inflammatory diseases in warm climates: 'we imagined that the world was persuaded, that the very reverse of this assertion was true; that northern constitutions are the most subject to fevers when transplanted into hot climates'. The reason being:

that all bodies are the best adapted, by nature, for that climate in which they are produced and have been resident: that the inhabitants of warm climates are remarkable for a lax fibre, hence their weakness, sloth, and effeminacy; and the women, and such as lead the most sedentary and inactive lives, are the most exempt from all feverish and inflammatory complaints.[70]

A new climate would exact a price for the discrepancy between the bodily constitution native to it and that of a stranger; a price particularly high for robust masculinity in a land suited for the effeminate and inactive.

Gendered weakness, then, provided a kind of strength, or at least protection. The young and robust, with the tensest fibres were the 'most obnoxious' to the bilious fever, wrote John Williams, while 'women and men of lax habits are seldom seized with it; or, when they are, come through with much less danger and difficulty'.[71] In 1783, Stephen Mathews added children to women and those of a 'lax and delicate texture' on his list of those 'seldom harassed' by bilious fevers, arguing that by the time of his writing the idea that the 'strength of the disease is par with the vigour of the afflicted' was an observation of such long standing and general acknowledgement that it would be a 'presumption' to disagree. Although some authors were more inclined to point to social and behavioural differences to explain relative susceptibility to the disease, most thus appeared to point to gendered anatomies.[72] Those who advocated bleeding as

the Measles, the Dry Belly-Ache, the Yellow, and Remitting, and Intermitting Fevers of the West Indies (London: J. Murray, 1778), 237.

[70] Reviewer, 'Essay on the Medical Constitution of Great Britain', *The Critical Review, or Annals of Literature* (1763): 188–9.

[71] Williams and Bennet, 29. See also Lind, who noted that European women were more subject to fatal fevers on the Guinea coast, but were 'not so subject' to the yellow fever of Jamaica. Lind, *An Essay on Diseases Incidental to Europeans in Hot Climates: With the Method of Preventing Their Fatal Consequences. To Which Is Added, an Appendix Concerning Intermittent Fevers*, 54, 117.

[72] Gilbert Blane, for example, blamed exercise in the sun and intemperance for bringing on fevers. 'It is in favour of this position', he stated, 'that women are not subject to the same violent fevers as the other sex, which is probably owing to their not being exposed to the same

a treatment for the illness often also added a physiological reason to their anatomical explanations. The problem, as John Williams noted, was that Northern
European bodies contained too much blood for their new climates, which then
exerted an excessive pressure on the body's vessels as the fluid warmed.[73] This
plethora had to be removed, a problem that nature took care of for women on a
monthly basis. In noting that European women in the East Indies seemed less
subject to hepatitis, Stephen Mathews could not quite determine whether the
cause was the 'delicacy of their formation' or the menses, but he did observe
that the greater the menstrual flow, the more relief the patient experienced.
John Tennent was more sure of himself. 'Women are seldom invaded with [the
yellow fever]', he asserted, 'which is owing to two reasons, 1. They have naturally a lax fibre. 2. They have the benefit of menstrual Discharges'.[74] Effeminate
men – like the women they resembled in their fibrous anatomical structure –
might be spared the most intense ravages of the illness, but they did not gain
the benefit of women's physiological distinction.

Women in these texts were not always, however, the sufferers of disease. On
many occasions they were deemed to be the cause. Willem Bosman devoted a
sizeable portion – he himself called it a 'tedious while' – of his twelfth letter
describing the Guinea Coast to the marital practices of the inhabitants, as well
as to revealing to his correspondent 'all our Venereal Ware-houses and their
contain'd Stores'. Bosman evinced some sympathy for the 'whores' that made
up the subject of part of his narrative, noting that their deaths were 'wretched
and miserable', being soon infected and dying young.[75] John Atkins had no
such sympathy in *The Navy-Surgeon*, laying the original cause of venereal disease at the feet of 'common women' (and women alone).

When the Venereal Appetite is jaded with the too intemperate Efforts of several Men, it
will be next to impossible for those Parts to suffer the continued frictions made there,

---

causes of illness'. Gilbert Blane, *Observations on the Diseases of Seamen* (London: Joseph
Cooper, 1785), 226–7. Hunter also pointed to 'the regularity and temperance of their living',
the avoidance of exertions in the open air, and the fact that they stayed indoors more, going out
only in the cool of the morning or evening 'and even then in a carriage' for women's longer life
expectancies. Hunter, *Observations on the Diseases of the Army in Jamaica; and on the Best
Means of Preserving the Health of Europeans, in That Climate*, 25.

[73] Williams and Bennet, 30. Similar arguments were made in the French colony of Saint
Domingue. See Weaver, 20–1.

[74] John Tennent, *Physical Enquiries Discovering the Mode of Translation in the Constitutions of
Northern Inhabitants, on Going to, and for Some Time after Arriving in Southern Climates ...
An Error ... In Recommending Vinegar to His Majesty's Fleet in the West Indies, to Prevent
the Epidemic Fever ... And the Barren State of Useful Physical Knowledge, as Well as the
Mercenary Practice of Physicians, by an Impartial State of Dr. Ward's Qualifications for
the Practice of Physic ... Illustrated with Remarks Upon a Printed Letter to a Member of
Parliament, Signed Philanthropos* (London: T. Gardner, 1742), 34. Tennent made a similar
argument in Tennent, 13–14.

[75] Bosman, 215.

(as common Women do) without excoriating and fretting the Membranes of the *Vagina*; and such Excoriations, how small soever in the Beginning, meeting with an ill habit of Body ... will soon degenerate to an Ulcer; which Ulcer will be the Distemper.[76]

This was a not uncommon etiological explanation and it was one that served to largely absolve men of guilt in the spread of diseases connected to the sexual act.[77] However promiscuous men might be, the fault lay with prostitutes that served as reservoirs of illness.

Racialised elements then entered this common discourse via claims that African women and their descendants were essentially all prostitutes. Thomas, for example, warned European ladies against using a 'negro, or mulatto woman' as a wet-nurse, for 'it is a great chance if she does not harbor in her blood the relics of many dreadful disorders, such as the yaws, leprosy, or a venereal taint; as all this race of people give themselves up to an unlimited prostitution'.[78] Long pointed to the excessive consumption of meat as one reason that Englishmen were more liable to bad fevers in the West Indies than the natives of other European countries, but he also emphasised their 'excessive indulgence in a promiscuous commerce, on their first arrival, with the black and mulatto women'. Ignoring the violence and compulsion involved in almost all instances of sexual contact between whites and blacks in a slave society. Long argued that black women, whether free or enslaved 'are few of them exempt from this *virus*'. But they kept their affliction secret 'by every artifice in their power, that no delay may happen in their business; for a hindrance in this respect would be a certain loss of profit to them'.[79] In this way, black women with venereal diseases became part of the trope of the 'scheming black

---

[76] John Atkins, *The Navy-Surgeon: Or, a Practical System of Surgery. Illustrated with Observations on Such Remarkable Cases, as Have Occurred to the Author's Practice in the Service of the Royal Navy. To Which Is Added, a Treatise on the Venereal Disease, the Causes, Symptoms, and Method of Cure by Mercury: An Enquiry into the Origin of That Distemper; in Which the Dispute between Dr Dover and Dr Turner, Concerning Crude Mercury, Is Fully Consider'd; with Useful Remarks Thereon. Also an Appendix, Containing Physical Observations on the Heat, Moisture and Density of the Air on the Coast of Guiney; the Colour of the Natives; the Sicknesses Which They and the Europeans Trading Thither Are Subject to; with a Method of Cure*, 2nd ed. (London: W. Warner, 1737), 208.

[77] Burnard and Follett argue that there was little social or even medical stigma, for men, associated with sexually transmitted diseases, for 'venereal infection was thoroughly embedded within the prevailing discourse of masculinity and empire'. Trevor Burnard and Richard Follett, 'Caribbean Slavery, British Anti-Slavery, and the Cultural Politics of Venereal Disease', *The Historical Journal* 55 (2012): 430.

[78] Thomas, 315. Contradictorily, however, slave-owners who forced females slaves into prostitution, 'did not accept that prostitution had adverse effects upon slaves' domestic relationships or their fertility'. Hilary McD. Beckles, 'Property Rights in Pleasure: The Marketing of Slave Women's Sexuality in the West Indies', in *West Indies Accounts: Essays on the History of the British Caribbean and the Atlantic Economy, in Honour of Richard Sheridan*, ed. Roderick A. McDonald (Kingston, Jamaica: University of the West Indies Press, 1996), 175.

[79] Long, II, 535, 36.

Jezebel', a bondswoman generally understood to be a prostitute who initiated a relationship with a white man 'solely to obtain material favours' and who then 'did everything possible to hurt her white partner immediately after he gave her money or gifts'.[80] Perhaps the most striking (if bizarre) version of this trope may be found in Robert Robertson's *Physical Journal Kept on Board his Majesty's Ship Rainbow, During Three Voyages to the Coast of Africa and West Indies, in the Years 1772, 1773, and 1774*. Robertson related the story of Charles Duplassey, a butcher, who presented himself to Robertson in pain and with a penis and scrotum considerably enlarged. Duplassey would die a few days later and after his death, Robertson was informed – although he had 'no great faith' in the information – that the butcher had been drunk the day before he had been taken ill and had lain 'with a black woman that night, who had *blown* him'. Robertson professed to being ignorant 'of what was meant by his having been *blown* by the woman' but called in another man from the ship who, apparently, 'had formerly sustained a like injury from a whore'. The informant claimed to have noticed nothing unusual in the act of coition, but felt certain that the woman was at fault, since she ran away as soon as she left the bed and never approached him again. As motive, he noted that both he and Duplassey, with whom he had conversed, had beaten the women before having sex with them, and that the butcher's partner had also fled afterwards. Radically playing down the violence committed against the women, Robertson treated the case as one almost supernatural, crediting the prostitutes (if such they were) with powers positively diabolic and used against men who had done little to earn their ire. '[I]t would appear', he noted with some relief, 'that only some prostitutes have this infernal act of *blowing* a man in the act of coition'. He confessed himself still 'perfectly ignorant of it; but if it really is in the power of a prostitute to commit so hellish a trick, I think it very providential that so few of them know the art, otherwise I may venture to say, that they would treat men in that abominable manner for every slight offence'.[81] The Jezebel would seem to merge here with the figure of the witch, able to

[80] Henrice Altink, 'Deviant and Dangerous: Pro-Slavery Representation of Jamaican Slave Women's Sexuality, C. 1780–1834', *Slavery and Abolition* 26 (2005): 274. See, more generally, *Representations of Slave Women in Discourses on Slavery and Abolition, 1780–1838* (New York and London: Routledge, 2007). Bush notes that opponents of slavery, on the other hand, 'saw the black woman not as a scheming black Jezebel, but as an innocent victim of the unholy lust of callous and brutal white men ... Abolitionists did not deny that black women were promiscuous, or that slaves in general lacked a moral code, they merely represented the latter as corrupted innocents'. Thus, contemporaries 'presented two conflicting images of the black woman, the abject creatures subjected to harsh patriarchal rule and the wanton woman who flouted all codes of accepted morality, neither of which was accurate'. Bush, 18, 21.

[81] Robert Robertson, *A Physical Journal Kept on Board His Majesty's Ship Rainbow, During Three Voyages to the Coast of Africa, and West Indies, in the Years 1772, 1773, and 1774* (London: E. & C. Dilly, J. Robson, T. Cadell, and T. Evans, 1777), 122–3.

cause harm not only by the transmission of infection, but also via practices that seemed to elude rational explanation.

As with the relationship between race and climate, that between sex and climate was complex. One might observe claims of the radical difference between the sexes, the pain of childbirth introduced as a punishment for Eve at the Fall, yet that proved to be modifiable according to whether one was in temperate or tropical climes. There were also more relative differences, where climate exacted a price from those whose British masculinity differed too much from the requisite effeminacy of their surrounds, and where specifically female processes, such as menstruation, could provide a kind of doubled protection. And there were cases where climate seemed to matter little against tropes that portrayed black women as collectively emblematising the worst of all feminine subversions, with elements that allowed their transposition from realms of natural affliction – perhaps worthy of sympathy, perhaps worthy of condemnation – to realms of supernatural and vindictive maleficence.

5.3   Race and Medicine, 1679–1740

The number of texts that discussed both medical matters and the physical variety to be found among different peoples was small in the late seventeenth and early eighteenth centuries. The most detailed comments, unsurprisingly, are to be found in location-specific medical tracts, such as those by Trapham, Sloane, and Towne on the West Indies, or Aubrey and Atkins on the Guinea Coast. One finds some material, but considerably less, in what might be considered travel narratives, such as Bosman's account of the time he spent in Africa, or Ovington's *A Voyage to Suratt*. A final set of sources is comprised of metropolitan works of medicine and natural philosophy, such as those by Arbuthnot and Huxham, which took the relationship between place, disease, and appearance as a central question. With such small numbers, trends are difficult to identify, but one can point to a change over time. Particularly from the 1720s onward, we shall see, one finds an increasing Hippocratic bent, with *Airs, Waters, and Places* taken as a paradigmatic text in framing a problematic that related location, diet, physical features, behaviour, and forms of governance.

We should begin by indicating what a racialist approach to medicine in this period might look like. Based on the materials, two kinds of arguments seem to have been plausible. The first looked at diseases that might be caused by, or (more weakly) related to, physical differences between the races. The second studied diseases that could be passed from generation to generation and that were particularly associated with the inhabitants of a specific part of the world. Arguments of the first type gained a certain degree of plausibility with Malpighi's studies. The difference between white and black could be seen as a (relatively) fixed one – at least one inherited by the next generation – and was a physically identifiable trait. Sloane explored the possibility that one particularly unfortunate affliction was caused by a physical difference in black bodies. In his account of the diseases of Jamaica he included the case of a female slave, brought to him by her owner, with many ulcers on her fingers and toes and 'several Bladders fill'd with *Serum* on several of her Joints'. Most peculiarly, these bladders appeared to fill with a periodicity tied to the cycle of the moon. Sloane was informed that the disease could be fatal and 'was peculiar to Blacks'. The doctor's treatment secured relief for a little time, but the disease returned quickly. Sloane mused over its possible cause: 'So soon as this Disease again appear'd, I thought, that perhaps, this was proper to Blacks, and so might come from some peculiar indisposition of their black skin'. Not only a disease peculiar to one race, then, this affliction was regarded as possibly the result of specific elements of a racial make-up.[82]

Sloane's tentative (and rather vague) suggestion is the only example of the first kind of racialist argument that I have been able to find. More common (if still rare) were arguments of the second type. Perhaps unsurprisingly, all of these hereditarian aetiologies concerned venereal disease, particularly syphilis. Unknown in Europe until the late fifteenth century, the new venereal disease quickly became associated with the inhabitants of the New World. And as Anna Foa has noted, associating a dread novel affliction with Indians was 'clearly not an innocent act'.

It meant searching for the origin of a sickness/evil of this kind, a sickness/evil tied to sexual excess and located as far from oneself as possible in the absolute Other, the person who had never known Christianity. This was an extreme projection: the disease was thrown back onto the 'nonhuman', onto the totally alien. To attribute it to a people outside the Revelation of Christ served to attenuate the impact of the debates on blame and divine punishment which had been encouraged by endogamous theories of the origin as the result of lasciviousness.[83]

One finds precisely this logic played out in Trapham's (bizarre) account of the origin of the disease known as Yaws, although he extended the argument to include not only 'the animal Indians' but also Africans, or, as he phrased it, 'the cursed posterity of the naked *Cham*'.[84] All venereal diseases, however various, Trapham argued, found their origin in the Yaws. And the cause was the same as that which produced 'strange, monstrous mixtures of animal shapes, more than ordinarily imitating the actions as well as the shapes of mankind'.[85] Baboons,

---

[82] Sloane, cvi. On Sloane's interest in the causes of blackness, see Malcolmson.

[83] Foa, 33.

[84] Trapham, 113. See also Londa Schiebinger, 'Scientific Exchange in the Eighteenth-Century Atlantic World', in *Soundings in Atlantic History: Latent Structures and Intellectual Currents, 1500–1830*, ed. Bernard Bailyn and Patricia L. Denault (Cambridge, MA: Harvard University Press, 2009), 309.

[85] Trapham, 114.

drills, pongoes, monkeys, and malmasets all arose, Trapham claimed, from unnatural and sinful acts of bestiality. Human semen was corrupted within the animal that received it. The progeny that resulted was of an 'anomalous Breed' and the tainted matter made its way back to the 'spermatick vessels of the more noble unlading Animal'.[86] For this 'sin against the principles of our Being', offenders were therefore punished with the Yaws.[87] Indians and Africans, by this logic, were inclined to such forbidden acts and had populated their native lands with new (quasi-human) beasts. They had also passed on the loathsome disease they had acquired to Europeans. Yet non-Europeans had been punished twice, in Trapham's account.

Whereas should he descend to an unsutable communication, and such but generally obtain, he must quickly quit his Royalty, if not to the beastly herd itself, yet to whose retains entire Humanity. Hence the Black may well become naturally Slaves, and the vast Territories of the Indians be easily invaded, and kept in subjection by inconsiderable force of the Spanish Tyranny. And even those Conquerors through mixture with these animal people, reap their infirmity of body and mind.[88]

As one can see, monogenism hardly stood as a bulwark against hateful depictions of non-European peoples. Certain races had, in Trapham's account, acquired bestial natures after the first and common creation. Indians and Africans had produced people-like animals, but they had become animal-like people, and had thus contributed to their own oppression.

Syphilis' modes of spread could do double duty in connecting the disease to certain peoples. As a venereal illness, it was associated with the lascivious – Indians, Africans, Jews and others.[89] Gabriel Dellon, for example, noted in his *A Voyage to the East Indies* that venereal disease 'is as common, and appears with the same Symptoms among the *Frenchmen* living in those Parts, as among the *Negro's*, they being equally given to Debauchery'.[90] The affliction was also, however, regarded as one that could be passed to future generations.[91] It could thus be imagined as both proper to a certain people, and also dangerous to those who associated with them. Yet such people did not need to be racialised, for one might also regard the distemper as proper to a certain *place*.

[86] Ibid., 115–16.
[87] Ibid., 115.
[88] Ibid., 117.
[89] Foa.
[90] Gabriel Dellon, *A Voyage to the East-Indies: Giving an Account of the Isles of Madagascar, and Mascareigne, of Suratte, the Coast of Malabar, of Goa, Gameron, Ormus: As Also a Treatise of the Distempers Peculiar to the Eastern Countries: To Which Is Annexed an Abstract of Monsieur De Rennefort's History of the East-Indies, with His Propositions for the Improvement of the East-India Company* (London: D. Browne, A. Roper, D. Leigh, 1698), 231.
[91] Sydenham, 248.

Sydenham, more critical than Trapham of 'that barbarous Custom of changing Men for Ware', also associated the disease with lands outside Europe, but argued against those who claimed that its native seat lay in the Americas, suggesting that the disease was born in Africa, and had been spread through the slave trade.[92] The fact that it had declined in virulence over the years, however, seemed to suggest an environmental cause. '[L]ike vegetables, being as it were transplanted from its own Country into another', he wrote, 'it does not so much flourish in Europe, but languishes daily, and the *Phenomena* grow milder'.[93] Although communicated by people, then, the disease seemed produced or shaped not by the characteristics of a race, as Trapham had claimed, but by the characteristics of a climate.

The majority of authors tended to follow Sydenham in ascribing the cause of illnesses to climate, environment, or diet, rather than innate racial difference. Sloane, Sydenham's protégé, observed only one disease out of scores that seemed related to the physical peculiarities of black bodies. Otherwise, his emphasis was on similarities. Venereal diseases, for example, 'had the same symptoms and course among Europeans, Indians, and Negroes'.[94] Indeed, the similarity of bodies led to an uncharacteristic rebuke of white Creole custom. Black wet-nurses, he noted, were used as often as white ones, being much more common, but were 'not coveted by Planters, for fear of infecting their children with some of their ill customs, as Thieving &c'. Sloane remarked that he had never observed such a consequence 'and am sure a Black's milk comes much nearer the Mother's than that of a Cow'.[95]

Few other authors had much good to say about the natives they encountered, yet they did not phrase their hostility in racialist terms. Bosman, for example, claimed that the inhabitants of Africa were 'all without exception, Crafty, Villanous, and Fraudulent, and very seldom to be trusted', but he did not ascribe this character to a physical cause.[96] Medically, he noted that the characteristic diseases of the region were the small pox and worms. The former, of

---

[92] Ibid., 247.
[93] Ibid., 248.
[94] Sloane, cxxviii.
[95] Nonetheless, he acknowledged that 'yet in Jamaica some Children are bred up by the Hand very well'. Ibid., cxlviii.
[96] Bosman, 117. The only other group of people who seem to come close to Negroes in baseness for Bosman were Muscovites. See, for similar levels of disdain, James Houston, who wrote of the natives of the Guinea Coast: 'I shall say only in one Word, that their natural Temper is barbarously cruel, selfish, and deceitful, and their Government equally barbarous and uncivil; and consequently, the Men of greatest Eminency amongst them, are those that are most capable of being the greatest Rogues; Vice, being left without any Check on it, becomes a Virtue. As for their Customs, they exactly resemble their fellow Creatures and Natives, the Monkeys'. Houstoun, 33–4.

course, was the scourge of Europe, the latter afflicted Negroes most, but not exclusively. In terms of their afflictions, then, Negroes and Europeans were not remarkably different.[97] Towne made the same point even more explicitly in discussing a disease apparently unknown in Europe yet common among blacks, namely 'Elefantiasis under the circumstances it occurs in the West Indies'.[98] Towne made clear that the predisposing causes of the illness were not specific to any one group. It struck those who had suffered through tedious illnesses and were then 'constrained to subsist upon bad diet and undigestible unwholesome food' or exposed to inclement weather.[99] 'Sometimes', he noted, 'white people, whose unhappy circumstances have reduced them to hardships but little inferior to what the Blacks are obliged to undergo, have given us proof that this disease is not limited to one colour'.[100]

Other than Atkins, the most detailed account of racial difference in a medical text before 1740 is to be found in T. Aubrey's *The Sea-Surgeon, or the Guinea Man's Vade Mecum*.[101] A subtitle of the work noted that it was intended 'for the Use of young Sea Surgeons', and Aubrey offered particular advice for those given the charge of maintaining the health of slaves bought on the coast of Guinea. Reasons of both economy and morality, Aubrey suggested, should lead to better treatment of Negroes, which better treatment could be supplied by limiting the number of ignorant surgeons and curbing the abuses of sailors, 'who beat and kick them to that Degree, that sometimes they never recover, and then the Surgeon is blamed for letting the Slaves dye, when they are murthered, partly by Strokes, and partly famished'.[102] One of the surgeon's roles, Aubrey argued, was to convince captains that slaves be better treated, if only out of the latter's financial self-interest. Such cynicism might well work on captains who cursed slaves for dying, but Aubrey himself put forward a remarkable position that promoted equality of medical treatment on theological grounds while simultaneously advocating for a more profitable form of slavery.[103]

[O]ne ought to please and flatter them as much as one can, because the more you preserve of them for the Plantations, the more Profit you will have, and also the greater Reputation and Wages another Voyage; besides it's a Case of Conscience to be as carefull of them, as the white Men; for altho' they are Heathens, yet have they a rational

---

[97] Bosman was, however, scathing about Mulattoes: 'This Bastard Strain is made up of a parcel of profligate Villains, neither true to the Negroes nor us ... [w]hatever is in its own Nature worst in the *Europeans* and *Negroes* is united in them'. Bosman, 141.

[98] Towne, 184.

[99] Ibid., 185.

[100] Ibid., 188.

[101] T. Aubrey, *The Sea-Surgeon, or the Guinea Man's Vade Mecum* (London: John Clarke, 1729). A *Vade Mecum* is, essentially, a handbook.

[102] Ibid., 128.

[103] Aubrey noted that his captain had asked 'what a Devil makes these plaguey Devils dye so fast?', ibid., 132.

Soul, as well as us; and God knows whether it may not be more tolerable for them in the latter Day, than for many, who profess themselves Christians.[104]

It was in the context of a discussion of improved care for the property of slavers that Aubrey introduced his comments on the physical and medical differences of different inhabitants of the African coast. 'It is highly necessary for you to endeavour to be acquainted with the Nature and Constitution of these People', he wrote in a chapter entitled 'Of the Negroes', 'together with their accustomed manner of Living, which will the better qualify you for preserving their Health, and also restoring them when afflicted'.[105] Aubrey divided Negroes into four groups, organised by colour, relative presence of 'aerial Spirit', and characteristic afflictions. The first were of 'a kind of Chocolate Colour; their Hair is commonly very short, crisped, and of a dark Russet'. Such people were, in terms of temperament, 'most commonly surly, proud, haughty, vain-glorious, quarrelsome, revengeful, implacable, yet commonly very valiant, and much given to Venery'. Possessed of the greatest amount of aerial spirit, the blood in such bodies was greatly inclined to inflammation and common illnesses included erysipelas and ardent fevers. The second group were 'natural Black, and are commonly lusty, strong, vigorous, cheerful, merry, affable, amorous, kind, docile, faithful, and easily diverted from Wrath, their Hair is very black, and may be drawn out to a great Length'. With less aerial fluid than the first group, their bodily fluids circulated less rapidly. Their characteristic illness was the pleurisy. With an eye to a key element of his occupation, Aubrey noted that these people, of all he would discuss, were the best tempered and made the best slaves. The third group he described as 'yellow, and for the most Part dull, heavy, sluggish, lazy, idle, stupid, timorous, and easily impos'd on; their Hair is of a dark brown, and may be drawn out to a great Length'. Their fluids moved even more slowly than the first two peoples', containing still less aerial fluid, and their characteristic afflictions were diarrhoea and, among women, the Fluor Albus or the Whites. The fourth group were those for whom Aubrey had the greatest distaste and 'are of a dark russet Colour, their Hair black and crisped, and very thin, which never grows to any great Length; they are naturally sad, sluggish, sullen, peevish, forward, spiteful, fantastical, envious, self-conceited, proper at nothing, naturally Cowards, very indecent, and nasty in all their Transactions'. Their appalling character was matched by the diseases with which they were most commonly afflicted. With the least amount of aerial spirit in their fluids their humours circulated slowly and were inclined to corruption, leading to leprosy, scurvy and 'schirrhous Tumours'. They were, moreover, 'the worst of Slaves, and very few of them

[104] Ibid., 121.
[105] Ibid., 102.

can be brought to Decency, or any tolerable Subjection, either by Flattery, or Austerity'.[106]

That we should not understand these divisions in racial terms is fairly obvious. There was a common cause of both physical differences and the body's tendency to be afflicted by certain diseases: the relative presence or absence of aerial fluid. Such a presence or absence was not a racial trait so much as a constitutional one. Europeans could be divided into four groups as well, and those groupings precisely mirrored those of Aubrey's 'Negroes'. Where one found the most aerial spirit, skin was swarthy, the hair brown or black, the inclination to venery high, and the intellect witty; where there was less, the skin was florid and hair usually brown, and 'the Disposition cheerful'; less still and the complexion was pale, the hair whitish or yellow-brown, 'the Sleep sound and long in Duration'. Once again, the last group was the least appealing: the complexion 'duskish livid', the temperament 'peevish and sullen'.[107] Aubrey made the obvious connection: 'These are the several Constitutions which the Ancients call Choleric, Sanguine, Phlegmatic and Melancholy'.[108] Unlike the ancients, however, Aubrey denied that one could find any of these humours in the blood, pointing to air as the elemental difference. One can thus see that rather than describing four African races, he had merely described choleric, sanguine, phlegmatic, and melancholic constitutions in Africa. Of the reason that natives of the Guinea coast were, in general, darker than whites, Aubrey said nothing, although given the emphasis throughout the text on climate and diet, one suspects that he would offer a fairly conventional environmentalist explanation.[109]

One can see in both Aubrey and Towne evidence of the neo-Hippocratism described in some detail in Chapter 2. Hippocrates was the first source cited in either man's work and one might see each of them as exemplars, in the periphery, of a movement also occurring in the metropole, which wedded the questions and approaches of *Epidemics*, and *Airs, Waters, and Places* with natural philosophical investigations of the weather and air more generally. Of the metropolitan works, the most systematically Hippocratic was almost certainly John Arbuthnot's *Essay Concerning the Effects of Air on Human Bodies*.[110] The sixth chapter, 'Concerning the Influence of Air on Human Constitutions and Diseases' began with a five page summary of *Airs, Waters, and Places,* noting

---

[106] Ibid., 104–5.

[107] Ibid., 10.

[108] Ibid., 11.

[109] 'I am persuaded', he declared, for example, 'that there is no Disease of whatsoever kind it be, but is either generated from a Deficiency of insensible Transpiration, or vitious Food; or inquinated Air'. Ibid., 22.

[110] Arbuthnot.

that 'this great Man' explained not only the relationship between diseases and the weather, but also ascribed the various complexions, temperaments, and governments of mankind to the different constitutions of the air in which such people lived.[111] Climate generally, and the air specifically, was thus responsible for geographically specific distempers and the physical appearance of the natives of given lands. 'There are Faces not only individual', Arbuthnot wrote, 'but gentilitious and national; *European, Asiatick, Chinese, African, Grecian* Faces, are characteris'd'.[112] And while he acknowledged that part of this commonality of features within nations was due to 'propagation' from the same stock, he also argued, again following Hippocrates, that air had a role to play: 'That the Complexion depends much upon the Air, is plain from Experience; the Complexion of the Inhabitants of several Countries being fair, swarthy, black, and adust, according to the Degrees of Heat, Drought, Moisture, or Coolness of the Air'.[113] Perhaps most telling, however, Arbuthnot insisted that climate would trump race when it came to 'Temper and Genius', given only a few years. Those who lived in the same countries at different times, he claimed, would come to possess the same character, 'even tho' the Race has been changed'.[114] Today's Frenchmen were largely the same as the Gauls in the time of Caesar, he asserted, adding his belief that 'if a Race of *Laplanders*' were today transported to Paris, they would rapidly become much like the men in that location described by the Emperor Julian in the fourth century.[115] John Huxham would make similar claims about the common cause of racialised physical differences and disease, in his *Observationes de aëre et morbis epidemicis*, suggesting that a Hippocratic orthodoxy had taken hold on the issue by the 1730s.[116]

To summarise, then, it might be suggested that medicine and 'science' (meaning natural philosophy and natural history) were in a rather similar

---

[111] Ibid., 123.
[112] Ibid., 146–7.
[113] Ibid., 148.
[114] Ibid., 149.
[115] Ibid., 149–50.
[116] John Huxham, *Observationes de Aere et Morbis Epidemicis: Ab Anno MDCCXXVIII Ad Finem Anni MDCCXXXVII, Plymuthi Fact. His Accedit Opusculum de Morbo Colico Damnoniensi* (London: S. Austen, 1739). Huxham thus writes: 'The great Dictator in Medicine, *Hippocrates*, asserts that not only the Diseases, but also the Temperatments and very Manners of Men, depend greatly on the various Constitutions of the Air, in his most elegant Book on Air, Water, and Situations'. On the relationship between physical difference and endemic diseases, he wrote: 'The Heat of the torrid Zone so exhausts the Liquids of the Inhabitants, and so crisps up their Fibres, that they look as if quite burnt up. – From the Relation of Physicians, who have practised in these Parts, their Blood is found much more thick and black than that of the *Europeans*; hence most ardent and pestilential Fevers are endemic in such Climates, the Humours growing putrid on the slightest Occasion'. *The Works of John Huxham, M. D. F. R. S. In Two Volumes*, I, xxvi, xxv.

position at the beginning of the eighteenth century. One finds a few isolated flirtations with racial logics in each realm. Such flirtations would continue in race-science, with Voltaire and Hume's polygenism (from the 1730s and in the 1750s, respectively) suggesting that race was beginning to function as causal explanation and not merely a climatic or special creative effect. The same was not true in medicine, where an environmentalist Hippocratic orthodoxy after the 1720s twinned race and disease together, as common effects of a much more important set of causes: location, diet, and – most importantly – air. It is with this growing separation between 'science' and medicine on the subject of race in mind that we turn to John Atkins: polygenist surgeon.

5.4   A Little Heterodox: John Atkins, Polygenism, and African Diseases

Born in 1685, Atkins began his medical training as a surgeon's apprentice and then joined the navy, serving in multiple locations. In 1721, he sailed for the Guinea Coast, with two ships sent to suppress piracy there. After meeting with moderate success, but suffering significant casualties, the ships sailed to Brazil and the West Indies before returning to England in 1723. Failing to find another position at sea, Atkins turned to writing. In 1724, he published *A Treatise on the Following Chirurgical Subjects*, the fifth chapter of which was concerned with 'some *African* Distempers'.[117] The *Treatise* was restructured and republished in 1734, as *The Navy-Surgeon*, with the section on African diseases moved to an Appendix. Atkins expanded on this material the following year, in an account of his journeys in the early 1720s, *A Voyage to Guinea, Brasil, and the West-Indies; in His Majesty's Ships, the Swallow and Weymouth*. Second, unaltered editions of both texts appeared in 1737, and a substantially modified third edition of *The Navy-Surgeon* was published in 1742.[118]

The *Treatise* began with a defence of surgery against the pretensions of the modern physician. Before the present degenerate age, Mankind had lived longer, healthier lives. Physic had largely been limited to the preservation of health through attention to the six non-naturals, particularly diet, rather than 'the various and inexplicable Prescriptions of Physick as it now stands'.[119]

---

[117] There is no date given on the text. The *Daily Journal* of 21 December 1724, however, lists the text as 'To Morrow will be publish'd'. The copy located in the Beinecke library at Yale appears to have been given to Yale College by the author in 1729. My thanks to the research librarian, Elizabeth Frengel, for confirming this for me.

[118] For biographical materials, see N. M., 'Atkins, John (1685–1757)', *Dictionary of National Biography* 2 (1885); F. Tubbs, 'John Atkins: An Eighteenth-Century Naval Surgeon', *British Medical Bulletin* 5 (1947–8).

[119] John Atkins, *A Treatise on the Following Chirurgical Subjects* ... (London: T. Warner, 1729), Preface, i.

Surgery, Atkins claimed – citing the wounding of Abel – had preceded physic in the cure of maladies, and it was Chiron the centaur, skilled in the surgical treatment of ulcers, who had taught medicine to Aesculapius. Followers of Aesculapius in the present, however, had vastly and unnecessarily multiplied diseases, hypotheses, and prescriptions 'that the Age of Man is scarce sufficient to make a Disquisition into'. The surgeon, on the other hand, required relatively little theoretical knowledge to practice his craft: anatomy; 'the different secretions of the Body'; the use of a small number of basic *materia medica*; and knowledge of the non-naturals supplied almost everything that could be necessary, beyond extensive practical study. It was the fruits of such practice that Atkins offered the reader, with chapters on ruptures, fractures, amputations, dislocations, and (with separate pagination) that scourge of the military man: venereal diseases.[120]

All of the above topics can be considered basic knowledge for the naval surgeon at any location, so one may understand why, in the next version of his text, Atkins should move the section on venereal disease within the main body of the work and remove his 'Journal of the Sick on the Coast of Guiney' to an appendix. Where all military surgeons should be familiar with the treatment of ruptures and gunshot wounds, for example, Atkins recommended his diary to 'those whose Fortune may carry them in the same Tract'.[121] Beginning with a characterisation of the climate – very warm (but with cooling breezes) and with thick, moist air that could 'rust your Pocket Instruments, Swords, or any Kind of Steel Implements in a Day's Time' – Atkins soon turned to a discussion of the cause and treatment of the illnesses suffered by his crew in 1722. The death rate, as he would note in *A Voyage to Guinea*, was almost unimaginable. The *Weymouth*, for example, left England with a complement of 240 men: by the time the ship returned – having picked up more men along her journey – she had lost a total of 280.[122] At one point in his travels, Atkins was made purser, since everybody else who might take up the position had died.[123]

Atkins blamed the climate and the dubious morality of the men. The heat of the sun was near overpowering, vastly worse on land than at sea, and when the

[120] Discussing the last, Atkins denied that the disease was a new one, brought back from the Siege of Naples. The affliction arose, he argued, first in women who had received too many partners. Excessive friction, coupled with an 'ill habit of body' produced ulcers, 'which Ulcer will be the Distemper'. Since this vice had existed long before the Siege, Atkins argued, so too had the disease, 'as Antient as corrupted Nature, it being irrational, either to suppose a World drowned for their Sins, Strangers to the Vice that contracts it, or that their Wickedness any more than ours deserved Exemption'. Ibid., Appendix, 4, 1.

[121] Ibid., 177.

[122] *A Voyage to Guinea, Brasil, and the West-Indies; in His Majesty's Ships, the Swallow and Weymouth*, 139.

[123] Ibid., 196.

sun set the air cooled and was filled with vapours, leading to dews that soaked beds through. Drunk on palm wine by the end of the day, men would fall asleep in the open air, their perspiration suddenly checked by the chill, which led almost inexorably, in Atkins' telling, to fevers 'more or less Malignant'. Even when sober, however, the men were not to be trusted. Sent on shore, where they were harder to manage than within the confines of the ship, they were 'ungovernable in their Actions and Appetites', stealing from the locals 'and debauching their wives' while eating and drinking whatever they pleased 'without any Enquiry how proper or wholesome for Food, or having any Regard to Custom and Manner of Living'.[124] Medical treatment availed of little and the crew eventually pushed out to sea, hoping (rightly, as it turned out) that a change of location and concomitant alterations of behaviour might halt the 'epidemical rage'.[125]

Having explained the diseases of European sailors in terms of their environment and behaviour, Atkins turned finally to the diseases that afflicted Africans, dividing these into two groups: 'Coast Negroes' and 'Inland Negroes', the latter of whom made up the bulk of those taken for the slave trade. Coastal Negroes, he asserted, were untroubled by many of the chronic and acute European illnesses because they were spared a luxurious way of life, subsisting largely on vegetable matter, bathing occasionally, and exercising enough to expel the recrements of their food. These coastal dwellers, he claimed, 'were abundantly more sprightly and active than the Inland Natives' who had not been 'mended' by their interactions with Europeans and 'are to appearance but a few Degrees in Knowledge above Beasts'. Some distempers – smallpox and sore eyes, for example – were clearly common to Europeans and Africans alike, but Atkins focused his discussion on four that were distinctive to Negroes: the sleepy distemper, the croakra, the yaws, and the chicoes.

Although he declared all four diseases 'more properly their own', the latter three were barely peculiar to a given people, let alone to be explained in racialist terms.[126] The yaws was the local term for venereal disease and was so similar to 'our Pox and Clap' that Atkins deferred further discussion to a subsequent chapter, where he would treat the subject in its generality. Chicoes were what had been known for a long time as 'Guinea' worms and were 'common with them, tho' not so properly said to be peculiar', since one also found them in the West Indies. If they afflicted Africans more often than Europeans, it was presumably because locals more often walked barefoot in the waters where the eggs of the 'insects' were found. The croakra, Atkins explained, was a skin

[124] *A Treatise on the Following Chirurgical Subjects*, 185–6.
[125] Ibid., 192.
[126] Ibid., 197.

disease, brought on by a change of diet and possibly by carelessness in drying the skin when it had been wet by salt water.

It is worth emphasising the dietetic and behavioural aetiology for croakra that Atkins supplied because it was in the context of his discussion of 'the distempered skins of *Africans*' that he turned to a consideration of the cause of their skin's colour. His polygenetic views would follow, but he did not adopt a racialist explanation of the disease: black skin might be peculiar to Africans, who had been created separately to all other humans, but the diseases of that skin were to be explained not by originary physical difference, but by the fact that – on slave ships – they were constantly in contact with sea water and were forced into 'a sudden Change to an unusual and coarse, if not a salt, Diet'.[127]

The natural cause for the dark skin and woolly hair of the inhabitants of much of Africa, Atkins declared, 'must ever perplex Philosophers to assign'.[128] Malpighi, it was true, had located the cause in the colour of a subcuticular mucus, but that had merely pushed the question back a step: why was the mucus differently coloured in different peoples? One could explain tanning under a hot sun by suggesting that the lightly coloured mucus of fine European skin was warmed until its thinner parts were eliminated, leaving 'the Remainer dark, as the clearest Liquors, they say, will leave some sediment'.[129] But Atkins doubted that the darkness of Africans could be explained through this mechanism, offering five reasons for thinking that such mechanical explanations would be inadequate. First came the argument by analogy with animals. Atkins noted that the sun did not seem to have the same effects on other animals in Guinea as it was assumed to have on humans. If the sun were responsible for producing the woolly hair characteristic of Africans, why did local sheep 'have hair contrary to that closer Contexture of the Skin, which is supposed to contribute to the Production of Wool in the humane Species'? The second argument involved a comparison with Europeans. Why did white skin never turn black and why did the skin of Mulattoes remain intermediary in colour between the two extremes? Third, Atkins observed that one could not explain African skin colour entirely by pointing to the tint of a sub-cuticular mucus, for the colour of black skin changed as the higher layers of skin altered. Black feet and hands gradually whitened, Atkins claimed 'by Friction and constant use' and the cuticle paled after the skin was burnt or scalded. Fourth, one might compare Africans to Americans, the latter of whom lived under an equally burning sun, but were not as black. Fifth and finally, not all Africans – despite their residence under the same sun – were the same colour. 'I saw

[127] Ibid., 202.
[128] Ibid., 203.
[129] Ibid., 204.

one ... who was woolly and, in every Respect else, a Negro ... but in Colour', he reported. A conclusion seemed to follow by necessity. 'From the whole', he asserted, without seeming awareness of the radicalism of the claim, 'I imagine that White and Black must have descended of different Protoplasts [i.e. progenitors], and that there is no other Way of accounting for it'.[130] No more was said on the issue, and the discussion turned back to the diseases 'peculiar' to the Guinea Coast.

Despite the brevity of Atkins' polygenetic remarks, it seems a reasonable question to ask, as Norris Saakwa-Mante has, about possible connections between Atkins' racial theories and his understandings of African diseases.[131] Did the surgeon regard the distempers suffered by Negroes as a result of the originary difference between their physical frames and those of Europeans? For three of the four distempers he analysed, including the seemingly most obvious case, involving an affliction of the skin, the answer would appear to be no. The fourth case – the sleepy distemper – is more complex. Though the affliction was apparently common, the symptoms were unusual. It came on suddenly, prefaced only with a few days of reduced appetite. Most characteristically, it induced deep slumbers and reduced sensation. '[P]ulling, drubbing, or whipping', Atkins observed with a disturbing dispassion, 'will scarce stir up Sense and Power enough to move, and the Moment you cease beating, the Smart is forgot, and down they fall again into a State of Insensibility, drivling constantly from the Mouth as if in a deep Salivation'.[132] The immediate cause seemed obvious to Atkins. The sufferer's brains were filled with a surfeit of phlegm or serum, which obstructed the nerves. One found somewhat similar conditions in Europe, he noted, among the elderly. Those who, during a long lifetime had indulged too much in food and drink, found themselves eventually with a brain the tone of which was significantly weakened, which could lead to habitual sleepiness. And yet, Africans were largely strangers to luxury and the Sleepy Distemper in Africa seemed to afflict the young and those 'destitute of the Means of Surfeiting'.[133] Whatever the cause of excessive drowsiness might be in Europe, the same causes seemed not to be in operation in this disease.

Atkins, in fact, pointed to three causes for the Sleepy Distemper: 'Cold and Immaturity'; 'Diet and Way of Living'; and 'the natural Weakness of the Brain'. In this edition of the text, neither the first nor the second were racialised.

---

[130] Ibid., 204–5. Atkins would seem here to be explicitly referencing Giordano Bruno, who had written in his own polygenetic musings, that: 'Aethiopum/genus ad illum protoplasten nemo sani iudicii referet [No one of sound judgment will trace the nation of the Ethiopians to that first man.] Quoted in Malcolmson, 192.

[131] Saakwa-Mante.

[132] Atkins, *A Treatise on the Following Chirurgical Subjects*, 197–8.

[133] Ibid., 199.

That the young seemed to suffer disproportionately from the disease made some sense, for in youth, Atkins noted, the elements of the body 'have not yet attained their due Spring and Perfection' and the body produced more phlegm and other drossy matter. In the 1734 version of his remarks, Atkins added a single half sentence to this discussion: 'and it is only supposing the *Africans* continue longer Children than the Europeans'.[134] Whether this extended youth was a result of the climate or was inherited from a different protoplast, Atkins did not say. The inadequacies of the local diet meant that the blood produced from such nutriment declined in quality while the indolence characteristic of native Africans meant that waste matter that resulted from the concoction of food into blood was not adequately disposed of during exercise. As a result, this waste matter found its way to the brain, which Atkins declared to be the weakest part to be found among Negro slaves.

It was this 'natural Weakness' of the African brain that Atkins thought was 'the principal Cause' of the sleepy distemper.[135] And where neither youth, diet, nor way of life seemed to point to any fundamental or original difference between the bodies of Negroes and Europeans, Atkins did suggest that Africans were 'hereditarily ignorant'. Brains, he argued, were like muscles, which gained in strength through exercise. Africans were 'destitute of all Art and Science, or any mechanical Knowledge to exercise the Brain'.[136] In consequence, that organ became ever weaker over time and from this weakness flowed the disease: 'the Brain must grow weak, and such a State of Thoughtlessness and Inactivity, dispose it for the Reception of Serosities'.[137] Saakwa-Mante has argued that this claim about the weakness of African brains 'is clearly intended as a racial characteristic'.[138] I remain unsure. The muscular metaphor is unclear, for it seems to suggest that Black and White brains begin in similar states and that – over a lifetime – the brains of Africans atrophy for lack of significant use. Weakness would appear to be acquired rather than innate. Moreover, the language of hereditarianism, which would in most cases be the most convincing evidence for racialist thought, here applies not to physical characteristics, but to knowledge (or its lack). Two factors would seem, in fact, to speak against a racialist reading, both concerning the distinction Atkins drew between Coastal and Inland Negroes. While both groups, one assumed, derived from the same co-Adamic original, each was not equally afflicted by the sleepy distemper, which seemed particularly to strike slaves, who were drawn from 'Country

---

[134] *The Navy-Surgeon: Or, a Practical System of Surgery*, 1st ed. (London: Caesar Ward and Richard Chandler, 1734), 20.
[135] *A Treatise on the Following Chirurgical Subjects*, 201.
[136] Ibid.
[137] Ibid., 202.
[138] Saakwa-Mante, 44.

People', rather than those from the coast.[139] Coastal people were less ignorant (thus overcoming their heredity?) and exercised more, allowing the expulsion of recrementitious humours. Were the sleepy distemper a racial trait, derived from structures of the brain passed down from a protoplast, one would expect that the disease – like skin colour or hair type – was essentially fixed. Fixity, after all, was one of Atkins' strongest arguments against a climatic explanation of the hue of African skin. Yet susceptibility to the sleepy distemper was anything but fixed: contact with Europeans had apparently produced African peoples who were not habitually plagued by the affliction, even if their Country brethren remained so.

Later texts only seem to emphasise the disconnect between Atkins' polygenetic theories and his medical explanations.[140] With few changes, *The Navy-Surgeon* reproduced the claims of *The Treatise*. The *Voyage to Guinea*, however, considerably expanded upon them. The 'colour, language, and manners' of Africans, Atkins observed, was as different 'as we may imagine we should find in the planetary Subjects above, could we get there'.[141] And the difference in physical features led one, again, to an assumption concerning separate creations:

The black Colour, and woolly Tegument of these *Guineans*, is what first obtrudes itself on our Observation, and distinguishes them from the rest of Mankind, who no where else, in the warmest Latitudes, are seen thus totally changed; nor removing, will they ever alter, without mixing in Generation. I have taken notice in my *Navy-Surgeon*, how difficultly the Colour is accounted for; and tho' it be a little Heterodox, I am persuaded the black and white Race have, *ab origine*, sprung from different-coloured first Parents.[142]

As in the earlier works, however, fixity seemed limited only to the skin and hair. Even other physical features were deemed changeable. 'Their flattish noses', for example, came about 'owing to a continued grubbing in their Infancy against their Mother's Backs'.[143] And levels of intelligence or civilisation were eminently improvable: ignorance may have been inherited, but it was not a permanent condition. 'That these people could arrive to better Knowledge by the use of proper Means and Instruction, there is no manner of doubt', Atkins declared. 'They give proof enough that their natural Endowments are

---

[139] Atkins, *A Treatise on the Following Chirurgical Subjects*, 198.

[140] The first edition of *The Navy-Surgeon* (1734) added only an ambiguous half line to the arguments offered in the section on the Guinea Coast in the 1724 *Treatise*, even as it restructured the latter text and made additions to the Preface.

[141] Atkins, *A Voyage to Guinea, Brasil, and the West-Indies; in His Majesty's Ships, the Swallow and Weymouth*, 34.

[142] Ibid., 39.

[143] Ibid., 180.

capable of following any pattern'. Although incapable of advance on their own, they could be led: 'when the Seeds and principles are laid by letter'd Nations, it is not then nigh so difficult to improve'.[144] The 'muscle' of the brain was capable of further exercise, in other words. What was now weak could become stronger.

It is hard, in general, to determine what drew Atkins to his polygenetic ruminations, or why he should have felt the need to publish views so heterodox. Cristina Malcolmson has placed Atkins toward the end of a lineage of authors responding to the set of questions posed in Robert Boyle's 'General Heads for a Natural History of a Counterey', published in the first volume of the *Philosophical Transactions* in 1666.[145] A paragraph of Boyle's queries asked after the inhabitants of new lands:

And in particular their Stature, Shape, Colour, Features, Strength, Agility, Beauty (or the want of it) Complexions, Hair, Dyet, Inclinations, and Customs that seem not due to Education. As to their Women (besides the other things) may be observed their Fruitfulness or Barrenness; their hard or easy Labour, &c. And both in Women and Men must be taken notice of what diseases they are subject to, and in these whether there be any symptom, or any other Circumstance, that is unusual and remarkable.[146]

The similarities to the issues discussed by Atkins seem self-evident. Yet both Boyle himself and the vast majority of those who took up his queries were committed to monogenism. It has sometimes been suggested that polygenism could function as a defence of slavery, but Atkins was deeply critical of that institution; considerably more so, indeed, than Boyle.[147] A theme running through *A Voyage* involves the debunking of the idea that Africans were cannibals. Tales about anthropophagy, he suggested, proceeded from the attempt 'to magnify the Miracle of escaping an inhospitable and strange Country' and also by design, in order 'to justify Dispossession ... Conquest and Cruelty' from those who convinced themselves that they were 'only subduing of brutish Nature'.[148] Hardly enthusiastic about Africans, who he described as cowardly, thievish, and lazy, Atkins was nonetheless near absolute in his hostility to the slave trade. Highly critical of the natives of the Guinea Coast, then, Atkins was well aware that much harsher positions than his own existed, and a proportion of his text sought to push back against this harshness. In fact, one of

---

[144] Ibid., 82–3.
[145] Atkins, Malcolmson argues, 'writes for the Royal Society, since he constructs his narrative in terms of the "General Heads", comments on Boyle's experiments on the air, and mentions a wealth of articles from the *Philosophical Transactions*'. Malcolmson, 191. See also 62.
[146] Robert Boyle, 'General Heads for a Natural History of a Countrey, Great or Small, Imparted Likewise by Mr. Boyle', *Philosophical Transactions* 1 (1666): 188.
[147] On Boyle's support for slavery and defence of monogenism, see Malcolmson, e.g. 15.
[148] Atkins, *A Voyage to Guinea, Brasil, and the West-Indies; in His Majesty's Ships, the Swallow and Weymouth*, xxiii.

the most remarkable parts of *A Voyage* – and one of the few where polygenism was explicitly invoked in support of another contention, rather than simply for its own sake – involved the deployment of the doctrine of separate creations as a *defence* of Africans against those who would criticise their lack of true religion. Having never received the benefit of revelation, how could they be judged for their heathenism?

They are set down as from the Clouds, without Guide, Letters, or any means of Cultivation to their better Part, but what immediately strike their Senses from beholding this Universe and the Beings contained in it; their Deductions from whence, as to a Deity devoid of Matter, is next to impossible, therefore we say mean and pitiful.[149]

Atkins polygenetic remarks remained unchanged in the second edition of *The Navy-Surgeon* and *A Voyage to Guinea*, both of which appeared in 1737. *A Voyage* would not be published again, but *The Navy-Surgeon* appeared in a third edition in 1742 and (posthumously) in 1758. And in these two last, Atkins completely retracted his polygenism while keeping unaltered his descriptions of diseases 'peculiar' to Africans. We shall get to Atkins' new racial views in a moment, but it is worth noting that the third edition of *The Navy-Surgeon* was, most generally, a very different book from its earlier versions. All of those had pitched themselves as practical works; guides to the day to day tasks of a surgeon at sea and in foreign lands. The 1742 edition, by contrast was considerably more scholarly. Loaded with many more quotations and references to classical and modern works, the book now opened not by getting straight into a discussion of fractures, but by considering the general question of the nature of sensation. Atkins added a 'dissertation' on cold and hot mineral springs and the introduction now included a disquisition on the life and changing fortunes of medical men in the Navy, covering many of the same issues that would reach a much larger audience with the publication of Tobias Smollett's *The Adventures of Roderick Random* in 1748. It was once easy to gain a berth as a naval surgeon, Atkins noted ruefully, 'when the Sea and the Gallows were said to refuse none'. Now, however, competition was fierce and seemed to turn not on the question of qualifications, but on personal wealth and powerful patronage.[150]

One finds multiple additions, small and large, even within the Appendix on Guinea.[151] In part, presumably, because the *Voyage* had covered not only Africa, but the West Indies and Brazil, and partly also because British troops had recently suffered such losses due to disease in the New World, Atkins now

---

[149] Ibid., 82.

[150] *The Navy-Surgeon; or, Practical System of Surgery with a Dissertation on Cold and Hot Mineral Springs; and Physical Observations on the Coast of Guiney* (London: J. Hodges, 1742), 1.

[151] Among the more minor, but still intriguing, is the addition of a name for the people living in Africa near the Southern latitude of 34 degrees: 'Hotmentotts'. Ibid., 367.

added several remarks about the West Indies. In the brief discussion of the Yaws, for example, he now noted that the word was used commonly in both places and that the disease might be more prevalent in the New World, 'where the Sexes not being balanced, may give greater Occasion for Infection'. In spite of a long tradition that sought to portray Africans and their descendants as promiscuous and immoral, Atkins argued that the opposite was true. The Yaws was uncommon on both the Guinea Coast and Inland, he observed. 'Nature perhaps repays their Ignorance of Means to cure, by a stronger Love and Inclination to Continency'. It was true that their women were almost always naked, but Atkins took this as a positive development. As a result, their 'Lust is glutted', and when they married, their friendships were stronger and more lasting, 'as not founded so much in Concupiscence'.[152] The section on Chicos, or worms, was also expanded, in this case dramatically. Natural Historical questions about the origin of Guinea worms segued into Natural Philosophical questions about the origin of life, the cause of the earth's rotation, and the nature of the soul and consciousness. In the previous two editions the text had concluded with remarks on removing worms from the skin. Now the final paragraph was pious and elegiac, Atkins 'advising all ... who wish for Immortality, to cast their Sheat-Anchor on Revelation', and commending 'one Faith, one Baptism, and one Lord Jesus Christ'.[153]

One must suspect that such seemingly new-found piety lay behind Atkins' decision to abandon views that were more than 'a little heterodox'.[154] In considering the differences between black and white bodies, the surgeon did not back off his criticisms of explanations that relied on the action of the Sun. All five objections to climatic causality were reproduced verbatim. But Atkins now excised his conclusion: there was no mention of different protoplasts. Instead, he offered a different explanation, and an environmental one at that. His 'Guess on this abstruse question' was now that differences in skin colour and hair type were due to differences in the soil in which generations had been bred.[155] Expanding his geographical perspective, Atkins acknowledged that it was not only blacks and whites who seemed utterly different. Brazilians were

---

[152] Ibid., 370.

[153] Ibid., 378.

[154] Another textual addition now offered an argument by design to explain the difficulties involved in navigating the Guinea Coast. 'If it be lawful to investigate the final Cause of such Obstacles as above to Navigation; one would think they had been set as a Guard to the Inability and Ignorance of the Natives, to protect them from the Cheat, Insult, and Slavery of Trading Nations'. Ibid., 351. The critique of slavery continued later: 'The Company mark [slaves] still *D. Y.* Duke of *York*, to perpetuate the Ignominy of his Headship to that Trade'. Ibid., 364.

[155] Ibid., 368. On seventeenth-century attempts to explain racial difference by pointing to differences in the soil of various locations, see Malcolmson, 58.

a different hue to Northern American natives, East Indians were different from each of these again, 'and all as distinct as black and white, which happens I imagine chiefly, on account of the Soil each is bred and nurtured in'. The soil changed the taste of plants when they were transplanted to different countries and 'Men by a like Analogy, change considerably by removing, even in their own Lives, and were they to marry and abide there'. Imagining earlier humans spreading across the globe, Atkins seemed to suggest that environs differing from that of their homelands could eventually turn even the whitest men as black as the African natives among whom they now found themselves and could make the English – a mixture of many peoples – into a single nation, physically distinguishable from its neighbours:

Particularly in those great Transmigrations of *Goths* and *Vandals*, quite to *Africa*, who are now without any Distinction from the ancienter Natives; so are the Moors in *Spain*. Ourselves are a Mixture of different Nations and *Complexions*, and 'tis the Soil has united them *English*, so as by that alone almost, to be distinguished from our nearest transmarine Neighbours.[156]

Having treated of plants and men, Atkins turned lastly to the animal kingdom, finding evidence there as well for the effects of transplantation. He had personally observed, he noted, that dogs, cocks, and sheep changed in both their 'Nature and Looks', and some animals simply could not be bred in regions of the earth far removed from their original.[157] Man was not so limited, but the price of his mobility was the alteration of his frame, not by the action of the sun in the heavens, but by the soil of the earth.

Atkins' case is a fascinating and revealing one, although it tends to trouble easy classification. For David Livingstone, Atkins' polygenetic utterances are evidence that '[p]lainly, the idea of multiple Adams was now receiving a more widespread airing'.[158] Yet Atkins published considerably earlier than all the other examples to whom Livingstone points and his 'airing' of co-Adamite ideas lasted only thirteen years before it was rejected in favour of a more orthodox environmentalism. If there was an opening for polygenetic views in the 1730s – Voltaire's comments suggest that this might have been so – it was narrow and, for Atkins at least, rapidly closed, opening again in the 1750s in the work of men such as the Reverend Hughes and David Hume. Perhaps the most interesting thing about Atkins' polygenism while it lasted, however, was its limitations. Co-Adamitism did virtually no *work* for Atkins. Unlike L. P., Voltaire or Hume, Atkins was seemingly uninterested in a critique of

---

[156] Atkins, *The Navy-Surgeon; or, Practical System of Surgery with a Dissertation on Cold and Hot Mineral Springs; and Physical Observations on the Coast of Guiney*, 368–9.

[157] Ibid., 369.

[158] Livingstone, *Adam's Ancestors: Race, Religion, and the Politics of Human Origins*, 61.

the Church or intellectual orthodoxies more generally. Polygenism was not part of a larger iconoclastic project. Nor, as we have seen, did Atkins' views on race inform his medical theories. If there is some little ambiguity about the connection between Atkins' posited aetiology for African sleepy distemper and his theories of originary physical differences, any supposed connection evaporates in later editions, which retain the former and abandon the latter.

Yet the conclusions that we may draw from a close reading of Atkins are not all negative. Indeed, the opposite is true, particularly when we compare his case to that of later polygenists (see Chapter 6). Virtually the sole target for ruminations about separate creations until the 1770s was the Church (Hume is an interesting exception). Apparently uninterested in an argument with clergy, Atkins' naturalistic heterodoxy went nowhere. In the latter part of the century, however, a second target emerged: the abolitionist movement. And one increasingly finds naturalistic arguments that apparently saw little value in a critique of literalist readings of biblical narratives turning their guns, instead, on a more secular vision of the brotherhood of Man and natural rights. Reading Atkins' earlier texts, then, helps us remember a time when medical environmentalism persisted, even while anti-climatic physical fixity was being posited, and when polygenism could, indeed, be only a 'little heterodox' (although even that little would prove too much), in the hands of a surgeon with seemingly no axe to grind against established theology.

6   Race, Slavery, and Polygenism: Edward Long and *The History of Jamaica*

Of all the Enlightenment figures to take up the question of race, there is perhaps none so infamous today as Edward Long, the Jamaican planter whose three-volume *History of Jamaica* appeared in 1774.[1] The notoriety is not undeserved. Long's racial calumnies stand out in a period where even those committed to monogenesis – the idea of the fundamental, original unity of humankind – stressed the bodily stench of 'Negroes' as an important, hereditary racial characteristic.[2] Hottentots, Long claimed, were 'a people certainly very stupid and brutal'.[3] So similar were they to orangutans that a Hottentot woman should regard it as no dishonour to be wedded to a simian husband. He suggested that the African slaves who worked sugar plantations in the West Indies were a different species from their white masters and denied that, in most cases, the offspring of white and black coupling could be fertile. Mulattoes were further analogised to mules.

Polygenism – the belief in separate creations for different human races – was, in the eighteenth century, a position both heterodox and unpopular.[4] Yet even among the radical racialist minority that adopted and promoted the position, Long's arguments were the most detailed and, frankly, the most odious. Hume's claim that nature had made an 'original distinction' between the various 'breeds of men', while oft quoted by pro-slavery advocates, was only to be found in a footnote to the second edition (1753) of his 1748 essay on 'National

---

[1] Edward Long, *The History of Jamaica, or, General Survey of the Antient and Modern State of the Island: With Reflections on Its Situation Settlements, Inhabitants, Climate, Products, Commerce, Laws, and Government: Illustrated with Copper Plates.*, 3 vols. (London: T. Lowndes, 1774).

[2] See, for example, Immanuel Kant, 'Von Den Verschiedenen Racen Der Menschen', in *Der Philosoph Für Die Welt*, ed. J. J. Engel (Liepzig: Dr Stintzings Bibl.,1777); Buffon.

[3] Long, *The History of Jamaica*, II, 364–5.

[4] That said, national distinctions mattered. Polygenism was more popular in France than Britain, where 'coy monogenism' dominated. Kidd refers to polygenism as a 'controversial fringe viewpoint in the British world', Kidd, *The Forging of Races: Race and Scripture in the Protestant Atlantic World, 1600–2000*, 85. As Stepan has noted, polygenism 'remained a minority strand of British racial thought' into the 1860s. Stepan, 3.

Characters'.[5] Lord Kames, whose polygenist views appeared the same year as Long's, found himself unable to commit completely to contradicting Biblical testimony on the unity of man, even as he denied that any natural cause could produce current racial diversity from the supposition of a single creation.[6] Voltaire, of course, had no such qualms in refuting Biblical claims, yet his heresies seem rather tame compared to Long's vicious racialism. 'Few eighteenth-century writers', David Brion Davis noted in 1966, 'could equal Edward Long in gross racial prejudice'.[7]

Even Long's contemporaries found his racialist views reprehensible, or at least (when they felt some sympathy towards them) requiring public repudiation. The polygenist portions of his *History* were overwhelmingly more likely to be cited by abolitionists – who must have been delighted to find a straw man come to life – than by the pro-slavery advocates among whom Long numbered himself.[8] Among the reasons it proved easy to dismiss Long's arguments was the fact that they reeked of special pleading. As a Jamaican planter and owner of slaves, Long could not pretend to any objectivity on the questions of Negro inferiority or the permissibility of the slave trade. Presumably, this is why we possess no detailed account of Long's arguments across the three volumes of his *History of Jamaica*, nor even an answer to what would appear to be the most basic question: What is the relationship between Long's defence of slavery and his advocacy of polygenism?

We do not have such an answer, I would suggest, because we believe that we already know it. Yet if Long's motives appear transparent, his arguments are not.[9] One might, for example, imagine that, since Long advocated the idea of special creations, he was free to claim that Africans (and their descendants in

---

[5] David Hume, 'Of National Characters', in *Hume: Essays, Moral, Political, and Literary*, ed. E. F. Miller (Indianapolis: Online Library of Liberty, 1987), 197–215, on 8, discussion of variant readings on 629–30. On the relation of this footnote to the remainder of the essay, see Kidd, *The Forging of Races: Race and Scripture in the Protestant Atlantic World, 1600–2000*, 93–4.

[6] *The Forging of Races: Race and Scripture in the Protestant Atlantic World, 1600–2000*, 95–9.

[7] David Brion Davis, *The Problem of Slavery in Western Culture* (Ithaca: Cornell University Press, 1966), 459.

[8] Seymour Drescher, *The Mighty Experiment: Free Labor Versus Slavery in British Emancipation* (Oxford: Oxford University Press, 2002), 76–7. The situation may have been different in the United States. Curtin argues that 'Long's greatest importance was in giving an "empirical" and "scientific" base that would lead on to pseudo-scientific racism. The part of the *History of Jamaica* dealing with race was reprinted in America in the *Columbia Magazine* of 1788, where it became support for later American racism'. Curtin, *The Image of Africa: British Ideas and Action, 1780–1850*, 45.

[9] On this point, and on Long more generally, see Anthony J. Barker, *The African Link: British Attitudes to the Negro in the Era of the Atlantic Slave Trade, 1550–1807* (London: Frank Cass and Company, 1978). Barker notes: 'Long's ulterior motives seem obvious. And yet there is just enough about the man and his work to raise doubts as to whether his racism meant something more', 41–2. For an excellent and sophisticated take on Long, one that is also attuned to the complexities of his positioning, see Wheeler.

the West Indies) were subhuman: essentially a kind of animal. Since it was perfectly legal to own animals, human chattel slavery would be justified. Yet, this is precisely *not* what Long argued. Rather than reducing Negros to the level of beasts, Long raised the Orang-Outang to the level of men, offering a three-level ranking of human species within *genus Homo*. His claim naturalised Negro inferiority, of course, but it did not do so by literalising the claim that Negroes were beasts of burden.[10]

The aim of this chapter is both to explicate and situate Long's arguments, in order to answer the question posed above. Or, rather, to explain why Long himself never quite answered it. For there is no point in the more than 1500 pages of his *History* where Long explicitly invoked his racial theories to justify or excuse his anti-abolitionism. I am thus focused here on Long's understanding of racial anatomies, leaving, for the most part, his claims about racial pathologies for Chapter 7. Of the three axes on which Part III seeks to re-locate race, this chapter emphasises two: period and location. In terms of the former, it is useful to contrast Long's Enlightenment racialism with forms more familiar from the nineteenth century. Heterodox as he was, there were still limits to iconoclasm. Yet Long was idiosyncratic even compared to many of his contemporaries, for reasons related to his geographical position. As previously noted, many if not most intellectual histories of race have (for a variety of reasons) focused upon metropolitan figures.[11] By contrast, my own attention has largely been on men who lived or worked in locations far from Britain. Long was one such figure. By re-locating race discourse to the colonies, by situating Long in the context of West Indian debates over slavery and meanings of physical difference, and by contrasting his forms of racialism to ostensibly similar figures in Britain and Europe, this chapter aims to provide a nuanced account of the relationships between slavery, race, and place.

That such relationships must be understood as nuanced and complex should be stressed. I noted in Chapter 5 that there was no necessary connection between Atkins' polygenism and his understandings of diseases he deemed to be characteristic of Africans. A close study of Long's writings makes clear that we should be equally cognisant of the subtleties connecting race and slavery. The intellectual history of the former, of course, cannot be written independently

---

[10] *Contra* Barker, who has claimed that both Estwick and Long 'suddenly declared the Negro sub-human'. Barker, 58. The views described in this chapter are closer to the majority position. See Philip D. Curtin, *The Image of Africa; British Ideas and Action, 1780–1850* (Madison: University of Wisconsin Press, 1973), 44. Even earlier was Jordan, who notes: 'Long did *not* imply that the Negro was actually a beast ... It is of the utmost significance that the most virulent traducers of the Negro were forced to wildly strenuous and preposterous attempts at proving that the orang-outang was nearly human'. Jordan, 493.

[11] An important exception is Delbourgo's study of the 'imperial creole', John Mitchell: Delbourgo, 'The Newtonian Slave Body: Racial Enlightenment in the Atlantic World'.

of the intellectual history of defences of the latter. Beliefs in racial fixity (and concomitant assertions of unchangeable racial inferiority) first became fully viable elements of public discourse in the 1760s and 1770s in response to strident criticisms of the slave system. Natural equality had been an easier position to hold when the slave system was largely unthreatened and anti-equality arguments followed quickly and reactively in the face of abolitionist critiques and – eventually – victories. Long's case provides a clear example of this reactive racialism, as he enunciated his positions, in 1772 and 1774, in direct response to a court ruling (the Somerset Case of 1772) which was read as negating the legitimacy of slavery on British soil. Yet Long's example also makes clear that the connection between defences of racial fixity and defences of slavery were not straightforward. Indeed, Long's arguments on these issues tended to point in opposite directions: legal arguments in defence of slavery posited a kind of equivalence between Africans and Britons; polygenism denied such equivalence outright. Forms of racialism and anti-abolitionism were related, then, but they were not necessarily connected in simplistic, instrumentalist ways.

The chapter is divided into four sections. The first two consider the justifications Long *did* offer for the necessity of the slave trade in the Americas. Almost all of these were presented in a legal register and need to be read as a response to the judgement delivered by Lord Mansfield in the Somerset case (1772), a decision that appeared to outlaw slavery on British soil. Section 6.1 discusses Long's criticisms of Mansfield's decision in 1772. The arguments in Long's *History* two years later must be read as a continuation, refinement, and elaboration of these criticisms. Many of these arguments, I show in Section 6.2, require the assumption not only of a bare humanity for Africans, but for the legitimacy of their legal systems, so that contracts entered into on African soil must be honoured.

Section 6.3 examines Long's articulation and defence of polygenism. Having done so, however, I point to the fundamental ambivalence of Long's position. It is an ambivalence that provides one of the major reasons – despite contemporary refutations – that we should pay attention to Long's claims. For Long was one of very few eighteenth-century writers on 'race science' with an extensive lived experience in and with political sympathies toward a part of the world that was both outside the bounds of the European metropole and which also contained a majority black population.[12] This ambivalence in Long's writings

---

[12] Long was born in England, but his family had strong connections to Jamaica. His great grandfather had served with Cromwell's army in 1655, his wife descended from an officer in the Penn and Venables expedition of the same year, and his family owned a large estate in Clarendon, Jamaica, known as Longville. It has been noted that the publication of his *History* 'marked the first occasion on which an extended historical narrative was undertaken by an author with a prolonged association with the island'. Howard Johnson, 'Introduction', in *The History of Jamaica* (Montreal: McGill-Queens University Press, 2002), 1. For other examples

on race, I show, stemmed directly from his desire to manage social relations and political systems in a slave society. Metropolitan figures who believed in the fixity of race (regardless of the question of origin) made a cornerstone of their position the essential identity of newly arrived African slaves and their descendants. If race were truly fixed, then the new environment of the New World could have little effect on the mental endowment, moral character, or physical features of the offspring of slaves born in Africa. For Long, however, the difference between 'salt-water' and 'creole' Negroes was to be the solution to the most pressing social problem of the sugar islands: slave insurrection. Where newly arrived slaves were believed to be the most likely protagonists in a future uprising, Long hoped that a selectively gentler slavery might win mulattoes and creoles to the side of plantation owners. This understanding of the (potential) political and social differences between generations of slaves, I argue, required a physical corollary: Long's polygenism presumed less fixity than the monogenism of a figure like Immanuel Kant.

If the realities of the Jamaican slave system provide one reason that Long's racialism is somewhat 'softer' than one might expect from a polygenist slave owner, Long's theology provides another. Long's, I argue in Section 6.4, was a physical rather than a mental racialism. Physical traits – skin colour foremost among them – were fixed; mental traits were far more subject to climatic and social influence. That this was a permissible distinction flowed from Long's dualism, for he refused to accept that the physical structures of the brain were responsible for human reason. Unlike Voltaire or Hume, then, Long was a polygenist who was not a materialist, willing to buck Biblical orthodoxy on one position while firmly rejecting heterodoxy on another.

In the conclusion, I reflect on two rather broader lessons to be drawn from Long's case. First, the need to pay more attention to the disjunction between the colonial practice of race science and its metropolitan theory; and second the need to distinguish, from Long's work onwards, between the registers in which proponents and opponents of polygenism spoke. Long's was the first major text, I would suggest, where polygenism was put forward, not as a minority position in theology, but rather as a minority position in natural history and physiology. It marks the point at which polygenism, and race theory more generally, became a claim about the racial present, rather than the biblical past.

of authors writing in a scientific register about race outside of Europe see, most famously, Thomas Jefferson, *Notes on the State of Virginia* (1781). See also Mitchell. On Mitchell, see Delbourgo, 'The Newtonian Slave Body: Racial Enlightenment in the Atlantic World'. Stepan's classic work is almost exclusively devoted to major metropolitan figures. This was, no doubt, part of a conscious choice to emphasise 'the main figures in science rather than the minor ones'. Stepan, xix.

6.1   Anti-Abolitionism and The Somerset Case

Candid Reflections

In March, 1749, James Somerset was purchased as a slave in Africa and transported to Virginia, where he was sold to Charles Steuart on 1 August. Twenty years later, in 1769, Steuart made a business trip to England and took Somerset with him, planning to stay for as long as necessary and then return to America. In 1771, Somerset fled Steuart's service, at which point Steuart tasked James Knowles, the Captain of a ship bound for Jamaica, to seize and imprison Somerset before taking him to the West Indies for sale. When news of Somerset's capture reached several prominent abolitionists, including the lawyer Granville Sharp, they brought a writ of *habeas corpus*, which Lord Mansfield, Chief Justice of the Court of King's Bench, granted. On 9 December, Knowles gave Somerset over to the custody of the court.[13] Mansfield delivered his judgement, in favour of Somerset, in June the next year

'Perhaps no 200 words', Dana Rabin has noted, 'have been subject to closer scrutiny'.[14] Mansfield's reported language left his ruling open to both narrow and expansive readings:

The state of slavery is of such a nature, that it is incapable of being now introduced by Courts of Justice upon mere reasoning, or inferences from any principles natural or political; it *must* take its rise from *positive* law; ... and in a case so odious as the condition of slaves must be taken strictly: the power claimed by this return was never in use here: no master ever was allowed here to take a slave by force to be sold abroad because he had deserted from his service, or for any other reason whatever.[15]

---

[13] This description of events derives from Captain John Knowles' testimony, quoted in Francis Hargrave, *An Argument in the Case of James Sommersett, a Negro, Lately Determined by the Court of King's Bench: Wherein It Is Attempted to Demonstrate the Present Unlawfulness of Domestic Slavery in England. To Which Is Prefixed a State of the Case* (London: W. Ostridge, 1772), 4–8. The classic discussions of the case are William M. Wiecek, 'Somerset: Lord Mansfield and the Legitimacy of Slavery in the Anglo-American World', *The University of Chicago Law Review* 42, no. 1 (1974); David Brion Davis, *The Problem of Slavery in the Age of Revolution, 1770–1823* (Ithaca: Cornell University Press, 1975), 469–522.

[14] Dana Rabin, ' "In a Country of Liberty?": Slavery, Villeinage, and the Making of Whiteness in the Somerset Case (1772)', *History Workshop Journal* 72 (2011): 19. For an excellent discussion of the relationship between the Somerset case and that of Mary Hylas in Hylas v. Newton, see Katherine Paugh, 'The Curious Case of Mary Hylas: Wives, Slaves, and the Limits of British Abolitionism', *Slavery and Abolition* 35 (2014). *The Politics of Reproduction: Race, Medicine, and Fertility in the Age of Abolition* (Oxford: Oxford University Press, 2017).

[15] Taken from the report of the case given in *The Scots Magazine* 34 (1772): 297–9. There is considerable disagreement today over the precise wording of Mansfield's decision. The *Scots Magazine* version has been described as 'probably the most accurate account of the judgment' by George van Cleve, 'Somerset's Case Revisited: Somerset's Case and Its Antecedents in Imperial Perspective', *Law and History Review* 24, no. 3 (2006): 632. It is also the version reproduced by Samuel Estwick, although Estwick altered the punctuation in ways that slightly alter its meaning.

Today, most scholars tend to support the notion that Mansfield intended something quite narrow in his ruling. His decision did not outlaw slavery in England, although it did forbid the forced removal of slaves from England and granted that a writ of *habeas corpus* applied to such cases of removal. Yet, as Seymour Drescher has shown, many slaves and masters at the time read Somerset's case as the end of English slavery.[16] Certainly Long, claiming to speak for West Indian planters, read Mansfield's ruling broadly, as asserting 'That the laws of *Great Britain* do not authorize a master to reclaim his fugitive slave, confine, or transport him out of the kingdom. In other words; that a Negroe slave, coming from the colonies into *Great Britain*, becomes *ipso facto*, Free'. Lawyers, Long noted, had succeeded in 'washing the black-a-moor white'.[17]

If they were unhappy with Mansfield's decision, it was nonetheless clear that the specific ruling in Somerset would have little effect on the day to day life of West Indian planters. It would surely be no more than an inconvenience to be unaccompanied by a slave while spending time in England. Far more ominous for slave holders in the Americas were the implications of the ruling, for almost every colonial constitution included a clause that forbade local legislatures from enacting a law deemed 'repugnant' to the laws of England. If slavery was unlawful and even 'odious' in the mother country, what could its status be at the reaches of the Empire?[18] One can thus understand both why Long should think it worthwhile to publish a tract debating Mansfield's decision and also why his pamphlet on the 'Negroe cause' was structured as it was. Only the latter part of Long's text dealt with the perceived injustice and potential consequences of the Somerset ruling. The first half offered a more general legal defence of slavery within the British Empire. Long's arguments were threefold. First, there was nothing new about African slavery. In the language of Mansfield's decision, 'immemorial usage' condoned the practice, which Long likened to an earlier form of unfreedom: villeinage. Villeinage, Long acknowledged, no longer existed. Not because it had been abolished, but because it had grown into 'desuetude' on English soil. 'On the decline of

---

[16] Seymour Drescher, *Capitalism and Antislavery: British Mobilization in Comparative Perspective* (Oxford: Oxford University Press, 1987), 36ff.

[17] Edward Long, *Candid Reflections Upon the Judgement Lately Awarded by the Court of King's Bench in Westminster Hall, on What Is Commonly Called the Negroe-Cause, by a Planter* (London: T. Lowndes, 1772), 56, iii.

[18] As Long phrased it, the doctrine in Somerset's case 'maintains, that Negroe slave-holding is inconsistent with the laws of *England*; and if it be so, this plain conclusion follows, *viz.* that every colony law which has been enacted touching this supposed property, whether by securing it to the planter, by making it deviseable in last wills, inheritable by his heirs, liable as assets for payment of his debts, subject to mortgage or other grants and alienations, are entirely void and null in themselves, to every intent and purpose, *as being repugnant to the laws of England'.* Ibid., 58–9.

villeinage within the realm', however, 'a species of it sprang up in the remoter parts of the English dominion, the *American plantations*'. The vision of the torch of unfreedom being passed from metropole to periphery was powerful both in its general argument, which suggested a continuity of laws, and in its specifics. For an English villein, while enjoying the rights of a free man in relation to others, was essentially the property of his lord, who owned the rights to his labour and that of his posterity. Among the very few rights of the villein with respect to his master was that to *Habeas Corpus* – a right that protected against imprisonment without trial and hence unlawful incarceration. According to Long, however, villeinage laws deemed the mere refusal to serve one's master sufficient cause for imprisonment. By analogy, then, the only rights available to a Negroe slave were those available to 'a similar class of inhabitants', namely villeins. Hence 'a right to his *Habeas Corpus cum causa*, yet neither bailable nor deliverable, if the cause returned should be, *his refusal to serve his Planter-master*, in any lawful employment'.[19]

Long's second argument was perhaps less legal than it was political and economic. The West India colonies, he claimed, were simply not viable if they were not worked by those born in and inured to hot climates. The argument was not necessarily a racialist one, for Long acknowledged that white creoles made up a potential workforce. But, he claimed, few white workers would agree to take on the laborious tasks of clearing land and planting crops unless compelled to do so by indigence. Under such circumstances, slavery was a necessity.[20]

Long's third and perhaps most convincing argument charged the English state with hypocrisy for a ruling that outlawed slavery in England while passing legislation that regulated the slave trade in Africa so as to maximise English profits. Numerous statutes could be found that had decreed Negroes, in the colonies, to be a form of property, liable to be seized, for example, for the payment of debts. With some justice, Long pronounced it 'preposterous' that the same state that had passed laws declaring Negroes to be commodities could then say that 'Negroe slaves emigrating from our plantations into this kingdom are to be deemed *free subjects of the realm*'.[21]

To these three general defences of the legitimacy of West Indian slavery, Long next appended two arguments that ostensibly treated the Somerset case alone. One of these amounted to little more than racialist scare-mongering, raising the prospect that the promise of emancipation would bring thousands of former slaves to British shores. The ruling, he asserted, was 'a direct invitation

---

[19] Ibid., 13.
[20] Ibid., 21.
[21] Ibid., 29, 33.

to *three hundred thousand blacks*' who could only make worse the dreadful situation in which 'the nation already begins to be embronzed with the African tint'. Sounding somewhat hysterical, he alluded to the possibilities of miscegenation, made possible by the fact that 'The lower class of women in *England* are remarkably fond of the blacks, for reasons too brutal to mention; they would connect themselves with horses and asses, if the laws permitted them'. Negroes, Long suggested darkly, might even be able to exploit a system of rotten boroughs and buy their way into a parliamentary seat.[22]

Rather more intellectually serious were Long's arguments about the question of compensation for the loss of property represented by slaves emancipated by English courts. The imperial state had allowed a situation where its laws were 'inconsistent with itself; there appears a direct collision between one part and another'. The planter who legally purchased a slave as a form of property in the colonies could then be deprived of that property in England. The responsibility for ameliorating this seemingly obvious injustice, Long argued, lay firmly at the feet of the English state, who 'should make him some requital, and by a fair purchase ... redeem his Negroe from bondage'.[23] An apparently reasonable response to the specificities of the Somerset case, this argument must surely also have functioned as a shot across the bow for those who might hope, post-Somerset, to convince the English state to suddenly outlaw slavery in its colonies. Were slavery indeed to be deemed 'repugnant' to English law, the English state would be responsible, Long implied, for the losses experienced by colonial planters. Abolition was unlikely to harm planters alone.

Race Theory and Slavery: Samuel Estwick and Considerations on the Negroe Cause

I have spent some time in elaborating Long's multiple arguments against Mansfield's ruling and the possibility of abolition for three reasons. First, as we shall see, because we find in them the germs of several of the claims made in *The History of Jamaica* two years later. Second, because the differences between the arguments made in the *Candid Reflections* and the *History* are then revelatory of the specific effects of Long's responses to reading other tracts dealing with the Somerset case. We can assume, for example, that by 1774 Long had read Francis Hargrave's *An Argument in the Case of James Sommersett* (1772).[24] Hargrave had delivered what were among the most convincing arguments in favour of Somerset during the trial, and published a

---

[22] Ibid., 59, 54–5.
[23] Ibid., 44.
[24] Hargrave.

version of those arguments soon afterward. Chief among them was his rejection of the analogy between villeinage and slavery with which Long had opened his *Candid Reflections*.[25] Whether Long accepted Hargrave's arguments or not, his own claims concerning the analogy between slavery and villeinage – although they did not disappear – nonetheless declined in importance in his *History*.

The third reason for paying close attention to the arguments in Long's *Candid Reflections* is the most important for this chapter. In spite of the clear bigotry on display in the tract from 1772, Long made no use there of theories of polygenism or even racial fixity. Indeed, the opposite was true. Although 'unseasoned' whites were incapable of labouring in Jamaica's climate, the same was not true of white creoles. The most important issue with regard to the question of whether an individual could withstand the rigours of plantation labour was not race but nativity. White or black, the only way to withstand the West Indian climate was to be born in it, or one very like it.

The source for many of Long's initial ideas on polygenesis appears to have been another pamphlet written in opposition to Mansfield's judgement, penned by the assistant colonial agent for Barbados, Samuel Estwick. Long read Estwick's text while his own was in proofs.[26] Long claimed to identify a number of similarities between the two documents, but the central arguments were, in fact, strikingly different. Estwick began by agreeing with Somerset's allies that African slavery bore little connection to villeinage.[27] In Estwick's view, however, slavery – novel or not – was not the point. For Negroes, according to English law, were not slaves: they were property. The argument was counter-intuitive, but in a sense it needed to be. Like Long, Estwick emphasised the apparent contradiction in English laws that regulated slavery in Africa and the colonies while declaring it illegal on English soil. Like Long, too, he noted that no law could be allowed in the colonies that contradicted fundamental tenets of the legal system of the mother country. Unlike Long, however, he did not conclude that the contradiction in metropolitan and peripheral laws was simply a matter of hypocrisy. Instead, he sought to resolve the contradiction by arguing

[25] Cf. Granville Sharp, *A Representation of the Injustice and Dangerous Tendency of Tolerating Slavery; or of Admitting the Least Claim of Private Property in the Persons of Men, in England* (London: Printed for Benjamin White, (no. 63) in Fleet-Street, and Robert Horsfield, (no. 22) in Ludgate Street, 1769). To my mind, Davis overemphasises the intrinsic implausibility – in the 1770s – of the analogy between villeinage and slavery. See Davis, *The Problem of Slavery in Western Culture*, 483.

[26] Long, *Candid Reflections Upon the Judgement Lately Awarded by the Court of King's Bench in Westminster Hall, on What Is Commonly Called the Negroe-Cause, by a Planter*, 75–6. Estwick had intended to submit his remarks to Mansfield prior to the decision, but the text had been held up, and was published a month after the ruling. Samuel Estwick, *Considerations on the Negroe Cause, Commonly So Called, Addressed to the Right Honourable Lord Mansfield, Lord Chief Justice of King's Bench, &C. By a West Indian* (London: J. Dodsley, 1772), 45–6.

[27] Estwick, *Considerations on the Negroe Cause, Commonly So Called, Addressed to the Right Honourable Lord Mansfield, Lord Chief Justice of King's Bench, &C. By a West Indian*, 5.

that the objects of legislation in each place were different. In regulating the sale of Negroes, Estwick argued, Parliament had declared them non-human property, like any other goods. If they were not human under the law, they could not be slaves.

The case is this, my Lord: seeing that Negroes are human creatures, it would follow that they should be allowed the privileges of their nature; which, in this country particularly, are in part the enjoyment of person and property. Now, my Lord, from hence a relation is inferred, that has not the least colour of existence in law. A Negroe is looked upon to be the servant of his master; but by what authority is the relation of *servant* and *master* created? Not by the authority of law, however it may be by the evidence of reason. By the law, the relation is, as *Negroe* and *Owner*: he is made matter of trade; he is said to be property; he is goods, chattel, and effects, vestable and vested in his owner.[28]

If Somerset was property, Estwick concluded, then the writ of *Habeas Corpus* could not apply, and Steuart should have his property returned to him.

Estwick's argument thus turned on the non-humanity of Negroes under English law. The second edition of his text – much extended and offered at a price sixpence higher than the first – elaborated on this claim. What was largely implicit in the first edition now became explicit, as in the following definition of slavery:

Slavery, my Lord, is that state of subjection, which mankind, by force or otherwise, acquire *the one over the other*. In every society therefore where this state of subjection prevails, the object and subject of those laws necessary for the regulation thereof are, what? *Human nature itself*. Let it be considered then whether *human nature* is either the object or subject of the laws of England, respecting the state and condition of Negroes.[29]

Answering his own question, Estwick claimed that it was both the will and the effect of 'the wisdom of parliament, that Negroes under the law should not be considered as human beings'. Rhetorically distancing himself from such an odious supposition, he then set himself the task of ascertaining why Parliament should have believed such a thing, dividing the putative arguments into two types: physical and political. 'Now the physical motive supposes a difference of species among men, and an inferiority of that species in Negroes: whereas the political consideration, on the other hand, infers a universal sameness in human nature; that is to say, in fact, that Englishmen are Negroes, and Negroes are Englishmen, to all *natural* intents and purposes'. Such a division, it will be noted, renders the political argument purely cynical, since it amounts to the following question: Given that Parliament believed that Negroes were fellow

---

[28] Ibid., 34–5.
[29] Samuel Estwick, *Considerations on the Negroe Cause, Commonly So Called, Addressed to the Right Honourable Lord Mansfield, Lord Chief Justice of the Court of King's Bench, &C*, 2nd ed. (London: J. Dodsley, 1773), 69–70.

human beings, why did it pass legislation that declared them not to be so? Estwick's answer charged the Government with explicit duplicity. Wishing to legislate to its own advantage, but fearing a public backlash to the legalisation of slavery, the state masked its real designs. 'Instead then of that Demon Slavery being called in to preside over Negroes, Trade, the guardian angel of England, was made the ruler of them'.[30]

Since the political argument accused the English state of intentionally misleading the public, Estwick's physical argument seems more palatable. This is no mean feat, given it was while explicating the latter that he came to posit polygenism. The differences between whites and Negroes, he claimed, were both corporeal and intellectual. Of the corporeal, he cited complexion and 'the wooly covering of their heads so similar to the fleece of sheep'. Of intellectual differences, Estwick pointed to what he described as savage forms of justice and other customs, and a 'barbarity' in their treatment of children which 'debases their nature even below that of beasts'.[31] The gulf between Africans and other humans, he suggested, was too large to be one merely of degree. Within the human *genus* one found not merely different races, but different species.

Like Long, who would follow him in this argument, Estwick made no explicit mention of the religious heterodoxy of his position. He made no reference to the Biblical passages usually cited by monogenists and their opponents: neither Adam nor Noah entered the discussion. Instead, he proffered a different kind of theological explanation, eschewing Biblical literalism in favour of an invocation of God's design in nature. In the vegetable and mineral kingdoms, as well as the animal kingdom excluding Man, one found 'these grand divisions of nature arranged in classes, orders, kinds, and sorts: we shall contemplate systems morally perfect'. Humanity – composed, it had been assumed, of a single, unified kind – stood alone in disrupting this ordered perfection. The assumption that Mankind was composed of multiple species, Estwick suggested, was one that exchanged the unity of a human brotherhood for a unity in God's design.[32]

Invoking the idea of a 'great chain of Heaven, which in due gradation joins and unites the whole with its parts', Estwick could then transform an originary difference into a natural inferiority.[33] Negroes were lower on the chain than

---

[30] Ibid., 88.

[31] Ibid., 80.

[32] Ibid., 72–3, 74.

[33] Estwick, *Considerations on the Negroe Cause, Commonly So Called, Addressed to the Right Honourable Lord Mansfield, Lord Chief Justice of King's Bench, &C. By a West Indian*, 74. The classic work on the chain is Arthur O. Lovejoy, *The Great Chain of Being: A Study of the History of an Idea* (Cambridge, MA: Harvard University Press, 1936). On its use in race-theory, see Stepan, 1–19.

whites, even if each could be considered 'wisely fitted' to its station.[34] And they would stay that way, for the boundary between species was fixed. From his own conclusions he inferred the logic of English lawmakers:

From this then, my Lord, I infer, that the measure of these beings may be as compleat, as that of any other race or mortals; filling up that space in life beyond the bounds of which they are not capable of passing; differing from other men, not in *kind*, but in *species*; and verifying that unerring truth of Mr. Pope, that
Order is Heaven's first law; and this confest,
Some are, and must be, greater than the rest:
The application of what has been said, is, that the Legislature, perceiving the *corporeal* as well as *intellectual* differences of Negroes from other people, knowing the irreclaimable savageness of their manners, and of course supposing that they were an inferior race of people, the conclusion was, to follow the commercial genius of this country, in enacting that they should be considered and distinguished (as they are) as articles of its trade and commerce only.[35]

Long's arguments on race in his *History* would borrow heavily – to the point of plagiarism – from Estwick's. But, as we will see below, his arguments concerning the legitimacy of West Indian slavery did not. The point is a crucial one. Estwick's polygenism and his defence of slavery were intimately and logically connected. The legal justification for slavery was that Negroes were non-human property. His polygenist arguments from natural history then buttressed that argument. Long, however, largely based his defence of slavery on notions of contract theory, which pre-supposed that both sides of the contract were human actors, even if one was inferior to the other. Taking part of Estwick's argument, but not its entirety, Long was left with contradictions that his own text was never quite able to resolve.

6.2   Slavery and *The History of Jamaica*

The History of Jamaica is a frustrating work. Lengthy, detailed, and – as Long himself admitted – digressive, it can read more like a series of discrete arguments than a coherent, single book. Long was magpie-like in his reading and would often crib and copy pages at a time from other texts, sometimes without fully digesting the arguments of his sources. This could lead to seemingly obvious contradictions, even within the same general set of claims. In a section of Volume II devoted to a description of the African slave trade, for example, the reader is told both that 'the slaves of a family are considered no mean part of it ... The owners are full as careful of bringing them up

---

[34] Estwick, *Considerations on the Negroe Cause, Commonly So Called, Addressed to the Right Honourable Lord Mansfield, Lord Chief Justice of the Court of King's Bench, &C.,* 74, 76
[35] Ibid., 81–2.

as their own children' and also that Africans 'consider their slaves merely as their necessary beasts'.[36] More common, however, were contradictions between distinct sections, since Long clearly had different axes to grind in each. Discussing the culture of 'Guiney Negroes', Long was scathing about their legal systems. Their laws were 'irrational and ridiculous'.[37] On the other hand, part of Long's defence of slavery required him to argue that Europeans should respect the right of African states to endorse and encourage slavery, framing that right not with ridicule, but in impressive eighteenth-century legalese: 'Africans having the right power of dispensing life or death; they are likewise empowered to regulate the conditions upon which life is granted, where it has been adjudged by their forms of proceeding to be forfeited to their laws, or customary usages'.[38]

It would be wrong, however, to dismiss the *History* entirely as a collection of incoherent, *ad hoc* arguments devoted to Long's particular interests. In most cases it is better, I would argue, to read the text as being in an almost inevitable tension with itself, brought about by Long's situatedness in several different contexts. One can see this by comparing arguments made in his *Candid Reflections* – addressed primarily to an English metropolitan audience – and those in the *History*, which was intended both to 'obviate slanders' from 'enemies of the West India Islands' and itself to criticise elements of Jamaican culture.[39] The argument Long made in 1772 for the necessity of slavery for the survival and economic prosperity of the sugar islands was straightforward: the climate was deadly for unseasoned whites. In his later and larger text, however, Long had much less interest in encouraging the vision of the West Indies as a death trap for new settlers. Both works cited James Lind's to buttress an argument for the necessity of using Negroes for the laborious and dangerous tasks of felling trees and clearing land. The *History* also cited Lind, however, for his claim that the West Indies was not the graveyard that many thought it was: 'The truth is, as Dr Lind has well observed, that every island in the West Indies, and other parts of the world, has its healthy and unhealthy spots'.[40]

The effort to de-emphasise the perils of the West Indian climate played into one of the *History's* largest themes: the stress on greater colonial self-sufficiency. Jamaican planter society was characterised by absenteeism. One-third of Jamaican planters were absentees in 1740; two-thirds in 1800.[41] Deeply critical of those who saw themselves as sojourners rather than settlers, Long

---

[36] Long, *The History of Jamaica*, II, 384, 89.
[37] Ibid., 378.
[38] Ibid., 391.
[39] Ibid., I: 6.
[40] This point would be oft-repeated. See, e.g. ibid., II: 506, 508.
[41] Andrew Jackson O'Shaugnessy, *An Empire Divided: The American Revolution and the British Caribbean* (Philadelphia: University of Pennsylvania Press, 2000), 4, 5.

wanted to encourage the establishment of local institutions – schools, medical colleges, local militia – and to promote white immigration. Obviously, claims that suggested that Jamaica's climate was deadly to whites were anathema to such aims and to efforts to keep British subjects in the West Indies for generations. At the same time, Long suggested that English illnesses in the colony were due, not to the climate itself (which was perfectly salubrious), but to the fact that settlers refused to adjust to their new living conditions. As a social practice, sojourning could lead to sickness. Englishmen sweltered in the hot tropical sun, dressed in tightly fitting coats and waistcoats, when they would be better off adjusting to the fashions of the East, and donning a 'Chinese Banyan'.[42] Most Europeans refused to adjust their diet, indulging in 'vast quantities of animal food' when a diet more appropriate to the climate would combine meat and vegetables, even 'inclining to the vegetable'.[43]

For much of the *History*, then, behaviour and custom trumped race or climate as an explanation for the health and well-being of the West Indian population. And even when there appeared to be racial differences in susceptibility to disease, Long was far more willing to incorporate social and cultural reasoning into the naturalistic explanations that had characterised his *Candid Reflections*. Making reference to the practices of slavery, for example, Long drew on the writings of the Revered Hughes, who had recommended that newly imported slaves be given only the 'gentlest' work during the first few years of their labour in the West Indies. They did not, that is, arrive 'seasoned' by virtue of their birth in the tropics. Like whites, they too required a period of adjustment.[44] And it was possible that race made no difference at all:

Their bodies and constitutions seem peculiarly adapted to a hot climate; yet, perhaps, they owe their health not more to this adaptation, than to their mode of living: since it is certain that the native Whites on this island, I mean such of them as are not addicted to drunkenness, nor have any hereditary distemper, are equally healthy and long-lived.[45]

Understanding Long's arguments, then, requires the realisation that there were often (at least) two distinct audiences for a given discussion: one in England, the other in the West Indies. This is certainly the case for Long's

---

[42] Long's discussion of the appropriateness of 'Eastern' dress was drawn from Hillary, *Observations on the Changes of the Air and the Concomitant Epidemical Diseases, in the Island of Barbados. To Which Is Added a Treatise on the Putrid Bilious Fever, Commonly Called the Yellow Fever; and Such Other Diseases as Are Indigenous or Endemial, in the West India Islands, or in the Torrid Zone.*

[43] Long, *The History of Jamaica*, II, 526.

[44] Ibid., 433, 28.Cf. Griffith Hughes, 'The Natural History of the Island of Barbados, Book II (1750)', in *On the Treatment and Management of the More Common West-India Diseases (1750–1802)*, ed. J. Edward Hutson (Kingston, Jamaica: University of the West Indies Press, 2005).

[45] Long, *The History of Jamaica*, II, 29.

defence of slavery, which is effectively divided into two parts. One deals with the trade in slaves in Africa, the other with the treatment and management of slaves in the West Indies. The former is legalistic and uncompromising – clearly written in opposition to abolitionists – the latter contains anti-abolitionist elements (refuting claims about the ill-treatment of slaves, for example), but is also, as we shall see, rather nuanced, offering prescriptions to ameliorate the practice of slavery on the island. In the end, *The History of Jamaica* would staunchly defend the legitimacy of the slave trade on legal grounds while criticising Parliamentary laws governing the trade on grounds that were at once moral and locally particular.

Long's opening salvo in defence of African slavery took on the question of its antiquity. Writing against prominent abolitionists like the 'Father of Atlantic Abolitionism', Anthony Benezet, Long asserted that a trade in slaves had been carried on by Africans for 'some thousand years'.[46] Although Europeans obviously profited by a trade in slaves, they could hardly be held responsible for creating the trade in the first place. Moreover, Long argued, European participation, far from ruining African lives, had improved them. Portuguese slavers, he suggested (while relying on the most critical accounts of African societies), may have thought it a 'meritorious act' to send slaves to work in their mines, thus saving them from the death, torture, cannibalism, and human sacrifice that characterised day to day life on the Guiney coast, 'thus mak[ing] their private gain compatible with the suggestions of humanity or religion'.[47] Regardless of motive, however, economics alone had lessened the savagery of African customs. Criminals and those captured in war were now worth far more alive than dead. It was those who sought to abolish the trade, Long argued with cynical cunning, who were without sufficient humanity, for to do so 'is therefore no other than to resign them up to those diabolical butcheries, cruelty, and carnage, which ravaged their provinces before the European commerce with them began'.[48]

Long's humanitarian defence of slavery stemmed from more than the desire not to immediately cede the moral register to his opponents. His moralising also drew the reader's attention to a more significant part of his argument: the character of those sold as slaves and, more particularly, the idea of slavery as punishment for legal infraction. Long suggested that those slaves sold to Europeans came from four distinct groups: war-captives; those sold 'by brutal parents, or husbands'; native slaves sold for some crime; and the free born, punished with slavery for a particularly egregious offence.[49] Ignoring the second category

---

[46] Ibid., 386; Maurice Jackson, *Let This Voice Be Heard: Anthony Benezet, Father of Atlantic Abolitionism* (Philadelphia: University of Pennsylvania Press, 2009).

[47] Long, *The History of Jamaica*, II, 387.

[48] Ibid., 391–2.

[49] Ibid., 388.

and minimising the impact of the first, he concentrated his attention on the two kinds of criminals. Citing a figure he had only recently read, Long claimed that it was 'well-known' that 99 per cent of slaves shipped from Africa were felons, their sentences commuted from death to exile and servitude.[50] Accepting this fact as true licensed a comparison both easy and powerful, for the British state had few qualms about the use of transportation as a punishment for criminals; fewer still about using such criminals as an indentured work force. Long had only to forget that he had recently condemned African laws as 'ridiculous' and to argue instead for an equivalence between the rights of African and European states to dispose of their unwanted as they saw fit.

It may be said of our English transported felons, as of the Negroe criminals, that neither of them go into a voluntary banishment; but it must be allowed, that the Africans may with equal justice sell their convicts, as the English sell theirs; and equally well vest a legal right to their service in the purchasers.[51]

Of course, Long was well aware of the limits of his analogy. African states may well have had the right to sell both criminals and their labour to Europeans in Africa. But by what right could one keep an individual convicted of no crime by British law in servitude in Britain or its colonies? The right, Long answered, of an implicit contract. Those captured in war, he argued, submitted voluntarily to slavery, for they had known the consequences of their actions in going to war, and had sought to reduce their opponent to the same state. Other slaves accepted the right of their owner to sell them 'as part of the law or usage of his society' and that right, Long asserted, was transferred across the seas. 'Surely a voyage from Afric to any other country, where this claim of property is continued, cannot dissolve the bargain'.[52]

Long's 'surely' in the sentence above was disingenuous. Abolitionists argued precisely that the claim of property over another human being – whatever its presumed legality in other nations – was anathema in Britain. Here Long must have felt the force of the Somerset ruling keenly. If a claim over property could dissolve in moving from Britain's periphery to its centre, how could one argue that contracts had to be maintained in moving between nations? But Long thought Mansfield had made a poor ruling, and he believed more generally that abolitionists overstated what was often portrayed as an innate English opposition to any loss of liberty. The fact of the matter was that unfreedom was a basic part of social life. It was hardly restricted to Africans

---

[50] Ibid., 391. The figure is given in An African Merchant, *A Treatise Upon the Trade from Great-Britain to Africa. Humbly Recommended to the Attention of Government* (London: R. Baldwin, 1772), 12.

[51] Long, *The History of Jamaica*, II, 390.

[52] Ibid., 394.

and their progeny and could only be defended by the exertion of force. It was force alone that kept the convict transported to America from evading his sentence, the inhabitants of debtor's prisons in confinement, the sailor and soldier in service, and the labourer in his place.

A labourer in England never consented to the laws which impose restrictions upon him; but there is in every government a certain supreme controuling power, included in the social compact, having the energy of law, or published and declared as the law of the land; by which every member of the community, high and low, rich and poor, is respectively bound: it is in truth an association of the opulent and the good, for better preserving their acquisitions, against the poor and the wicked. For want, complicated with misery and vice, generally seeks relief by plundering from those who are better provided. An African is as much bound by this supreme power, as the English labourer.[53]

In Jamaica and the other West Indian colonies, this broad social compact was supplemented by a set of formal laws that constrained the liberty of slaves in particular ways. In turning to an examination of such laws, Long also turned away from a discussion of the African slave trade and toward the management of slaves on British colonial soil. In general, his arguments now took a particularist turn. No longer concerned with the general right of another nation to make its own laws, or the transfer of property rights between nations, Long focused instead on the specific legal framework for enslavement on the sugar islands.

The Jamaica *Code Noir*, Long claimed, had been based on the model used in Barbados, itself drawn from English villeinage laws. As he had in his *Candid Reflections*, Long sought to establish a temporal and legal continuity between metropolitan and colonial forms of unfreedom. 'At the time we first entered on the settlement of Barbadoes', he noted, 'the idea of slavery could hardly be extinguished in England'. However, villeinage also had another role to play in the argument of the *History*. Here it was a potent symbol of the savagery of English laws, compared to the leniency of West Indian practice. Villeinage laws were characterised by 'severity', which was the source for the inclemency of the original laws governing slaves in the West Indies. Nor was legislative barbarity limited to those formally denoted as slaves. Long had compared Africans to English labourers on the grounds of their shared subordination to a 'social compact'. Now he did so on the basis of the punishments incurred for infractions. 'The penal laws in England', he wrote, 'were always sanguinary, and still retain this savage complexion'.[54]

If English laws thus provided clear models for harsh treatment, the characters of African slaves, claimed Long, appeared to require it. '[W]ild and savage to

---

[53] Ibid., 392–3.
[54] Ibid., 495, 96.

an extreme: their intractable and ferocious tempers naturally provoked their masters to rule them with a rod of iron; and the earliest laws enacted to affect them are therefore rigid and inclement, even to a degree of inhumanity'. Long equivocated over whether the cause for African depravity was due to nature or custom. Whatever its cause, however, it resulted in the treatment of slaves as 'brute beasts' rather than men. Now taking up Estwick's major theme, Long suggested that this attitude on the part of the early settlers in the West Indies – the attitude of a harder and less enlightened age – had been shared by Parliament, who 'fell in with the general idea and considered Negroes, purchased from that continent, as a lawful commercial property'.[55]

At this point in his argument, Long sprang a trap, one that had been some time in the making, and which deflected one of the most stinging criticisms of planters and slave owners back onto the law makers of the mother country. Long had spent some time, in a discussion of the character of white creoles, defending them from the charge that they sorely mistreated their slaves. Citing Granville Sharp by name, Long noted that abolitionists had compared the overworking of slaves to the 'merciless usage practiced in England over post-horses, sand-asses, &c'.[56] Long's response was both to deny the veracity of such a charge and to indulge in his now familiar ploy of invoking the treatment of British labourers and prisoners.[57] The careful reader of the entire text, however, could note that Long did not deny that some people *did* treat African slaves as mere beasts. Their fellow Africans did so, which was why transportation to the West Indies was, by comparison, 'perfect freedom'.[58] The original white settlers had also done so, a century earlier. This placed the English parliament, which had legislated to create an equivalency between Negroes and other property, in unpleasant company. And where neither Africans nor long-dead settlers could have any effect on the contemporary practices of slavery in Jamaica, Parliament's decisions, Long claimed, made it legally impossible for planters to do as they wished and to improve the lot of many of their slaves. '[T]he greatest oppression, under which our Negroes in the islands at present labour, arises materially from that statute, which declares them as houses, lands, hereditaments, assets, and personal estate, transferrable, and amenable to payment of debts due to the king and his subjects'.[59]

The problem, as Long saw it, was that Parliamentary statutes made no distinction between Creole slaves and those who had arrived directly from Africa.

[55] Ibid., 497.
[56] Ibid., 268.
[57] Ibid., 269–70, 400.
[58] Ibid., 399.
[59] Ibid., 497.

New slaves probably still required the draconian laws on the books. But Long asserted that the majority of Negroes, particularly on the older islands, were now Creoles and bore a more 'humanized' aspect than their ancestors. As a result, in practice at least, laws now wore a 'milder aspect'. Long suggested that this distinction between kinds of slaves be formalised in law, to make the servitude of Creoles 'approach near to a well-regulated liberty' and to 'make them forget the very idea of slavery'.[60]

Some *medium*, it is said, might be struck, between liberty, and that absolute slavery which now prevails; in this *medium* might be placed *all Mulattos*, after a certain temporary servitude to their owner; and such *native Blacks*, as their owners, for their faithful services, should think proper to enfranchise.[61]

For Long, the only barrier in the way of striking this medium between liberty and slavery was Parliamentary law. It was Parliament that treated Negroes as chattel and Parliament that must newly model its laws to raise the status of black Creoles 'some degrees above sheep and oxen'.[62]

In spite of their shared condemnation of Parliament, Long and Estwick's arguments on legal questions were significantly different. Estwick had set himself the task of explaining and justifying what he represented as the logic behind the English State's legislation; Long found himself deeply critical of that logic. Estwick's defence of slavery relied on the presumed inhumanity of slaves; Long's – with its emphasis on contract law and his constant comparisons between Negro slaves and members of the English lower classes – presumed that Africans (however 'depraved' their customs) were men. The differences between the two strident critics of Lord Mansfield's Somerset decision are perhaps nowhere clearer than in their treatment of the fixity of race. Long suggested that the savage manners of newly arrived African slaves may have led early settlers and then Parliament to see them as subhuman. Unlike Estwick, however, Long met every such suggestion with equivocation. Above all, whatever customs were carried from Africa, these were not racial traits. Estwick made no distinction between African and native slaves. For Long, it was of the essence and important enough to require a modification of the Negro Code to reflect it. African 'savagery' was a product of Africa and was not transmitted to African progeny born and raised in the West Indies. Racial fixity, put simply, was not part of Long's defence of slavery. What role(s), then, did it play in the *History of Jamaica*?

[60] Ibid., 498–502.
[61] Ibid., 503.
[62] Ibid., 500.

6.3   Special Creation and the Problem of Race

Fixity

The central issue in Long's discussion of race – as for those of his contemporaries interested in the question – was the relative effect of climate and innate, heritable racial characteristics. Which aspects of physique and behaviour were malleable under different skies (given enough time), and which were not to be changed? For most monogenists – Kant was a rare but important exception – climate (understood broadly) explained everything. At some point in the past, humanity had looked similar. If Biblical narratives were taken literally, the resemblance was a familial one. Human groups spread from a common centre through different climatic zones until their physical and intellectual features displayed the myriad diversity of the human species today.

As we saw in the last chapter, Buffon had enriched this rather simplistic explanation by expanding upon the ways in which climate could affect the body. Kant's theory of the origins of human racial difference was a response to another criticism of what we might call naïve monogenism. By the late 1700s both the slave trade and settler colonialism had encouraged the conviction that skin colour and other features did not change nearly as quickly as had once been imagined. Neither black slaves in the Americas, nor white settlers in the tropics had altered their skin tone perceptibly over the course of several generations. Kant sought to reconcile the contradiction between monogenism and this apparent racial fixity in a manner directly opposed to Buffon's and played down the possible effects of climate, direct or otherwise. Human races, he claimed, did indeed share a common origin and Mankind had spread to the various regions of the earth, changing by small amounts in direct response to their new environments. Members of that original common race, however, carried with them seeds of change.[63] In the right climate, those seeds had come to fruition and the four major races were born. Further dramatic change was now no longer possible. New races could only be born from the original stock and that was now largely extinct. Kant thus replaced a mechanical explanation with a teleological principle, while at the same time defending monogenism from one of its most pertinent critiques.

No polygenist, of course, denied the effect of climate (most, in fact, granted it more agency than did Kant). They argued merely for its limits. Thus, Long

---

[63] 'Human beings', he argued, 'were created in such a way that they might live in every climate and endure each and every condition of the land. Consequently, numerous seeds and natural predispositions must lie ready in human beings either to be developed or held back in such a way that we might become fitted to a particular place in the world'. Immanuel Kant, 'Of the Different Human Races', in *The Idea of Race*, eds. Robert Bernasconi and Tommy L. Lott (Indianapolis: Hackett, 2000), 8–22, 14.

noted of white Jamaican Creoles that the shape of their eye sockets had changed to protect them in the strong sunlight of the West Indies. 'Although descended from British ancestors, they are stamped with these characteristic deviations'.[64] Invoking a common trope, Long suggested that native women, like tropical plants and animals, 'attain earlier to maturity' in the West Indies. They married young, and bore children at age twelve. Like hothouse flowers, they also faded fast, but 'console[d] themselves, however, that they can enjoy more of real existence here in one hour than the fair inhabitants of the frozen, foggy regions do in two'.[65] Climate had its effects on behaviour and intellect, too. The warm weather 'rouzed the passions', so that chastity was to be all the more admired. And nativity could even trump race. Creole blacks and whites, Long noted, shared a common fondness for music and an 'exceedingly correct' ear for melody.[66]

If climate could change much, however, it could not change all. Those in England who believed that birth in Jamaica had turned the children of English parents tawny-skinned had been deceived. Encountering planters' children in the most expensive public schools of the mother country, they had assumed that the progeny were legitimate. Instead, Long asserted, the swarthy West Indian offspring were, in fact, the product of English men indulging in 'goatish embraces' with black women.[67] Generalising from his Jamaican experiences to the broadest question of human malleability, Long denied that any external effects could explain the most pertinent differences between black and whites.

Climate, perhaps, has had some share in producing the variety of feature which we behold among the different societies of mankind, scattered over the globe: so that, were an Englishman and woman to remove to China, and there abide, it may be questioned, whether their descendants, in the course of a few generations, constantly residing there, would not acquire somewhat of the Chinese cast of countenance and person? I do not indeed suppose, that, by living in Guiney, they would exchange hair for wool, or a white cuticle for a black: change of complexion must be referred to some other cause.[68]

To skin colour and hair, Long proceeded to add a raft of physical and intellectual differences that characterised blacks: the shapes of the features of their face; the colour of the lice on their bodies; their 'bestial or fetid smell'; the failure of Africans to make 'any progress in civility or science'; and the miserable state of their houses and roads. They were, as a people, 'brutish, ignorant, idle, crafty, treacherous, bloody, thievish, mistrustful and superstitious': characteristics

---

[64] Long, *The History of Jamaica*, II, 262.
[65] Ibid., 285.
[66] Ibid., 283, 63.
[67] Ibid., 328. Trevor Burnard, '"Rioting in Goatish Embraces": Marriage and Improvement in Early British Jamaica', *The History of the Family* 11 (2006).
[68] Long, *The History of Jamaica*, II, 262.

that were not the effect of climate.[69] Common climates, then, failed to eradicate essential differences between whites and blacks. And diverse climates, such as those found across Africa or the Americas, failed to produce racial diversity. America, for example, lay between 65 degrees North of the equator and 55 degrees South, with climates that encompassed those of all the known continents. Yet the complexion of its inhabitants was everywhere the same, 'only with more or less of a metalline luster'.[70] Distinctions between Whites and Negroes would appear, then, to be innate and permanent. To these anti-climatological arguments, which spoke to *racial* difference, Long then added one from his observations – such as they were – of interracial coupling, which suggested that the difference was even more profound. Mulattoes, he argued, were infertile with each other, but not necessarily with individuals from the races of their parents.[71] 'The subject', Long concluded, 'is really curious, and deserves a further and very attentive enquiry'.

[I]t tends, among other evidences, to establish an opinion, which several have entertained, that the White and the Negroe had not one common origin … For my own part, I think there are extremely potent reasons for believing, that the White and the Negroe are two distinct species.[72]

Marshalling a great deal more evidence – however questionable it may have been – Long had arrived at a position much like Estwick's. And, like Estwick, Long next proceeded from a natural historical to a natural theological defence of polygenesis. Diversity within *genus Homo* would bring Man within the compass of the great system God had produced, which divided and subdivided every other class of animal. Long's invocation of the racialised chain of being amounted to rank plagiarism of Estwick's language.[73] Yet, differences existed between Long and Estwick, and important ones at that. Long's chain included Mulattoes, placed between Whites and Blacks. More significantly, Long's argument was ultimately more consistent. Both men had argued that Mankind needed to be divided into a number of distinct species. Neither argued that whites were the only humans. Both established a system where Africans were lesser men, but men nonetheless. Estwick, however, ostensibly speaking for

---

[69] Ibid., 352–3, 54.

[70] Ibid., 375.

[71] Even by Long's standards, this was a weak claim. He claimed not to know of any counter-examples to his claims about Mulatto sterility, but quickly sought to deflect any produced by others by suggesting that any such were, in fact, likely the secret product of 'intrigue' with one of the parent races. Even more problematic for his case was his acceptance that, in some cases, Mulatto men and women did produce offspring. In such situations, he asserted, their young did not survive to maturity. This was not a case discussed by Buffon or other naturalists and would seem to significantly detract from the argument regarding distinct specieshood.

[72] Long, *The History of Jamaica*, II, 336.

[73] Ibid., 375.

Parliament in its defence of slavery, had argued that Negroes – being less than Whites – were therefore beasts, and hence property. Long's defence of slavery, on the other hand, required the assumption that Africans were capable of making and assenting to contracts and were hence men. And in Long's taxonomy, Negroes were indeed men, as were Whites, Mulattoes, and – most peculiarly – Orangutans.

The amount of space devoted to demonstrating the humanity of Orangutans in the *History* is at first baffling. One is tempted to read it as little more than a shallow attempt to be scandalous, and to allow Long to titillate and appal his readers with his obsessively repeated stories of 'amorous intercourse' between the male animal and Negroe women.[74] Closer attention to the text does not rid one of this impression entirely, but it becomes clear that the dozen pages Long dedicated to the topic are not without significance as part of his overall argument. His central aims in discussing the tripartite division of humankind were, first, to establish a ranking and, second, to insist that essential differences existed without physical causes. That is, the physical differences between Orangutans and 'other' men were minor; intellectual differences were merely of degree; and these intellectual differences could not be explained by differences in the structure of the body. Orangutans, wrote Long, 'have some trivial resemblance to the ape-kind, but the strongest similitude to mankind, in countenance, figure, stature, organs, erect posture, actions or movements, food, temper, and manner of living'.[75]

If Polygenism was a heterodox position, arguing that Orangutans were men might be called ultra-heterodox. Long had drawn the idea from James Burnet, Lord Monboddo, who had offered reams of evidence suggesting that certain apes were humans in a primitive state of development. Rousseau had also flirted with the notion.[76] Many naturalists, of course, had noted striking similarities between the physical structure of apes and men. Buffon and Long both cited Edward's Tyson's careful dissection of an Orangutan in 1699. Tyson had marvelled at the familiarity of the ape's anatomy, but refused utterly (as did Buffon later) to see this as evidence for the creature's humanity. 'Physical similarities', he wrote, 'merely emphasized the intellectual and spiritual gulf between man and chimpanzee'.[77]

For Long, on the other hand, the 'gulf' was not as wide as naturalists had imagined. Gathering as many travellers' accounts as possible, he provided

---

[74] Ibid., 370.

[75] Ibid., 358.

[76] Barker, 54. On Monboddo, see Alan J. Barnard, '*Orang Outang* and the Definition of *Man*: The Legacy of Lord Monboddo', in *Fieldwork and Footnotes: Studies in the History of European Anthropology*, ed. Han F. Vermeulen and Arturo Alvarez Roldán (London: Routledge, 1995).

[77] Quoted in Barker, 49.

a wealth of examples of Orangutans wearing clothes, building huts, making noises like children, being taught to drink wine, handling cutlery at the dining table, and understanding enough of the medical treatment given one during an illness to request the same again. Like Monboddo, Long compared Orangutans to children, and suggested that the only true test of the creature's natural inferiority (including the capacity for speech) would be to educate a specimen as a man, through school and university, up to the age of 20 or 25.[78] The example might seem farcical, yet it possessed rhetorical power. Few would imagine that such an education would produce a thinking, speaking man – white or black. Orangutans, most would be happy to conclude, were naturally inferior. But what, then, was the *cause* of such inferiority if the animal was, with regard to its physical structure and organisation, largely identical to the other species within *genus Homo*? It could only be an originary difference in mental faculties, created by the Deity:

[I]f we admit with Mr. Buffon, that with all this analogy of organization, the oran-outang's brain is a senseless *icon* of the human; that it is meer matter, unanimated with a thinking principle, in any, or at least in a very minute and imperfect degree, we must then infer the strongest conclusion to establish our belief of a natural diversity of the human intellect, in general, *ab origine* … the supposition, then, is well-founded, that the brain, and intellectual organs, so far as they are dependent upon meer matter, though similar in texture and modification to those of other men, may in some of the Negroe race be so constituted, as *not to result to the same effects*; for we cannot but allow, that the Deity might, if it was his pleasure, diversify his works in this manner, and either withhold the *superior principle* entirely, or in part only, or infuse it into the different classes and races of human creatures in such portions, as to form the same gradual climax towards perfection in this human system, which is so evidently designed in every other.[79]

What Buffon regarded as a gulf, in other words, Long portrayed as a graduated progression.

To this point in his argument, Long had attempted to demonstrate that enough differences existed to declare blacks and whites different species, while enough similarities existed to insist upon them being common members of the same genus. He had also, with his argument involving Orangutans, sought to make plausible the case that profound mental distinctions between the species might exist, even if their physical structure was essentially similar. To prove that point, however – and to establish the intellectual inferiority of Negroes *ab origine* – Long had also to show that a change in external circumstances could not efface the apparent mental failings of the darker races. This, after all,

---

[78] Long, *The History of Jamaica*, II, 359–61, 70.
[79] Ibid., 371.

was the claim of many abolitionists. Long had to envision an experiment for a Negroe that had a form like that earlier proposed for the Orangutan.

Long believed that such an experiment had already been tried. It was surely what he'd had in mind (and intended to mock) when he conjured for his readers the image of an ape at university. In the late eighteenth century, a story commonly told concerned Francis Williams, born in Jamaica the son of two freed slaves.[80] The Duke of Montagu, so the tale went (Long reproduced it) had sought to test the proposition that climate and external circumstances were vastly more important than any innate racial capacity, and had sent the young man to university in England. He returned to the West Indies and opened a school where he taught reading, writing, Latin, and mathematics. Williams' case would seem, on its face, to refute the claim that the difference in intellectual capacity between whites and blacks was due to race, rather than upbringing. As a result, those committed to the reality and permanency of race tended to try to dismiss the force of his example. Hume, for one, had mocked him in his infamous footnote. 'In Jamaica indeed', the Scottish philosopher had written, 'they talk of one Negroe as a man of parts and learning, but 'tis likely he is admired for very slender accomplishments, like a parrot, who speaks but a few words plainly'.[81] Long reproduced, translated, and annotated one of Williams' Latin poems in the *History*, so that his readers might judge its merits. He insisted, however, that appropriate criteria be used for that judgement. Critics were not to be impressed merely by the fact that a black man had produced a Latin poem at all. Instead, Long maintained, one had to determine the quality of the poem, given that Williams had the advantage of 'an academic education, under every advantage that able preceptors, and munificent patrons, could furnish'. In Long's judgement, the poem was 'a piece highly laboured; designed modeled and perfected, to the utmost stretch of his invention, imagination, and skill'. It was the kind of production one might expect from any 'middling scholar' who had attended one of England's elite institutions.[82] The implication, then, was that the best a Negroe could produce was equal only to (elite) white mediocrity. Long's conclusion, cribbed from Estwick and jumbling together two couplets from Pope, affirmed the humanity of all races – *contra* Estwick – while insisting upon rankings in the quality of men.

The Spaniards have a proverbial saying, *'Aunque Négros somos génte'* 'though we are Blacks, we are men'. The truth of which no one will dispute; but if we allow the system

---

[80] On Williams, see Vincent Carretta, 'Who Was Francis Williams?', *Early American Literature* 38 (2003).

[81] Hume, 'Of National Characters', 208, 629–30.

[82] Long, *The History of Jamaica*, II, 484.

of created beings to be perfect and consistent, and that this perfection arises from an exact scale of gradation, from the lowest to the highest, combining and connecting every part into a regular and beautiful harmony, reasoning them from the visible plan and operation of infinite wisdom in respect to the human race, as well as every other series in the scale, we must, I think, conclude, that,

'The general *order*, since the whole began,
Is kept in *nature*, and is kept in *man*.
Order is heaven's first law; and, this confest,
Some are, and *must be, greater* than the rest.[83]

Malleability

One might think that this was rather weak tea for a man who had been adamant about the radical inferiority of another race. Where Estwick had made Negroes beasts, Long was ultimately reduced, by Williams' example, to the anaemic insistence that the bounds of the race limited them to rising no higher than the average level of the best educated sons of England's elites. Long, however, had already called attention to what he portrayed as the deficiencies of the Duke of Montagu's experiment.

Considering the difference which climate may occasion, and which Montesquieu has learnedly examined, the noble duke would have made the experiment more fairly on a native African; perhaps, too, the Northern air imparted a tone and vigour to his organs, of which they never could have been susceptible in a hot climate.[84]

The objection seems peculiar: the point of the (thought) experiment had been to determine how much of the difference between whites and blacks was permanent and how much due to climate, education, and other factors. If Long and Estwick were right, and the Deity had imposed natural limits on the intelligence of Negroes, then no change in external circumstance could raise them beyond their pre-determined bounds. As Long noted, in his own version of Hume's remarks, changes in climate and training might produce the semblance of true intelligence, but not the reality.[85] In his contestation of the significance of Montagu's results, however, Long would seem to be admitting a far more important role for climate – and hence malleability, as opposed to racial fixity – in determining the intelligence and mental capacities of non-white

---

[83] Ibid., 484–5.
[84] Ibid., 476–7.
[85] 'The examples which have been given of Negroes born and trained up in other climates, detract not from the general idea of a narrow, humble intellect, which we affix to the inhabitants of Guiney. We have seen *learned horses*, *learned* even *talking dogs*, in England; who by dint of much pains and tuition, were brought to exhibit the signs of a capacity far exceeding what is ordinarily allowed to be possessed by those animals'. Ibid., 375.

races. As he noted explicitly, 'The climate of Jamaica is temperate, and even cool, compared to many parts of Guiney; and the Creole Blacks have undeniably more acuteness and better understandings than the natives of Guiney'.[86]

In his objection to Montagu's results, Long revealed not only the fundamental ambivalence of his arguments about racial fixity, but also the source of this ambivalence: the necessary difference between Creole and African Blacks. We have noted the stress placed on this difference earlier, when discussing Long's plans to produce distinct legal codes for Mulattoes and Creoles on the one hand, and newly arrived African slaves on the other. It is worth dwelling on this contradiction for a moment. Remember that within a framework that insisted upon the fixity of race, a key point of evidence (perhaps *the* key point) was that races did not change in significant ways as they moved from one climate to another. A great deal of Long's description of the native black inhabitants of Jamaica, however, concerns their radical differences from their African brethren. In terms of behaviour, where Africans were dirty, violent, and inclined to cruelty, even to their own children, Creoles were fastidious; could, with Christian instruction, 'be kept in good order without the whip'; and were good, if somewhat stern parents. Physically, Long noted that Black Creole women had more trouble during childbirth than those in Africa. Most generally, 'the Creole Blacks differ much from the Africans, not only in manners, but in beauty of shape, feature, and complexion'.[87] The last point is well worth emphasising, since it will be remembered that Long had been adamant that complexion could *not* change in different climates. Why, then, when the best argument in favour of racial fixity and separate creations was the essential sameness of Blacks born in Africa and Jamaica, did Long keep asserting the importance of their differences?

The simplest answer is fear. Long was quite explicit about his anxieties. The decade before the publication of the *History* had seen a large number of slave insurrections on Jamaica and other West Indian Islands. Barbara Bush puts the average at one significant revolt every two years between 1731 and 1823.[88] Vincent Brown estimates that rebellions and conspiracies occurred on average once a decade on Jamaica alone in the century after 1740.[89] A description of the most significant of these took up a sizeable number of pages in Long's *History*. What became known as Tacky's Revolt began on 7 April 1760, when

---

[86] Long, *The History of Jamaica*, II, 476–7.

[87] Ibid., 411, 10.

[88] Bush, 68.

[89] Brown, 3. 'Slave conspiracies and revolts were especially frequent during the "most troubled decade in Jamaica's long history as a slave society" – the 1760s'. O'Shaugnessy, 38.

ninety slaves (led by two Coromantees named Tacky and Jamaica) killed several whites and burned and looted a number of plantations.[90] By the time the Rebellion was quelled – in a particularly brutal fashion – an estimated 400 slaves, sixty whites, and sixty free blacks had been killed or committed suicide. One hundred slaves were executed and a further five hundred were exiled.[91] As savage as the response by white authorities was, rebellions by Coromantees and their allies occurred again in 1765, 1766, and 1767.[92]

As with so many of the problems of the slave system, Long laid part of the blame at the feet of absent landlords.[93] Solving the problem of sojourning planters might help reduce the risk of rebellions, but Long also had another solution: winning part of the slave population to the side of white residents. In his mind, the population was already divided, although those who lived outside of the colonies could not see it and insisted (as a true racialist might) that there was little difference between groups of slaves. 'The vulgar opinion in England', wrote Long dismissively, 'confounds all the Blacks in one class, and supposes them equally prompt for rebellion; an opinion that is grossly erroneous'.[94] It was 'imported Africans', he insisted, 'who are the most to be feared'.[95]

Long's suggestion that two legal codes be adopted instead of a single, draconian *Code Noir* was thus part of an overall argument that sought, for political and social reasons, to divide into disparate groups what a dedicated polygenist should have seen as an essentially indiscriminate whole. Long was utterly blunt in his logic: Whites could not withstand a fully coordinated rebellion from a population seasoned to its environs and outnumbering them ten to one. 'We are obliged to it, both from reason and self-interest; bodily strength and their adaptation to the climate, would enable them to pass from the lowest to the highest stations, and give the law to their masters, if they were willing unanimously to accept it'. Creoles and Mulattoes needed to be made use of as 'instruments ... to restrain one another within the bounds of their allotted condition'.[96] Complete consistency on the question of racial fixity, Long might have argued, was a luxury that West Indian planters could not afford. Whatever the arguments might be in favour of the identity of native-born and imported Negroes, social and political exigencies required that they be treated very differently. Facts and fears on colonial soil tended to trouble the simpler boundary-making of the metropole.

---

[90] Burnard and Garrigus, 125–6.
[91] Ibid., 122–3.
[92] Brown, 149.
[93] Long, *The History of Jamaica*, I, 389.
[94] Ibid., II: 444.
[95] Ibid., 309–10.
[96] Ibid., 503–4.

6.4   Polygenism, Theology, Materialism

Among the many striking aspects of Long's heterodoxy in espousing polygenism was his refusal to acknowledge it as such. The pages of the *History of
Jamaica* are more likely to vaunt Long's radicalism in Natural Philosophy –
comparing his racial theories, for example, with Copernican astronomy – than
in theology.[97] References to Genesis, or other relevant biblical passages are, at
best, oblique. One should probably read the following as a swipe at the story
given in Genesis, but it is to be noted that neither the book, nor the name of
God's first human creation is given.

Without puzzling our wits, to discover the occult causes of this diversity of colour
among mankind, let us be content with acknowledging that it was just as easy for
Omnipotence to create black-skinned, as white-skinned men; or to create five millions
of human beings, as to create one such being.[98]

Long's text does not mention the Fall, although that may well be what he
had in mind when he noted that childbirth was easy in Africa. If Negroes were
part of a separate creation, then it would follow that African women were not
punished for the sin of eating of the Tree of Knowledge. On the other hand,
Long noted that slaves in Jamaica had a harder time with delivery, implying
that climate, not divine justice, was the cause of labour pains.[99]

The few explicit Biblical references in the *History* show that Long had little
sympathy for literal readings of the Holy book, particularly when literalists
used their readings as a basis for contemporary policy. In general, the theological arguments of the *History* were based far more on the book of nature than
the book of God. The design involved in the Great Chain of Being was only
one instance of Long's natural theological leanings. Providence, he suggested,
had designed the vegetable products of the West Indian Islands to counteract
the potential ill effects of heat, humidity, and a poorly adapted diet. The local
succession of morning and evening breezes appeared, to Long as 'gracious
dispensations of the Ruler of the universe' and a prime reason that the plague
had never been known on the island.[100] Even seemingly negative aspects of
nature in the tropics, like hurricanes and earthquakes, were 'doubtless ...
destined to answer some wise and perhaps salutary purpose in the oeconomy of
nature'.[101] What may have happened in the Garden of Eden seemed to pale in
comparison to the evidence for God's beneficent plan through time and across
the globe.

---

[97] Ibid., 337.
[98] Ibid., 352.
[99] See Chapter 7.
[100] Long, *The History of Jamaica*, I, 372.
[101] Ibid., III: 619.

Keeping this in mind suggests that Long's seemingly radical polygenist heterodoxy may have flowed from (or at least been supported by) a rather more commonly unorthodox anti-literalism, one shared with many Enlightenment figures. It seems necessary to downplay Long's religious iconoclasm somewhat, since on other theological issues he was far from espousing any form of heresy. Compared to Voltaire, for example, who Long cited as a supporter of polygenism, Long was decidedly conservative, most clearly so in his rejection of even the hint of materialism. The brains, physical structure, and organisation of the three species in the human *genus*, Long had argued, were essentially identical. Not even the most skilful dissector could locate the source of the intellectual differences between orangutans and men in their material make-up. 'The sole distinction between [an orangutan] and man, must consist in the measure of intellectual faculties; those faculties which the most skilful anatomist is incapable of tracing the source of, and which exist *independent of the structure of the brain*'.[102] The difference was a spiritual one: the graded amounts of the 'superior principle' that God had allowed each species.

Long did not make the point himself, but it is worth noting that decoupling the connection between intellect and the physical body provides a way of reconciling his insistence on the reality and fixity of race with his equally adamant arguments concerning the important differences between Negroes born in Africa and Jamaica. One need only assume that he was willing to grant that the range of intellectual capabilities susceptible to climatic change (and other changes in external circumstances) was larger than the concomitant range for physical characteristics. Williams' case would seem to make this point immediately. Long knew of no black man who had – over any period of time, let alone a single generation – come to physically resemble the members of the British elite attending Westminster or Eton. Complexion, facial features, and the texture of hair appeared fixed enough for Long to think of them as largely incapable of variation, and hence evidence for separate creations in and of themselves. Training and a new environment, however, could change the behaviour, morals, and even intellectual level of slaves brought to Jamaica, and in that possibility for change stood also the hope that Whites could build alliances with their non-brothers to defend their mastery in the West Indies.

Conclusion

Long was willing to offer indirect criticisms of narratives given in Genesis. Materialism, however, was a bridge too far. His espousal of polygenesis was

---

[102] Ibid., II: 368–9.

heterodoxy, but Long was an orthodox enlightened Christian.[103] The best way to resolve this apparent contradiction, I would suggest, is by seeing the radicalism of Long's support of the notion of special creations as lying within the domain of politics or social theory, rather than theology. Such a claim requires us to read Long's polygenesis as written in a somewhat different register to that of Lord Kames, who published in the same year and fretted much more openly about the conflict between his position and that given in the Bible. It requires us to realise that all of those who argued against that brotherhood of man – whether they did so in a religious vein or not – risked social opprobrium. This was particularly true, of course, when their position appeared self-serving, as in Long's case. But even Georg Forster, who put forward the notion of special creations in the course of a debate with Kant in the late 1780s, acknowledged that opponents of his position had accused him of removing one of the few barriers still holding Europeans back from perpetrating horrors against Africans. (With some justice, Forster retorted that a belief in monogenesis had hardly stayed the whip in a slave owner's hand thus far.)[104] In the age of empire and slavery, polygenesis was no longer (if it had ever been) a purely theological heresy. It was, as Long's text showed, a question of profound scientific and political significance.

That said, nineteenth-century British polygenists and racial theorists found Long a problematic source. I have noted already that those who cited his work on race tended to be abolitionists, who mined the *History* for its viler comments, as evidence of the moral failings of their opponents. Those wishing to make serious scientific points on the nature of humanity probably shied away from an author who spoke credulously of Orangutans as part of the human species, capable of dressing and dining like Men, and indulging in illicit sexual relations with human women. Even beyond this, one suspects that Long would have seemed old-fashioned, with his refusal to accept that differences in the organisation and make-up of the brain caused differences in intellect. This supposition, drawn from phrenological research, formed the bedrock of nineteenth-century race science. Long's refusal to see significant differences in the brain structures of the races placed his ideas outside the realm of normal race science.

I began this chapter by asking about the connection between Long's polygenism and his defence of slavery. We can now see that the answer is that there wasn't really one, but that this absence was no mere oversight. Where Estwick was content to see Negroes as beasts and hence property, Long refused

---

[103] On enlightened Christianity in this context, see Kidd, *The Forging of Races: Race and Scripture in the Protestant Atlantic World, 1600–2000*, 79–120.

[104] Georg Forster, 'Noch etwas über die Menschenraßen. An Herrn Dr. Biester', *Teutsche Merkur* October and November (1786).

to deny slaves humanity, even as he maintained their natural inferiority. The assumption of humanity was central to a legal argument based on contract law, but it was also essential for a socio-political argument that saw a certain part of the slave population as potential allies against the insurrectionary remainder.

For the intellectual historian of race, it is the polygenist planter's insistence on these differences between Creole and newly arrived slaves that remains one of the most striking aspects of the *History of Jamaica*. In part, this surely flows from the logical oddity of the position. Yet is also derives from the fact that Long was one of the few racial theorists writing with a deep experience in a plantation colony. I am certainly not the first person to point to the ways that the colonial context shifted the terms of seemingly familiar debates about the nature of race. In a study of the medical construction of 'whiteness' in nineteenth-century Australia, Warwick Anderson noted that the very categories of race science seemed irrelevant to the concerns of most of his actors. Terms like monogenesis, polygenism and social Darwinism, he suggested 'may be malapropisms that distract us from working out how racial theory ... was produced and transacted among colonial scientists and ordinary doctors. In my experience, terms of this sort are at best blunt tools that tend to mutilate the racial thought of out-of-the-way intellectuals'.[105]

I have tried to show here, at least for the eighteenth-century Jamaican case, that terms like poly- and monogenesis *do* make sense, whether they were actors' categories or not. But we must also note – in agreement with Anderson's larger point – that the fact that race relations were lived on a daily basis, that race was more than mere theory for Long, that the survival of whites in close propinquity to an enslaved, majority black population appeared to require making alliances and accommodations, made his polygenesis seem convoluted, even contradictory. Ultimately, if we still regard Long's polygenism as the product of a rather transparent self-interest, we must nonetheless understand that the interests of those in the colonies were not always those of the metropole. Seemingly familiar structures of racial difference were made differently in the centre and periphery.

---

[105] Anderson, *The Cultivation of Whiteness: Science, Health and Racial Destiny in Australia*, 3.

7   Pathologies of Blackness: Race-Medicine, Slavery, and Abolitionism

In 1773, when he penned a brief and anonymous pamphlet entitled *An Address to the Inhabitants in America upon Slave-Keeping*, Benjamin Rush was twenty-seven years old and three years away from adding his name to the Declaration of Independence.[1] He had completed his MD in Edinburgh under William Cullen in 1768 and had returned to Philadelphia the following year to begin his own practice, soon thereafter taking up the professorship for chemistry at the University of Pennsylvania. A figure of no mean importance, then, in spite of his relative youth, it seems no surprise that Rush should have been approached, according to his own account, to write something in support of a petition to the Pennsylvania Assembly arguing for a higher duty to be imposed on the importation of slaves, and thus providing an economic impetus for the eventual eradication of what abolitionists called the 'man-trade'.

Less than thirty pages long, Rush's *Address* offered a crisp and scathing summary of the arguments put forward to defend slavery, rejecting each as only so much self-serving or simply wicked rhetoric. Proponents of slavery had declared Negroes to be the natural inferiors of Europeans in intelligence or morality: Rush denied it outright. Were slaves idle, treacherous, or inclined to thievery then this was a result of their enslaved condition and would end when they were free. 'The vulgar notion' that the colour of their skin was a mark of the curse on Cain, their forefather, Rush rejected as 'too absurd to need refutation'.[2] Indeed, black skin was no curse, but rather a blessing, for it 'qualifies them for that part of the Globe in which Providence has placed them. The ravages of heat, diseases, and time, appear less in their faces than in a white

---

[1] Benjamin Rush, *An Address to the Inhabitants of the British Settlements in America Upon Slave-Keeping (the Second Edition). To Which Are Added, Observations on a Pamphlet, Entitled, 'Slavery Not Forbidden by Scripture; or, a Defence of the West-India Planters'. By a Pennsylvanian* (Philadelphia: John Dunlap, 1773). On the local context for the debate that ensued, see W. Caleb McDaniel, 'Philadelphia Abolitionists and Antislavery Cosmopolitanism', in *Antislavery and Abolition in Philadelphia: Emancipation and the Long Struggle for Racial Justice in the City of Brotherly Love*, ed. Richard Newman and James Mueller (Baton Rouge: Louisiana State University Press, 2011).

[2] Rush, 3.

one'.[3] To the common economic defence of the trade – that one could not produce sugar, indigo, or rice without slave labour – Rush offered three retorts. First, were the claim true, economic necessity could hardly justify the violation of 'the Laws of justice or humanity'.[4] Second, the economic premise of the claim was, in fact, false: free labour in Cochin China produced sugar at prices lower than those gained from the use of slaves in the West Indies.[5] Third, and perhaps most interesting, there was something wrong with the assumption that only those born in climates like those of the West Indies could labour there.

I know it has been said by some, that none but the natives of warm climates could undergo the excessive heat and labour of the West-India islands. But this argument is founded upon an error; for the reverse of this is true. I have been informed by good authority, that one European who escapes the first or second year, will do twice the work, and live twice the number of years that an ordinary Negro man will do.[6]

Rush's argument was unusual, for he was suggesting that those born in Africa, where the soil supplied all that the human frame required with minimal effort, were not used to hard labour, however accustomed they might be to warm environs. A European, by contrast, could become seasoned to the climate in a year or so, and could then use their native capacity for labour to their advantage under a different sky.

More familiar were Rush's rejections of moralist and religious pro-slavery arguments. Claiming that the trade in men served a moral purpose by introducing pagan Africans to Christianity, for example, was 'like justifying highway robbery because part of the money acquired in this manner was appropriated to some religious use'.[7] Rush had no more time for positions holding that slavery had saved Africans from death (their lives forfeit as captives of war) or who found support for slavery in the Old Testament. There was nothing decent about slavery and much that was degrading and terrible. Taking a page from the book of his fellow Philadelphian, Anthony Benezet, Rush detailed the horrors of the torture inflicted upon slaves by brutish masters: 'Behold one covered with stripes, into which melted wax is poured – another tied down to a block or a stake – a third suspended in the air by his thumbs – a fourth – I cannot relate it'.[8] Magistrates and legislators, 'men of sense and virtue' and – above

---

[3] Ibid., 3–4.
[4] Ibid., 4.
[5] On the debate over the economic value of free v. enslaved labour, see Drescher, *The Mighty Experiment: Free Labor Versus Slavery in British Emancipation*. On the question of how 'free' some free labour was, see Andrea Major, *Slavery, Abolitionism, and Empire in India, 1772–1843* (Liverpool: Liverpool University Press, 2012).
[6] Rush, 8.
[7] Ibid., 14–15.
[8] Ibid., 23.

all – ministers all had to speak out to end a trade that violated every sense of justice, economic logic, and Christian benevolence.

The rejoinder from the pro-slavery camp was rapid.[9] Writing as 'A West-Indian', Richard Nesbit sought in *his Defence of the West-India Planters* to cast stories of horrific brutality as either outright falsifications – 'I never knew a single instance of such shocking barbarities' – or else the actions not of all planters, but of exceptional villains within their number.[10] Nisbet followed what would become the general trend of pro-slavery tracts in many of his other attacks and defences. He invoked 'self-interest' as a reason to deny that slave owners regularly damaged or destroyed their valuable human property. He cited the existence of slavery in the Old Testament to defend the practice today, suggesting also that one could not – as Rush had – use either the absence of such approval in the Gospels or Christ's 'general maxims of charity and benevolence' to condemn the trade.[11] And Nisbet pointed to the plight of others, closer to home, whom abolitionists should seek to protect before they pled the cause of Negroes in other lands. If the exigencies and necessities of states required a kind of slavery for soldiers and sailors, why could the same arguments not be made for labourers in sugar fields? Were Britain to give up on the sugar trade, the kingdom would soon be beggared and left defenceless, easy prey for the French or other powerful adversaries.[12]

As in Rush's case, however, the most unusual of Nisbet's arguments turned on the question of African physiology. Rush had attempted to turn two pro-slavery arguments against themselves, arguing that black skin was no curse, but rather an advantage in the warm climates of Africa, and also that African slaves were not the best labourers in the similarly warm climate of the West Indies. Nisbet was having none of it. 'The writer confesses, that hard labour within the tropics shortens human life, and that the colour of the negroes qualifies them for hot countries, yet he is desirous, that our white fellow subjects should toil in these sultry climates, that the Africans might indulge their natural laziness in their own country. The former are, no doubt, much obliged to him for his kind intentions'.[13] And Nisbet rejected completely Rush's claims for

---

[9] Rush's pamphlet in fact inspired three different rejoinders, which Tise has characterised as 'constitute[ing] the most acute formulations of traditional proslavery thought prior to the nineteenth century'. Larry E. Tise, *Proslavery: A History of the Defense of Slavery in America, 1701–1840* (Athens and London: University of Georgia Press, 1987), 28.

[10] Richard Nisbet, *Slavery Not Forbidden by Scripture. Or a Defence of the West-India Planters* (Philadelphia: 1773), 15.

[11] 'If the custom had been held in abhorrence by Christ and his disciples, they would, no doubt, have preached against it in direct terms'. Ibid., 8.

[12] By freeing Africans, Nisbet intoned, 'Britons, themselves, must become abject slaves to despotick power'. Ibid., 13–14.

[13] Ibid., 10.

African equality. Although he acknowledged that it was 'impossible to determine, with accuracy' whether European or African intellects were superior, since Africans 'have not the same opportunities of improving as we have', Nisbet determined the matter in favour of Europeans in any case. With a reference to Hume's infamous footnote as support, Nisbet declared that 'it seems probable, that they are a much inferior race of men to the whites, in every respect'.[14] Importing slaves to the New World appeared to improve both their work ethic and intellect, but Nisbet was wary of geographic explanations for what he suggested was African inferiority to all other peoples, both past and present. 'The stupidity of the native cannot be attributed to *climate*', he opined, for the nearby Moors and Egyptians were not so inferior.[15] Without advocating for polygenism explicitly, Nisbet opened the door to the position and similarly left it as merely implied that natural inferiority should serve as justification for African enslavement.

Rush would have the last word. To the planters' invocation of self-interest as a reason to doubt stories of brutality, he replied by questioning the applicability of such economic rationalities: 'It is to no purpose to urge here that Self Interest leads the Planters to treat their Slaves well. There are many things which appear true in Speculation, which are false in Practice. The Head is apt to mistake its real Interest as the Heart its real Happiness'.[16] He gave ground on the question of African inferiority even as he suggested that physical causes (i.e. climate) could explain the discrepancy. Yet, he questioned the import of this argument in the current debate. Let it be allowed, he suggested, that his opponent had made his case: 'Would it avail a man to plead in a Court of Justice that he defrauded his neighbor, because he was inferior to him in Genius or Knowledge?'.[17] Rush listed his extant allies ('Montesquieu, Franklin, Wallis, Hutchinson, Sharp, Hargrave, Warburton, and Forster') and sought to win more, by analogising the fight for African freedom to the fight against British tyranny in America.[18] 'Where is the difference', Rush asked, 'between the British Senator who attempts to enslave his fellow subjects in America, by imposing Taxes upon them contrary to Law and Justice; and the American Patriot, who

---

[14] Ibid., 20–1.

[15] Ibid., 23–4.

[16] Rush, 13. The British public would, in any case, increasingly fault slave-owners for their exclusively economic rationalities. The turning point may have been the infamous *Zong* incident in 1781, when 133 African slaves – insured as cargo – were thrown overboard as supplies of potable water ran low. 'The *Zong* affair', note Burnard and Garrigus, 'played a central role in making the abolition of the slave trade a matter of intense public interest in Britain. It served as a supreme example of the callous financial calculations on which the slave trade was based'. Burnard and Garrigus, 216.

[17] Rush, 33.

[18] Ibid., 18.

reduces his African Brethren to Slavery, contrary to justice and Humanity?'.[19] If the last argument seems something of a stretch to modern ears, it was not so at the time. As Larry Tise has noted, public champions of slavery were hard to find in the immediate aftermath of the American Revolution, when liberty for all was the byword.[20]

For our purposes, among the most interesting elements of Rush's response to Nisbet is the fact that the Philadelphian physician made use of his medical expertise in a way he had not in his earlier pamphlet. The first critique of the slave trade, once theological and economic apologies were dispatched, had tended to focus on individualised barbarisms perpetrated against the bodies of the enslaved. But Nisbet had made something of a tactical error in attempting to pre-emptively dispose of one of the most telling abolitionist arguments, one which pointed to the net decline of the native slave population in the West Indies as proof of the specific barbarity of the slave system there.[21] Nisbet termed it a 'common accusation' (albeit one which was 'very unjust') which held that 'the West-Indies are obliged to have supplies from Africa, to keep up their numbers'. Calculations were not straightforward, Nisbet argued: in any case, neither the failure to flourish nor the loss of African lives in the West Indies could be blamed on European owners. The slave population was 'checked by the irregularities of both sexes, and their carelessness in preserving their health'. And further misfortunes that slaves encountered, he added with galling insouciance, 'are mostly of their own seeking'.[22] Rush, unsurprisingly, disagreed, noting that African populations in Africa were hardly in decline and invoking both their 'Colour and certain Customs' to explain their ability to withstand diseases that crippled European populations. It was conditions in the New World, not native African weakness or behavioural flaws that led to populational decline. As we have seen, it had become a trope to note that childbirth was attended with less difficulty in warmer climates. Rush cited a Dr Bancroft who reported that 'Indian women in Guiana seem to be exempted from the Curse inflicted upon

---

[19] Ibid., 30.

[20] 'So long as Americans revered the revolution and its ideology, slavery was inseparable from evil. It was only when they thought of slavery outside the perspective of Revolutionary ideology that they ascribed good to it'. Tise, 37.

[21] On the natalist debate, see Sheridan, *Doctors and Slaves: A Medical and Demographic History of Slavery in the British West Indies, 1680–1834*, Chapter Eight; Michael Tadman, 'The Demographic Cost of Sugar: Debates on Slave Societies and Natural Increase in the Americas', *The American Historical Review* 105 (2000); Katherine Paugh, 'The Politics of Childbearing in the British Caribbean and the Atlantic World During the Age of Abolition, 1776–1838', *Past and Present*, no. 221 (2013). *The Politics of Reproduction: Race, Medicine, and Fertility in the Age of Abolition*; Bush; Bush-Slimani; Sasha Turner, 'Home-Grown Slaves: Women, Reproduction, and the Abolition of the Slave Trade, Jamaica 1788–1807', *Journal of Women's History* 23 (2011).

[22] Nisbet, 27.

Eve', and a Dr George Taylor, who served as physician and man-midwife on St Kitts, who observed that white women on the island gave birth easily.[23] Rush noted that far more children died in the West Indies soon after birth than elsewhere, due to the disease known locally as the Jaw-Fall (infant tetanus), and blamed the fact directly on 'their peculiar circumstances as Slaves'. And, like many abolitionists, Rush drew attention to the effects of the seasoning, which 'destroys many of the Negroes'. But he did specifically reject the common explanation for this massive death rate, arguing that the climate of the West Indies was not responsible. As before, he argued not for African weakness, but rather for a kind of relative strength: 'They are even exempted from the most fatal epidemic diseases to which the White People are subject'. It was, rather, their new diet, the hardships and suffering they were now forced to undergo, labour 'in a Climate not intended for it', and their intemperance with regard to liquor that was to blame for the 'immense Waste' of their lives. And all of this suffering was to be charged not to a curse, or innate debility, or African cultural failings, but to the evils of the slave system itself.

I have begun with a close of reading of the debate between Rush and Nisbet because their exchange brings to the fore a large number of the themes to be explored in this chapter on race, medicine, abolitionism, and slavery in the second half of the eighteenth century. The literature on the abolitionist debates is, of course, vast, but comparatively little attention has been paid to the role played – on either side – by medical men.[24] As we can see, however, medical arguments supplemented and were entwined within arguably more familiar moral, theological, and economic positions. The relationships between medicine, climate, and disease were critical for a debate that turned on who was to blame for the inhuman and near-unimaginable losses of human life due to the seasoning or whether black bodies were essential for the cultivation of sugar under a blazing New World sun. Medical men and medical logics were marshalled in arguments over African inferiority and the very question of their humanity. And doctors, surgeons, midwives and others all participated – as we have seen both here and in previous chapters – in ongoing discussions over the question of the single or multiple origins of different 'races'. As abolitionist critiques invoked changes – more or less cosmetic – doctors became even more

---

[23] Taylor noted, however, that 'Negro Women' had a much more difficult time, putting this down to the distortion of their pelvis by '[k]icks they get when young, and to the Hardships they undergo during their Pregnancy'.

[24] A recent and very welcome exception is Sean Morey Smith, 'Seasoning and Abolition: Humoural Medicine in the Eighteenth-Century British Atlantic', *Slavery and Abolition* 36 (2015). See also Sheridan, *Doctors and Slaves: A Medical and Demographic History of Slavery in the British West Indies, 1680–1834*. Quinlan.

thoroughly imbricated within the slave system. From the 1760s one begins to find medical texts written on ways to handle the initial seasoning and later care of slaves. From the 1780s, the writings of men who claimed to administer to the medical needs of thousands of slaves per year were cited, critiqued, and debated in parliamentary sessions devoted to the question of the continuation of the trade within the British Empire. Abolitionists excoriated planters for the death and suffering – from disease, neglect, and harsh treatment – of the slaves they owned, while some West Indian doctors used their experiences to offer *apologia* and negations of precisely these charges.

Before turning to the structure of this chapter, let me be clear about why the history of race-medicine should matter for the broader intellectual history of race, by looking at two forms of boundary-making that have helped to shape our understandings of that history. The first comes from one of the foremost analysts of Kant's theories on race. 'The fact that the scientific concept of race was developed initially in Germany rather than in Britain or America', Robert Bernasconi has written, 'suggests that it was not specifically the interests of the slaveowners that led to its introduction, but rather, as Kant's essays themselves confirm, an interest in classification and above all the attempt to provide a theoretical defence of monogenism'.[25] On the one hand, I share Bernasconi's scepticism with what are common lay beliefs, which suggest that scientific racism was invented largely as a justification for slavery and a rapacious colonialism.[26] If abolitionist debates are an important place for locating the rise of racial conceptions, such simple instrumentalism – as I noted in Chapter 6 – is nonetheless not adequate as a means of understanding the complexity of the issues involved. On the other hand, Bernasconi appears to leave as unconsidered the question of why, in 1775, monogenism should need such vigorous defence? Attention only to elite discourse – and hence to the provocations of Kames – ignores the fact that the Scottish jurist was only one of several polygenist authors in the second half of the century and that most others were directly responding to Benezet and his allies in the 1760s and the threat posed by the Somerset decision in 1772. Monogenism did, indeed, require defence, but it did so in part because of the attacks levelled by slave owners.

The second attempt at boundary-making comes from Blumenbach, whose history of previous thinkers on race has tended to shape the boundaries of many subsequent reconstructions. It was with some chagrin that Blumenbach

---

[25] Robert Bernasconi, 'Who Invented the Concept of Race? Kant's Role in the Enlightenment Construction of Race', in *Race*, ed. Robert Bernasconi (Malden, MA and Oxford: Blackwell, 2001), 21.

[26] This is, for example, the first answer my undergraduate students proffer when asked about the origin of scientific racism. Of course, from the end of the eighteenth century, scientific racism worked as a powerful defence of an already-established slave-trade.

lamented, in 1775, that some should try to allow pathology to 'obtrude' into the natural history of the varieties of mankind.[27] His aim, he suggested, was to restore each area to its natural place, assuming that separation was the original state. Like Bernasconi, Blumenbach's aim here was to offer a purified understanding of what the 'real' question of race was. For both, however, refusing the act of purification – rejecting it as poor history – pays dividends, for it insists on keeping power and politics in the story. Of course, it is not difficult to see power and politics in Kant's claim that 'all Negroes stink' or Blumenbach's studious examination of the skulls of peoples sent him by Europeans in far-flung lands. Yet attention to the history of medicine brings to the fore the immediate power-relations between, for example, a West Indian physician and the thousands of slaves nominally under his care, or the forms of authority that treated the melioration of pain and suffering as an issue requiring race as a category of analysis. A dual denial of boundaries is necessary, for we need to understand race in the later eighteenth century – even seemingly abstract, taxonomic and naturalistic understandings of race – as intimately related to the theories and practices of slavery. One way to do so is to broaden our understanding of what such naturalistic understandings were, and to insist, as I have throughout this part of the book, on seeing the pathologies and physiologies of race together with its anatomies.[28]

The chapter is divided into three sections. Section 7.1 explores the role of medicine in abolitionist debates. West Indian doctors and other men who claimed to possess medical understanding offered critiques or defences of slavery that relied on their own expertise and experience; they put forward their own practice as examples of the ways in which slavery might be meliorated or reformed; and some, as we shall see, even penned manuals that served simultaneously as propagandistic tracts that sought to demonstrate the existence of a humane slavery and also offered descriptions of the kinds of practices that would keep slaves healthy through the seasoning and beyond.

Section 7.2 continues and develops the arguments of Chapter 5, noting that climatic, cultural, and dietetic explanations of 'racial' disparities remained the orthodox position throughout the century.[29] While many writers noted that

---

[27] Johann Blumenbach, 'De Generis Humani Varietate Nativa (1775)', in *The Anthropological Treatises of Johann Friedrich Blumenbach*, ed. Thomas Bendyshe (London: Longman, Green, Longman, Roberts, and Green, 1865), 101.

[28] For the literature's near-exclusive focus on anatomy, rather than pathology, see, e.g. Curran. See also Wheeler. An exception, in spite of its title, is Hogarth.

[29] Much has been written about ongoing tensions between universalistic and racially particular medical theory and practice into the nineteenth century. See, for example, John S. Haller, 'The Negro and the Southern Physician: A Study of Medical and Racial Attitudes, 1800–1860', *Medical History* 16 (1972); Savitt; 'The Use of Blacks for Medical Experimentation and Demonstration in the Old South', *The Journal of Southern History* 48 (1982); 'Slave Health and Southern Distinctiveness', in *Disease and Distinctiveness in the American South*, ed. Todd

Africans, Europeans, and Creoles seemed to suffer from different afflictions, fixed physical attributes were rarely invoked as an explanation within medicine. Hippocratism, broadly construed, remained the standard paradigm for etiological claims. It is, however, useful to note a division *within* these Hippocratic causes that may be discerned in writings about the diseases of warm climates. Where the objects of comparison were different parts of the globe – and the different distempers characteristic of these parts – climate was invoked as the standard and primary explanation. Different diseases (or different manifestations of the same disease) were found in different climates. Where medical men were interested in understanding the cause of varying susceptibilities within the *same* geographic region, on the other hand, climate unsurprisingly played much less of a role.[30] As specific attention to the diseases of slaves rose in response to the pressures of abolitionist critiques, medical texts increasingly emphasised the diet, clothing, housing, and behaviour of slaves (and other members of non-white populations), rather than the impact of a common climate. Thus, if one does not find 'race' in these orthodox medical tracts, one does find increasing attention to the social and cultural differences between whites and others.

Section 7.3 continues the arguments of Chapter 6, in that it explores a number of the heterodox and racialist positions that were increasingly defining a real and significant minority in European conversations. Edward Long would not be alone in his polygenism in the last decades of the 1700s. Hard versions of racial thinking would play particular roles in a debate over whether free labour was a possible alternative to slave labour in the West Indies.[31] As we have seen in the exchange between Rush and Nisbet, this issue contained mine fields for both sides. Abolitionists tended to play down the intrinsic dangers of the warm climate in favour of trenchant critiques of the backbreaking and relentless labour slaves were forced to undergo. Pro-slavery advocates who were unwilling to simply describe Africans as animals, on the other hand, needed to portray the West Indian climate as deadly to whites, but seemingly innocuous to slaves, else they be charged with murder by forced labour. Medical and anatomical claims thus abounded in a discourse about an innate, physically-rooted capacity (or not) for those of African descent to endure that which could not be tolerated by Europeans. Just as significantly, by 1780 one can begin to locate precisely the sorts of arguments that had been absent in the first half of

---

L. Savitt and James Harvey Young (Knoxville: University of Tennessee Press, 1988); Martin S. Pernick, *A Calculus of Suffering: Pain, Professionalism, and Anesthesia in Nineteenth-Century America* (New York: Columbia University Press, 1985); Fett.

[30] This is in spite of a close attention to what today would be called 'micro-climates'. See Johnston.

[31] Drescher, *The Mighty Experiment: Free Labor Versus Slavery in British Emancipation.*

the eighteenth century, arguments where medical logics and racial logics were combined and where racialised physical differences were described as causing characteristically racial medical differences. At the end of the century, race-medicine was beginning to emerge.

7.1   Medicine and Abolitionism

In 1789, when the Jamaica House of Assembly published two reports on the slave trade, the abolitionist debate was coming to a head.[32] The year before, William Wilberforce had introduced a parliamentary resolution that would have committed the British House of Commons to a discussion of the trade in its next session. Petitions were already flooding in, from both sides. An investigatory report on the matter by the Privy Council was published in April 1789 and in May Wilberforce delivered an immediately famous speech describing the horrors of the middle passage and arguing that abolition would lead to a near-certain improvement of the situation of slaves in the West Indies.[33] The Committee of the Jamaican House responded in October and November, dividing the criticisms levelled in the many petitions before Parliament into those that concerned the African slave trade and those that concerned the treatment of slaves in the West Indies. On the first matter, they (disingenuously) suggested that 'the inhabitants of the West-India islands have no concern in the ships trading to Africa'. The African trade was a British interest. Jamaican planters were involved in the trade only as the buyers 'of what British acts of Parliament have declared to be legal objects of purchase'.[34] The crucial accusations, then, were those regarding the treatment of the enslaved within the island, which they divided into four charges: that the laws governing negroes were harsh; that the laws were executed with inhumanity and without mercy; that negroes were grossly overworked and were not granted sufficient days of rest; and that the decline in the numbers of slaves on the island was due to their poor treatment.[35] It is this last charge and the attempts at defences against it that should most

---

[32] Jamaica.

[33] '[H]is *speech* is circulated everywhere', wrote one pro-slavery writer with chagrin in 1792, 'and the cruelties recorded in it are becomes as familiar to *children* as the story of *Blue Beard* or *Jack the Giant Killer*'. Jesse Foot, *A Defence of the Planters in the West Indies; Comprised in Four Arguments* (London: J. Debrett, 1792), 75.

[34] Jamaica, 2–3. On medicine and the middle passage, see Sheridan, 'The Guinea Surgeons on the Middle Passage: The Provision of Medical Services in the British Slave Trade'. Latest estimates suggest that roughly one in seven of the 3.4 million African slaves taken by the British Empire died in the middle passage. Richardson. The proportion changed over time, however, with losses averaging roughly 20 per cent before 1600 and dropping to 12 per cent in the second half of the eighteenth century. David Northrup, *Africa's Discovery of Europe, 1450–1850* (Oxford: Oxford University Press, 2002), 118.

[35] Jamaica, 3.

capture our attention here, for it was on this issue that the Committee invoked the evidence of medical men.

Beginning with deeply suspicious exculpatory calculations that still indicated that there had been a net loss of more than 26, 000 lives among slaves on the island since 1655,[36] the report then listed the two main causes of slave mortality: 'The great proportion of deaths that happen among negroes newly imported' (that is, the seasoning), and 'The loss which prevails among the negro infants that are born in the country'.[37] The three medical men called to provide evidence to the committee (whose interviews were then published as appendices) came to the same broad conclusions on the question of the seasoning. Deaths were not to be laid at the doors of planters, they averred. Losses among newly arrived slaves were due to diseases from which they were suffering prior to landing, acquired either in Africa or on board ship. They differed more on the causes of the deaths of infants. James Chisholme and Adam Anderson both agreed that roughly one-quarter of all negro children died within two weeks of their birth. Chisholme ascribed this to the lack of cleanliness and care with which they were treated and dressed, a point that Anderson denied.[38] Neither, however, seemed to regard the issue as one that was easily solvable in practice. John Quier reported that the affliction was not common in the area of his practice and placed the blame for the island's declining slave population on the promiscuity of negro women, which led both to frequent abortions and to a lack of care for children, who were 'lost through neglect and the want of maternal affection, which the mothers seldom retain for their offspring by a former husband'.[39] Rehearsing standard tropes about the wickedness, ignorance, and wantonness of slaves, then, physicians lent their expertise to the apologist cause.

We shall return to some of these claims soon, but for us the most basic point to be drawn from the report of the Jamaican Assembly is the centrality of medical arguments to the abolitionist debate.[40] Reading abolitionist tracts,

---

[36] Burnard and Garrigus also call this figure 'highly improbable'. Burnard and Garrigus, 233.

[37] Jamaica., 15.

[38] Chisholme argued that paying greater attention to the sanitary conditions of newborns would thus, in principle, solve the problem quite easily. 'But, simple as this may appear in theory, those who are much conversant with negroes', he asserted, 'will be aware of the difficulty, if not impossibility, of putting it in practice, in a degree sufficient to answer the purpose. For, such is the ignorance, obstinacy, and inattention of negroes: so little regard have they for each other, and so averse are they to executing the directions of white people, when repugnant to their own prejudices', ibid., Chisholme, Appendix 6, 26–8, Anderson, Appendix 7, 28–30.

[39] Ibid., Quier, Appendix 8, 30–3.

[40] Beyond the specific elements cited below, I want to cite here my more general debts to Sheridan's coverage of the relationships between medicine and slavery in Sheridan, *Doctors and Slaves: A Medical and Demographic History of Slavery in the British West Indies, 1680–1834.*

the public was horrified by stories of torture and punishment and moved by descriptions of the backbreaking labour slaves were forced to undergo. Almost every island passed laws in response to such critiques, but it was hard to deny charges that such laws were mere unenforceable (and certainly unenforced) window dressing when faced with the brute fact of a decline in population. Claims like Rush's, which held the slave system responsible for a prodigious loss of life, required expert responses, which blamed not planters or their laws, but shipboard conditions and the practices of slaves themselves. Among the most trenchant critics of slavery were medical men – Rush and James Ramsay perhaps the most famous. As we can see, however, physicians and surgeons also argued for the other side. It was not slavery *per se,* that was to blame, they argued, for matters were complex. But the situation could be improved and, practiced properly, medicine could aid in melioration.

If we accept that medicine played a role in abolitionist debates, we should also acknowledge the role played by abolitionist debates in pushing certain medical issues to the fore. The Jamaican Assembly seemed to make it obvious that the profound losses due to the seasoning should be discussed in explicitly medical terms, but this had not always been so. Charles Leslie's *New History of Jamaica* (1740) did not shy away from describing some of the worst elements of life on the island: 'trivial errors' punished with brutal whippings, slaves treated cruelly simply for the pleasure of the overseer, and 'their Bodies all in a Gore of Blood, the skin torn off their Backs with the cruel Whip, beaten Pepper, and Salt, rubbed in the Wounds, and a large Stick of Sealing-wax dropped leisurely upon them'.[41] And yet, only a half-dozen pages after this horrific depiction, Leslie described the stunning number of deaths due to the seasoning without any of this emotion or empathy.[42] An Owner, he noted, must replenish 'his Stock ... every Year, or he would soon want Hands for his Work. Almost half of the new imported Negroes die in the Seasoning'.[43] One should compare this invocation of a numerical claim to that of Anthony Benezet, the French-born Quaker who has been called the 'father of Atlantic abolitionism'.[44] In 1762, Benezet, too, noted that roughly half of the slaves imported to Jamaica died of the seasoning, while a quarter perished in Barbados, bringing the total number

---

[41] Leslie, 305.

[42] As Delbourgo observes, discussions of the appalling treatment of slaves were not necessarily understood, in the first half of the eighteenth century, as 'self-evident horrors', but rather (as in the case of Sloane's descriptions, which were endlessly cited and reproduced by later abolitionists) as 'morally and politically indeterminate curiosities'. Delbourgo, 'Slavery in the Cabinet of Curiosities: Hans Sloane's Atlantic World'. 15.

[43] Leslie, 312.

[44] Jackson, David L. Crosby, ed. *The Complete Antislavery Writings of Anthony Benezet, 1754–1783* (Baton Rouge: Louisiana State University Press, 2013).

of deaths, including the passage, for a single year of British trading to the West Indies and colonies in North America to twelve thousand souls.

What a sad dreadful Affair then is this Man-Trade, whereby so many Thousands of our Fellow rational Creatures lose their lives, are, truly and properly speaking, murdered every Year; I do not think there is an Instance of so great Barbarity and Cruelty carried on in any Part of the World, as is this, Year after Year. It is enough to make one tremble, to think what a Load of Guilt lies upon this Nation, on this Account, and that the Blood of Thousands of poor innocent Creatures, murdered every Year, in carrying on this cursed Trade, cry aloud to Heaven for Vengeance.[45]

It is surely no coincidence that the first tract on how to properly season slaves to avoid such losses appeared two years later. James Grainger was born in Scotland around 1721 and graduated with a medical degree from Edinburgh in 1753, then moving in 1759 to St Kitts. In publishing his 'Essay on the More Common West-India Diseases' in 1764, Grainger registered his 'astonishment, that among the many valuable medical tracts which of late years have been offered to the public, none has been purposely written on the method of seasoning new negroes'.[46] This 'method' was fairly straightforward, involving gradual habituation to the work of the fields. Or, as he phrased it in his poem, 'The Sugar Cane': 'Let gentle work,/Or rather playful exercise, amuse/The novel gang: and far be angry words;/Far ponderous chains: and far disheartening blows'.[47] This was valuable counter-propaganda and signalled the beginning of medicine's involvement in a discourse about the development of a more benevolent slavery. The seasoning, in Grainger's work, was not a brutal statistical fact that underscored the fundamental inhumanity of the man-trade. It was, rather, a problem to be resolved by better and more medically informed management. Urging better medical treatment for the enslaved, the planter could be economically rational and take back the moral high-ground ceded to the abolitionist:[48]

But it is not enough to take care of Negroes when they are sick; they should also be well clothed and regularly fed. Neglecting either of these important precepts is not only

---

[45] Anthony Benezet, *A Short Account of That Part of Africa, Inhabited by the Negroes* (Philadelphia: William Dunlap, 1762), 39–40.

[46] Grainger, 6.

[47] 'The Sugar-Cane (1764). Book IV'., in *On the Treatment and Management of the More Common West-India Diseases (1750–1802)*, ed. J. Edward Hutson (Kingston, Jamaica: University of the West Indies Press, 2005), 62–3. On the poem, see Kelly Wisecup, *Medical Encounters: Knowledge and Identity in Early American Literatures* (Amherst: University of Massachusetts Press, 2013), 127–60. See also Smith.

[48] 'The antislavery movement, particularly in its evangelical Christian incarnation, drew strength from a new rhetoric about slave mortality; what had earlier been described principally in economic terms became a moral problems of vital importance to the "soul" of the British nation'. Brown, 157.

inhuman, it is the worst species of prodigality. One Negroe saved in this manner more than pays the additional expences which owners of slaves by this means incur. But, supposing it did not, it ought seriously to be considered by all masters, that they must answer before the Almighty for their conduct towards their Negroes.[49]

As Larry Tise has noted, pro-slavery writings tended to be reactive: a number appearing in response to the criticisms levelled by Benezet and others in the 1760s, another grouping, including those written against Rush, emerging after the Somerset case in 1772, and a third in response to a book written by the former surgeon, Reverend James Ramsay in 1784. *An Essay on the Treatment and Conversion of African Slaves in the British Sugar Colonies* excoriated planters for their treatment of the enslaved and drew bitter and often *ad hominem* replies. Ramsay covered some of the same ground as abolitionists before him, building before the reader's eye an image of the grossly excessive labour and brutal punishments to which slaves were subjected. He also added comparatively new elements, drawing on surgical knowledge gained first in his training under Dr George Macaulay, physician at the British Lying-in Hospital in London, and then his practice in the Navy and – even after his ordination – on the island of St Christopher.[50] Ramsay may have been the first major abolitionist writer to detail the system for caring for sick slaves. A poorly paid surgeon, he noted, was employed to care for sick slaves, with his income set at a certain amount per head per year. Some 'frugal planters' eschewed the services of medical men, dosing their slaves with commercially available powders and pills, calling in a practitioner only to 'pronounce them past recovery'.[51] Where the plantation manager was a steady, stable and married man, Ramsay suggested, one could count on better diets and treatment for the sick, with the manager's wife taking on a supervisory role. Yet the practice of hiring married men was becoming less common, and when such a figure was a 'gadding, gossiping reveller (a character sometimes to be met with)', the sick were very poorly served. 'Often, while the manager is feasting abroad, careless and ignorant of what has happened, some hapless wretch among the slaves is taken ill, and unnoticed, unpitied, dies, without even the poor comfort of a surgeon, in his last moments, to say, "It is now too late"'.[52] And it was not unusual for as many as one in eight (presumably seasoned) negroes to die of 'fevers, fluxes, dropsies' in a year as a result of excessive labour and minimal food and

[49] Grainger, 'An Essay on the More Common West-India Diseases, James Grainger, Md (1764), with Additional Notes by William Wright, MD, FRS (1802)', 51.
[50] James Watt, 'Surgeon James Ramsay, 1733–1789: The Navy and the Slave Trade', *Journal of the Royal Society of Medicine* 87 (1994).
[51] James Ramsay, *An Essay on the Treatment and Conversion of African Slaves in the British Sugar Colonies* (Dublin: T. Walker, C. Jenkin, R. Marchbank, L. White, R. Burton, P. Byrne, 1784), 70–1.
[52] Ibid., Note, 71–2.

care.[53] Even more disturbing than this portrayal of callous neglect may have been Ramsay's description of the treatment of pregnant and nursing women.[54] Plantation owners forced all who were deemed capable to work in the field gang, so that 'hardly any remonstrance from the surgeon can, in many cases, save a poor diseased wretch from the labour'. To this work were assigned even pregnant women in the last months of their term: 'and hence suffer many an abortion; which some managers are unfeeling enough to express joy at, because the woman, on recovery, having no child to care for, will have no pretence for indulgence'.[55] Were she to carry the child to term, Ramsay continued, the infant would be born in a 'dark, damp, smoky hut', which explained the loss of such infants to cramps and convulsions.[56]

Philip Gibbes published his *Instructions for the Treatment of Negroes* two years after Ramsay's *Essay*, although he was at pains in a later edition to stress that his 'sentiments were entertained and these instructions given, long before Ramsay wrote or Wilberforce spoke'.[57] His positive recommendations were fairly basic and involved allowing sufficient time for new slaves to become seasoned to the climate before they were put to strenuous labour and providing them with sufficient amounts of nutritious food, after the recommendations of Count Rumford.[58] Turning to the question of whether pregnant women should work in the fields, Gibbes agreed with Ramsay (albeit for somewhat different reasons): 'A small degree of the knowledge of the human frame', he asserted, 'will inform you, that laborious exercise obstructs procreation: for which reason it is extremely improper and ill-judged to make females carry

---

[53] Ibid., 83.

[54] Ramsay's interest in this topic no doubt derived from his time spent training at the British lying-in hospital. See Watt; Paugh, 'The Politics of Childbearing in the British Caribbean and the Atlantic World During the Age of Abolition, 1776–1838', 128.

[55] Ramsay, 75. Such critiques had some effect. 'Under the Leeward Islands Act of 1798, for instance, female slaves "five months gone" were to be employed only on light work and were to be punished by confinement only "under penalty of five pounds". Ameliorative legislation passed in the Leewards in 1798 and Jamaica in 1809 included provisions that female slaves "having six children living" should be "exempt from hard labour" and the owner "exempt from taxes" for such female slaves'. Bush, 29.

[56] Ramsay, 76.

[57] Philip Gibbes, *Instruction for the Treatment of Negroes &C. &C. &C.*, 2nd ed. (London: Shepperson and Reynolds, 1797), 132. That said, he did confess that his hope in originally publishing lay in 'repelling the illiberal attacks of dangerous and mistaken zealots'. Ibid., 68.

[58] Gibbes' *Instructions* are perhaps most remarkable for the execrable poetry they contain. Gibbes reproduced songs intended to be sung by slaves and written by 'a very ingenious Lady'. For example, this one, on labour: 'How useful is labour, how healthful and good!/It keeps us from mischief, procures wholesome food;/ It saves from much sickness and loathsome disease/ That fall on the idle and pamper'd with ease'. Or this one, on the curse of Ham: 'We're children of Cham! He his father offended,/ Who gave him the curse which to us is descended./ "A servant of servants" alas! is our curse;/ And bad as it is, it has sav'd us from worse'. Ibid., 107, 33.

canes to the mill or in uneven fields'.[59] Robert Thomas, writing in 1790, con-curred, suggesting that benevolence was already a part of the care provided by several proprietors, who did not assign women to the field gang after their first three or four months of pregnancy, demanded lighter work until the sev-enth or eighth month, when no further duty was required, and 'annually send out baby-clothes for the use of their breeding women'.[60] That position marked a difference from John Quier's, in his testimony to the Assembly. Quier had insisted that he had not known any cases of abortions to follow – as Ramsay had claimed – from excessive labour or 'ill usage', and averred instead that 'moderate labour is beneficial to pregnant women, as being the best means of preserving general health'.[61]

Where Gibbes, Quier, Thomas and other defenders of slavery were all in apparent agreement, however, was on the necessity to move the debate on the declining slave population away from the question of death rates and towards those concerning birth rates. For on the latter they could dwell on questions of the promiscuity of enslaved women and avoid many of the ugly questions about infant mortality that abolitionist authors were raising. Deploying a trope explored in Chapter 5, Gibbes thus claimed that 'Early prostitution is the cer-tain obstruction to population', offering a frankly graphic farming analogy (derived from a 'very sensible friend') to explain his logic:

When the earth is prepared and ploughed, and the seed, at the proper season, is cast into the furrows, if it be ploughed over and over again, would the seed thus, disturbed in its germination strike root deeply, or would it vegetate at all? If sowed with different seeds, inimical to each other, how weak and mingled would be the produce! Let the divine command be carefully observed as well in your care of the women as of the soil, *Sow not thy land with divers seeds.*[62]

More standard explanation connected Afro-Caribbean hyper-sexuality with a resultant venereal infection, leading to infertility, or else tied 'prostitution' to the procuring of abortions, which then led to medical difficulties.[63] Long, for example, stated simply that 'the women here are, in general, common

---

[59] Ibid., 86.
[60] Thomas, xi–xii.
[61] Jamaica., Appendix 8, 32.
[62] Gibbes, note, 125–6.
[63] 'Put simply', writes Katherine Paugh, 'many British authors believed that racially charac-teristic sexual promiscuity led to venereal disease and infertility, while they believed that Christian monogamy encouraged fertility'. Paugh, 'The Politics of Childbearing in the British Caribbean and the Atlantic World During the Age of Abolition, 1776–1838', 129. On hyper-sexuality, see Morgan, '"Some Could Suckle over Their Shoulder": Male Travelers, Female Bodies, and the Gendering of Racial Ideology, 1500–1770'. Altink, *Representations of Slave Women in Discourses on Slavery and Abolition, 1780–1838*; 'Deviant and Dangerous: Pro-Slavery Representation of Jamaican Slave Women's Sexuality, C. 1780–1834'.

prostitutes; and many take specifics to cause abortion'.[64] The Governor, Edward Trelawney, invoked abortions as the direct cause of low populations: 'what chiefly contributes to their being so few Children among the *English* Negroes', he asserted, 'is the Practice of the Wenches in procuring Abortions. As they lie with both Colours, and do not know which the Child may prove of, to disoblige neither, they stifle it at birth'.[65] Thomas insisted that the frequency, amongst Afro-Caribbean women, of cases of 'the whites' [probably Leucorrhea] was due to 'the frequent abortions they designedly bring upon themselves, in order to prevent their having the trouble of rearing their offspring, to which they are seldom bound by the same ties of maternal tenderness and affection that white women are'.[66] Thomas, in fact, offered a litany of reasons for the fact that 'not one estate in fifty can keep up its original number, even although the greatest humanity and lenity have been practice, and all possible pains have been taken for rearing the children that have been born', ranging from early promiscuity, prostitution, abortions, early loss of infant life, and diseases to which women in warm climates were more subject than in colder ones.[67] How powerful was this discourse may be gleaned from the fact that even an author profoundly critical of the Report of the Jamaican Assembly and of Quier's testimony in particular found himself in agreement with the doctor's claim that many abortions on the island were the result of 'promiscuous intercourse'.[68] Negative judgements about black female sexuality made unlikely bedfellows.[69]

Like many of the owners of plantations in the West Indies, Gibbes was an absentee landlord, living in Britain. Such owners were, as Sheridan noted, 'highly vulnerable to antislavery propaganda', and many pushed for measures to improve, although not abolish, slavery.[70] Where general problems with the treatment of slaves were acknowledged by this group, blame was placed largely on the backs of managers and overseers, who became the public face of the atrocities and neglect abolitionists had identified. Coupled with rising prices for slaves in the last decades of the century, the weight of public opinion pushed colonial legislatures to institute new laws and codes to protect slaves from the most brutal treatment and, eventually, to encourage an increase

---

[64] Long, *The History of Jamaica*, II, 436.

[65] Quoted in Sheridan, *Doctors and Slaves: A Medical and Demographic History of Slavery in the British West Indies, 1680–1834*, 224.

[66] Thomas, 279.

[67] Ibid., xix–xx, xvi.

[68] A. Jamaica Planter, *Notes on the Two Reports from the Committee of the Honourable House of Assembly of Jamaica* (London: James Phillips, 1789), 61.

[69] For more on this point, see Paugh, 'The Politics of Childbearing in the British Caribbean and the Atlantic World During the Age of Abolition, 1776–1838'.

[70] Sheridan, *Doctors and Slaves: A Medical and Demographic History of Slavery in the British West Indies, 1680–1834*, 230.

in their population.[71] In Jamaica, the Consolidated Slave Act of 1781, for example, introduced clauses requiring adequate clothing, the allocation of provision grounds and 'sufficient time to work the same', and prescribing the punishment for a master who mutilated or dismembered slaves. The Act of 1787 added further clauses, with medical elements that seem to have been a direct response to Ramsay's criticisms, allowing towns and parishes to levy taxes to provide 'food, medical care, and attendance' for slaves – too old or sick to care for themselves – who had been abandoned by their owners and requiring that a surgeon provide, under oath, an account of the increase or decrease of numbers on every plantation, with a description of the cause of each decrease, in order to 'prevent the destruction of negroes, by excessive labour and unreasonable punishments'. Critics noted, however, that many such laws were essentially toothless. As one writer identifying himself as a 'Jamaica Planter' put it: 'I have for many years been conversant with Jamaica, and know of but one instance of the law against mutilation being inforced, and that instance occurred since the people in Britain have interested themselves in favour of the poor negroes'.[72] The editor for that work put his finger on one of the most obvious intrinsic problems with legislation that pitted masters against slaves in the realm of the law: the testimony of slaves was not admissible against owners.[73]

Laws that mandated that medical men, dependent upon owners for their livelihoods, testify in cases of excessive neglect or unlawful deaths also seem impossibly naïve (assuming that they were intended to have real effects in the first place).[74] Indeed, the testimony of such practitioners seems to have largely served the opposite cause. Thus, Jesse Foot, who had served as a surgeon for three years in the West Indies, with the 'care of two thousand negroes annually' invoked his own experiences as part of his *Defence of the Planters in the West Indies*.[75] Foot declared that he had not seen 'any other treatment than that which humanity dictates', adding that 'during my practice I never was called

---

[71] Ramsay noted that 'slaves be now raised to a price that few old settled plantations can afford to give'. Ramsay, 76. On the new slave laws, see Goveia, 152–202. 'The West Indian Slave Laws of the Eighteenth Century', *Chapters in Caribbean History* 2 (1970). Similar logics applied in the French West-Indies. Weaver, 29.

[72] Jamaica Planter, 20.

[73] Ibid., i–ii.

[74] As Goveia notes, the position of a doctor 'was a difficult one, since he was himself an employee of the planter on whom he would be forced to inform if he took his responsibilities for his slaves more seriously than his loyalty to an employer and fellow inhabitant'. Goveia, *Slave Society in the British Leeward Islands at the End of the Eighteenth Century*, 198. 'Only with the Coroner's Act of 1817 did an actual law establish a clear and unambiguous requirement that coroners perform inquests into the deaths of slaves, also stipulating that slaveholders could not be jurors at inquests concerning their own slaves. A belated response to antislavery pressure, the act established that, in principle, the deaths of black people merited serious investigation' Brown, 80.

[75] Foot, 31.

to give *surgical relief* to any negroes who had suffered from the severity of chastisement'.[76] Robert Thomas drew on nine years of medical care for three thousand negroes a year to make a similar point: 'I never was called upon', he asserted, 'to administer assistance to a negro in consequence of any violence or cruelty exercised over him, either by the master, manager, or overseer'.[77] It is possible that one outcome of the new laws – coupled with the need to be seen to be responding to anti-slavery critiques and the economic incentives introduced by the increasing value of slaves – may have been a reduction in the number of planters who relied on their own judgement alone in treating sick or injured slaves. And yet, even though the number of practitioners rose, it should be clear from the sheer number of slaves under their yearly care the minimal attention each patient could receive. Foot and Thomas were hardly alone in having thousands of slaves under their charge.[78] In their testimony before the Jamaica Assembly, Chisholme, Anderson, and Quier detailed the size of their practices – around 4000 slaves a year – as part of their credentials. The 'Jamaica Planter' placed this number in some perspective by noting that a regiment or a ship of war of five hundred men was accorded a surgeon and perhaps several surgeon's mates. 'Once, twice, or thrice in a week, to gallop to a plantation, to take a peep into the hospital, or hot-house, as it is called, write in a book, "bleed this", "purge that", "blister another", "here give an opiate", "there the bark", is not, in my opinion, taking care of, though it may be called taking charge of, the healths of 4000 or 5000 negroes'.[79]

The abolitionist debate – spearheaded, in some cases, by those with medical training – managed to place the medical care of slaves near the forefront of public concern. As a measure of this, one might note that in 1789, the Privy Council Committee systematically asked witnesses about the care of slaves in sickness, the laws that existed to regulate such care, and the provision for slaves when they were old and infirm.[80] Colonial legislatures acted to place such laws on the books from the 1780s onwards. Yet much of the attention in the colonies had been reactive. Tracts about such medical care for the enslaved tended to dissipate after Wilberforce's bill – delayed until 1791 – sputtered in the House, the country's political mood swinging against radical reform in the aftermath of the French Revolution. In 1792 all Wilberforce was able to extract from his fellow parliamentarians was the agreement on a 'gradual abolition' of

---

[76] Ibid., 75–6.
[77] Thomas, xv.
[78] For average number of slaves per practitioner on different islands, see Sheridan, *Doctors and Slaves: A Medical and Demographic History of Slavery in the British West Indies, 1680–1834*, 302 ff.
[79] Jamaica Planter, 60.
[80] Sheridan, *Doctors and Slaves: A Medical and Demographic History of Slavery in the British West Indies, 1680–1834*, 271.

the slave trade. An Act to that effect would wait until 1807. Beyond legislation, it should be clear that medical logics were a key part of the discourse around abolitionism, with practitioners arrayed on either side of the debate. For every Rush or Ramsay who drew attention to the tremendous losses of life due to the seasoning or infant tetanus, or to the appalling treatment of pregnant and nursing women and sick or aged slaves, there was a Quier, a Foot, or a Thomas willing to testify to the exceptionality of horrific punishments, when they were meted out, or to the culpability of slaves in their own declining population. Medical expertise was a valuable commodity in a battle between melioration and abolition. It was no less so in the debates over relationships between disease and 'race'.

7.2   Race, Climate, Disease

It was not at all uncommon for medical men writing about the diseases of warm climates to discuss differences in susceptibilities and outcomes between the peoples native to different places. It was, however, very rare (at least until the 1780s) for anyone to explain these differences by invoking fixed physical characteristics as a cause. For roughly the first half of the eighteenth century, as I argued in Chapter 5, the standard element – with some striking exceptions – invoked to explain both seemingly geographically particular diseases and 'racial', political, and cultural variance was environment, broadly construed. The touchstone was Hippocrates' *Airs, Waters, and Places*, which had been the model for location-specific medical texts since the early 1700s. Neo-Hippocratism as 'anthropological' method reached new heights around mid-century, with the publication of Montesquieu's *Spirit of the Laws* in 1748.[81] Drawing on John Arbuthnot's equally Hippocratic *Essay Concerning the Effects of Air on Human Bodies* (1733), Montesquieu argued that cold air caused the body's fibres to contract, which increased their 'spring' and strength, while warmth relaxed and lengthened them.[82] 'Therefore', he wrote, 'men are more vigorous in cold climates'.[83] Indeed, 'The people in hot countries are timid like old men; those in cold countries are courageous like young men'.[84] More broadly, both large-scale modes of governance and smaller-scale social mores were rooted in climatic conditions.[85] The text was

---

[81] Anne M. Cohler, Basia C. Miller, and Harold S. Stone, eds., *Montesquieu: The Spirit of the Laws* (Cambridge: Cambridge University Press, 2010).

[82] Arbuthnot. Curran, 134.

[83] Cohler, Miller, and Stone, 231.

[84] Ibid., 232.

[85] We find it claimed in Book 17, on the relationship between climate and political servitude, for example, that '[P]ower should always be despotic in Asia', while Book 14, on the laws and the

to prove enormously influential in abolitionist discourse as well as many other sites. Rush was far from the only anti-slavery writer to invoke the authority of the French *philosophe* to bolster his claims about the non-essential, climatically variable differences between peoples, even as he avoided Montesquieu's more troubling suggestion that warm climates might provide the only locations where natural slavery could be countenanced.[86]

Within medicine, as within political writings, climate served to explain both differences and similarities. Where climates were distinct, one found people of different appearance and political systems, as well as different diseases. Where seemingly different peoples inhabited the same region, however, one would expect, over time, the emergence of common political and social orders as well as afflictions. Climatic similarity, that is, overpowered other forms of difference. It was climate that produced the unity that was England, for example, despite the variety of human stocks that made up the population. In an age that saw the emergence of European national states, such unities mattered, but they were far more fraught in the colonies, particularly those built on the binary distinction between the enslaved and the free. Montesquieu's equivocation over whether slavery could ever be tolerated was telling. I have found at least two medical texts from the 1750s and 1760s, however, that take climatic reasoning to its logical conclusion. In them, one finds whites and blacks, Europeans and Africans, the free and the enslaved, grouped together by a discourse about nativity and habituation. In Charles Bisset's *Treatise on the Scurvy* 'Negroes, Creoles, and seasoned Europeans' are grouped together by the fact that they rarely suffer from either the 'malignant Bilious Fever' or the scurvy.[87] What the three kinds of peoples have in common is a relative rigidity of the fibres internal to the body. To become seasoned to the climate is to acquire such rigidity and in such a way to have one's body 'become nearly assimilated to those of Creoles and Negroes'.[88] James Lind's essay on the health of seamen

---

climate argues that Mohammed's prohibition on the drinking of wine 'is a law of the climate of Arabia'. Ibid., 283, 39.

[86] Montesquieu vacillated on this point: 'But as all men are created equal, one must say that slavery is against nature, although in certain countries it may be founded on natural reason, and these countries must be distinguished from those in which even natural reason rejects it, as in the countries of Europe where it has so fortunately been abolished ... Therefore, natural slavery must be limited to certain particular countries of the world ... I do not know if my spirit or my heart dictates this point. Perhaps there is no climate on earth where one could not engage freemen to work'. Ibid., 251–3. Cf. Curran, 137. 'While Montesquieu clearly found the enslavement of any human to be antithetical to his overall philosophical project, his understanding of climate and the *nègre's* physiology produced a significant exception to this rule: although unfortunate, under certain conditions, enslaving the black Africa was a *reasonable* decision'.

[87] Bisset, *A Treatise on the Scurvy. Design'd Chiefly for the Use of the British Navy.*, 10.

[88] Ibid., 41.

similarly paired whites and blacks on the grounds of their shared habituation. 'The *Negroes* and *Creoles*, sleeping without Hurt in the Dews,' he wrote, 'is a proof how far the Constitution may be framed and accustomed to bear what otherwise is so highly prejudicial'.[89]

Climatic explanations applied *within* a given region thus tended to produce (perhaps unnerving) similarities. We should therefore not be surprised to find that, within a slave society like the West Indies or colonial settings like those in India, climate alone was more rarely invoked to explicate medical distinctions between blacks/Africans and whites/Europeans than other elements. Far more common were invocations of particularistic diets and behaviours, which served to re-affirm important differences without making such differences either essential or unchangeable. J. Z. Holwell, for example, offered a sympathetic *Account of the Manner of Inoculating for the Small-Pox in the East Indies* (1767), one that extensively praised and recommended the practices deployed by Bengali Brahmins. He was somewhat less enthusiastic, however, about the dietary habits of the natives of the Island of St Helena, whose overuse of yam, in particular, seemed to incline them to death when afflicted with the smallpox.[90] Writing about the dysentery as it appeared on the Bite of Benin on the Guinea Coast in the mid-1780s, Robert Atchison also pointed an accusatory finger at the use of yams or fish as a 'chief food' instead of grains. Coupled with a climate where labour was largely unnecessary to supply human wants, the result were slaves who were of a 'very weak habit of body, subjected to disorders in a most remarkable degree', in stark contrast to those found on the Windward Coast, where grain was plentiful and the enslaved were strong, hardy, and 'consequently less subject to disorders than any others'.[91] James Hendy paired the putrid dysentery with leprosy in 1784 in a discussion of the effects a change of diet had effected on Barbados in the last quarter century. Earlier, he suggested, Negroes had eaten a great deal of flying fish and salted fish. Now that their diet consisted largely of vegetables, both diseases were considerably less common.[92]

Perhaps as part of an indirect criticism of what was increasingly being cast as the gluttony and intemperance of white West Indian Creoles, some authors

[89] Lind, note, 69.

[90] 'African Coffries', he noted, appeared to have the same mortal susceptibility, 'altho' I know not what to ascribe it to, unless we suppose one similar to that above mentioned, to wit, some fundamental aggravating principle in their chief diet'. J. Z. Holwell, *An Account of the Manner of Inoculating for the Small Pox in the East Indies* (London: T. Becket and P.A. De Hondt, 1767), 6.

[91] Robert Atchison, 'Observations on the Dysentery, as it Appears among the Negroes on the Coast of Guinea', *Medical Commentaries* 9 (1785): 268–9.

[92] Hendy, note, 43–4.

saw fit to praise the sparse and limited diet forced upon slaves.[93] John Quier, in a letter written to Donald Monro in 1770, suggested that the small amount of meat available to the enslaved was probably partly responsible for the relative absence of bilious complaints among them.[94] The anonymous author of a 1776 text providing *Practical Remarks on West India Diseases* similarly lauded the food customarily eaten by slaves in the context of a broader social taxonomy of West Indian life based on diet. People living in warm climates, the author claimed, could be divided according to whether they ate mostly animal food, a mixture of animal and vegetable food, or mostly vegetable food. This tripartite division mapped onto social distinctions between European men of all classes, women and Creoles, and Negroes. Upper class Europeans in the tropics, it was argued, indulged in plentiful quantities of meat and strong liquor, while lower class Europeans ate animal food of lower quality, such as salted provisions, and drank substantial quantities of new rum. As a result, both fell victim to bilious complaints. Women and creoles moderated their consumption of meat with 'various salads, fruits and vegetable compounds of the country' and displayed an admirable temperance with regard to drink.[95] Negroes, finally, had meals that were largely vegetable, with some small portion of salted animal food. The medical outcome of this diet was, according to the author, straightforward. 'To their food alone it is they are indebted for an exemption from the variety of diseases arising rather from a superabundance or acrimony of the bilious fluid; insomuch that acute bilious disorders are to be met with in no negroes'. The only exceptions to this rule allowed by the author – and that with a more than somewhat moralising edge – were when slaves were, though their connections with white people, allowed to 'indulge in luxury and idleness, and that kind of living which more properly place them in the first class'.[96] That said, a vegetable diet had its own problems, leading to worms, jaundice, and stomach-complaints, such as pains, diarrhoea, and constipation.

Other authors were thankfully either more equivocal or straightforwardly critical of the limitations of slave diets. In his *Essay on the More Common West-India Diseases*, James Grainger argued that the excessive consumption of 'new fiery spirits' by slaves resulted in more cases of the distemper known as the 'dry belly-ache'.[97] One might expect blacks to suffer more from

---

[93] Christer Petley, 'Gluttony, Excess, and the Fall of the Planter Class in the British Caribbean', *Atlantic Studies* 9 (2012).

[94] Monro et al., 192–3.

[95] Anonymous, *Practical Remarks on West India Diseases*, 8.

[96] Ibid., 9.

[97] Grainger, 'An Essay on the More Common West-India Diseases, James Grainger, MD (1764), with Additional Notes by William Wright, MD, FRS (1802)', 27–8. The intemperance of slaves was a complaint made by several authors. See also Anonymous, *Practical Remarks on West India Diseases*, 10.

heartburn as well, given that they ate far more vegetable matter than whites. That they were spared this discomfort, Grainger put down to well-salted and – seasoned greens and the fact they 'drink little punch and no wine'.[98] William Chamberlaine also pointed to the downsides of a mainly vegetable diet, in an account of the efficacy of cowhage as a treatment for worms. 'Very little animal food comes to the share of a negro slave', he noted, and what was available was 'of the most indigestible kind', such as salted fish and cured meat. Almost sole reliance on vegetable food meant that it was rare to see a negro child, Chamberlaine claimed, without a swollen belly or other symptoms due to worms.[99] Writing from Demerary almost at the end of the century, William Macbeth pointed not to food as the cause of 'a singular affection of the urinary organs', but to drink. Negroes, he claimed, had to drink 'bush-water', while whites did not, which led to the discrepancy in susceptibility to the affliction. Macbeth strengthened his case by noting that the two cases of whites suffering from the illness came about when rain-water was scarce, and that there were very few cases among black 'domestics', who drank the same cistern water as white plantation owners.

Of course, not all afflictions seemed to have dietetic causes. While the author of *Practical Remarks on West-India Diseases* argued that a want of luxury in diet meant that blacks were spared some diseases, he noted that they were plagued by many due to their occupations, 'which expose them to every change and inclemency of the weather'.[100] In this way, he suggested, they were like European sailors and soldiers, although their disorders were probably even more acute. Lewis Rouppe, who had practiced both medicine and surgery in the French army and Dutch navy, made a similar observation in his doctoral thesis, completed in Leiden in 1764, on the diseases of seamen. Rouppe seemed astonished by the fact that West Indian slaves did not suffer from scurvy, while European sailors did.[101] Rouppe's best guess was that slaves did better from the fact that they ate fruit unavailable to men at sea. It was, in fact, a commonplace to point to slaves' exposure to the elements and environment – either through poor housing or clothing – as the cause of multiple distempers. C. Chisholm reported on a West Indian liver disease to which all 'people of

---

[98] Grainger, 'An Essay on the More Common West-India Diseases, James Grainger, MD (1764), with Additional Notes by William Wright, MD, FRS (1802)', 37–8.

[99] William Chamberlaine, *A Practical Treatise on the Efficacy of Stizolobium, or Cowhage, Internally Administered, in Diseases Occasioned by Worms. To Which Are Added, Observations on Other Anthelmintic Medicines of the West Indies* (London: J. Murray, 1784), 3–4.

[100] Anonymous, *Practical Remarks on West India Diseases*, 10.

[101] 'But whosoever considers the situation of the negroes, who are slaves to the Europeans in the West-Indies, and compares their food with that of the sailors; the huts in which they dwell, their want of cloaths and covering, and the miserable life which they lead, will wonder that these unhappy creatures can escape the scurvy'. Rouppe, 133–4.

all colours, sexes, and ages' were subject, but to which blacks and the young were particularly liable. 'The distinction', he argued, 'appears to have chiefly arisen from the greater exposure of the negroes to the cold dews of the night, and their habitations more readily admitting the cold northerly winds which generally blow at that time'.[102] Quier blamed the frequency of stomach and bowel disorders among negroes to their greater exposure to the 'vicissitudes of the weather than white people', while Hendy argued that negroes in Barbados suffered from a glandular disease there because of their poor clothing, although wealthy white inhabitants were also victims, because of their foolish insistence on sleeping with their windows open to the night air.[103] Lack of adequate shoe-wear led to chigoes and sores.[104]

In amongst all of these differences between the kinds of illnesses that troubled blacks and whites, the degrees of their severity, and the capacity to recover, one finds – for most of the eighteenth century – little talk of innate, *racial* distinctions. Chamberlaine may have observed that the blood of negroes was different to that of white people – thinner, for example, and 'less disposed to coagulate' – but this was due to hard labour in a hot climate, to a lack of time to rest, and a vegetable diet.[105] Quier similarly argued that negro constitutions were 'more robust' than that of whites, and hence less inclined to bilious diseases, but this robustness was not given from birth, but gained 'on account of the labour and hardships they go though'.[106] The broadest statement of the inessentiality of the differences that divided white and black patients came from the author of the *Practical Remarks*. Variety in food and forms of labour, he argued, led to different diseases, but if one held all such changeable causes equal, then all peoples were equally liable to the same afflictions: 'for though these various circumstances have most undoubtedly an effect on the constitution, so as to make it more susceptible of certain diseases, yet that can by no means imply the impossibility of the like symptoms, and being, *caeteris paribus*, equally contingent to the whole race of mankind in these climates'.[107]

7.3   Racial Pathologies

It was the central contention of Chapter 5 that 'race-medicine' as I have defined the term did not really exist prior to at least the 1750s. Even a polygenist such

---

[102] C. Chisholm, 'The History of a Singular Affection of the Liver, Which Prevailed Epidemically in Some Parts of the West Indies', *Medical Commentaries* Second Decade, Vol. 1 (1787): 357.
[103] Monro et al., 192–3. Hendy, 31–2.
[104] Hendy, 32.
[105] Chamberlaine, 7.
[106] Monro et al., 193.
[107] Anonymous, *Practical Remarks on West India Diseases*, 30.

as John Atkins did not make use of conceptions of intrinsic racial difference in his explanations of the causes of diseases common among the inhabitants of the Guinea Coast. I show here that matters would be different in the last decades of the century, with at least half a dozen writers from the mid-1770s to 1820 putting forward medical theories of the difference between black and white bodies. Such theories, I show, can be divided according to the dominant medical logics of the day. Those up until the mid-1780s tended to work within what I have called the 'putrefactive paradigm', stressing the ability of African skin to throw out the putrid matter that was so easily produced in warm climes. Dark skin was thus an advantage, but one that was put to work in defending the use of black enslaved labour in the colonies against the charges of abolitionists. From the late 1780s, putrefactive theories were increasingly replaced by the nervous theories most commonly associated with Haller and Cullen. Within the nervous paradigm, more emphasis was placed on the differential 'sensibility' of black and white bodies. Moving inward, physicians found race to be more than skin deep, and black bodies were less able to feel pain or discomfort, for putatively physiological reasons. What would be deemed poor treatment or neglect if endured by whites, then, could be deemed appropriate for slaves and the sharp critiques of abolitionists might be blunted. For a group of writers committed to claims about the essential differences between black and white bodies, paradigms might change, but medicine remained in the service of slavery.

'So Far From Suffering an Inconvenience': Medicine, Climate, and Labour

The sixth chapter of the second volume of Edward Long's massive *History of Jamaica* was concerned with 'Regulations for Preserving Health' on the island. Long had worked through the major authors on the diseases of warm climates, citing Pringle, Huxham, Bisset, Hillary, Rouppe, and De Monchy (among others), and at times resorting to near-plagiarism of the various works of James Lind. Long recommended gradual habituation to the new climate and the avoidance of swampy areas, 'infested with muskeetos, which seem as if placed there by the hand of Providence, to assault with their stings, and drive away every human being, who may ignorantly venture to fix his abode among them'.[108] Long also advocated wearing the loose garb of the 'Mandarin', rather than the heavy clothing favoured by Europeans, and the consumption of sugar – 'so welcome and necessary a substance' – as well as the 'mild vegetable acids' and peppers that grew locally, in order to combat the body's

---

[108] Long, *The History of Jamaica*, I, 506.

putrefactive tendencies.[109] When it came to the diseases customary among slaves, Long pointed to the standard causes: climate, diet, and behaviour. Negroes, for example, were the first to be afflicted with epidemic distempers because they indulged 'too liberally' in fruits and roots after the heavy rains that followed a long drought.[110] On the positive side, however, the 'custom of the negroes' to light fires in their dwellings in order to drive away mosquitoes 'has another good effect, the correcting of the night air, and disarming it of its damp and chill, which might be prejudicial to their healths'.[111] And, erasing putative racial distinctions, Long contrasted the diseases characteristic of those born on Jamaica – regardless of colour – to those of newly arrived Europeans.

The natives, black and white, are not subject, like Europeans, to bilious, putrid, and malignant fevers: they are not only habituated to the climate, but to a difference in respect to diet and manners; which works no small change in men's constitutions. A Creole, if he was to addict himself to that kind of diet which is known to have a tendency to produce disorders, or an acrid, corrupt bile, would no more be exempt from them, than an European.[112]

In most cases, then, broadly Hippocratic conceptions, coupled with an emphasis on nativity, served to explain the diseases of all groups on the island. I can, in fact, find only one part of this chapter in which Long emphasised intrinsic physical differences between black and white bodies. It came, tellingly, in a discussion about the relative capacity to labour in tropical climates and invoked Benjamin Franklin as its authority. 'Dr Franklin very properly concludes', he noted, 'that the quicker evaporation of perspirable matter from the skin and lungs of Negroes, by cooling them more, enables them to bear the sun's heat so much better than the Whites can do; though, abstracted from this, the colour of their skins would, otherwise, make them more sensible of that heat'. Franklin, who had made these observations in a letter to the South Carolinian physician John Lining in 1758 had made clear his awareness of the stakes of this question: 'if this is a fact, as it is said to be', he noted parenthetically, 'for the alledg'd necessity of having negroes rather than whites, to work in the West-India fields, is founded upon it'.[113] Long had, in fact, invoked a more explicitly medicalised version of this argument earlier in his text, precisely to defend black slavery (and simultaneously taking the opportunity to critique

---

[109] Ibid., 549–50, 28.

[110] Ibid., II: 614.

[111] Ibid., I: 510.

[112] Ibid., 534.

[113] In Benjamin Franklin, *Experiments and Observations on Electricity* (London: Printed for David Henry, 1769), 363–8. The same claims were made in the United States, of course. Curtin notes that 'some believed that whites could not even do hard labour as far north as South Carolina'. Curtin, *The Image of Africa: British Ideas and Action, 1780–1850*, 85.

slaves for their promiscuity). 'Negroes', he asserted, so far from suffering an inconvenience, are found to labour with most alacrity and ease to themselves in the very hottest part of the day ... The openness of their pores gives a free transpiration to bad humours; and they would enjoy robust health, under the hardest toils expedient here, if they were less prone to debauch, and venereal excess'.[114]

As Jordan observed in *White over Black,* the trope that held that black skin conferred advantages when labouring in warm climates was very common in the eighteenth century, but also usually 'formless and imprecise'.[115] One can see, however, that medical discussions formed one site for a general claim to acquire form and precision. In 1780, the physician Johann Peter Schotte had his weather diary for a year spent on the island of St Lewis, in the river Senegal, communicated to the Royal Society by Joseph Banks.[116] In 1782, he reproduced that letter in a larger book dedicated to the analysis of a fever that had broken out in Senegal at the beginning of August 1778 and had raged until the middle of September.[117] Counting those who survived the initial onslaught, but relapsed later, 59 of 92 white people were dead at the end of January the next year.[118] Schotte offered no precise count of native deaths, but he did note that 'Europeans suffered much more by it, in proportion, than the mulattoes, and those much more, than the blacks'.[119] Increasing darkness of skin (or at least decreasing admixture of 'European' characteristics), in other words, seemed to offer some protection, but only once the disease struck. 'The blacks are almost as subject to it as white people', Schotte observed, 'but in them it is not so violent'.[120] Interestingly, he did not put this differential mortality down to diet, although he noted that brackish water and a diet consisting overwhelmingly of animal food, as well as excessive sweating seemed to produce a disposition to the disease, which then required only the addition of 'human contagion' to become manifest. Nor did Schotte suggest that blacks were proportionately spared because of their nativity or seasoning. Indeed, Schotte argued that those

---

[114] Long, *The History of Jamaica*, II, 412.

[115] Jordan, 261. See also 526–7.

[116] J. P. Schotte, 'Journal of the Weather at Senegambia, During the Prevalence of a Very Fatal Putrid Disorder, with Remarks on That Country', *Philosophical Transactions* 70 (1780). Schotte communicated a second letter, via Banks, three years later. 'A Description of a Species of Sarcocele of a Most Astonishing Size in a Black Man in the Island of Senegal: With Some Account of Its Being an Endemial Disease in the Country of Galam', *Philosophical Transactions* 73 (1783).

[117] *A Treatise on the Synochus Atrabiliosa, a Contagious Fever, Which Raged at Senegal in the Year 1778, and Proved Fatal to the Greatest Part of the Europeans, and to a Number of the Natives.* (London: M. Scott, 1782).

[118] Ibid., 40.

[119] Ibid.

[120] Ibid., 108.

who had been in the country longer were 'more subject to some disorders, and have less chance of recovering from them, than fresh people from Europe'.[121] Instead, just as Long had, the physician pointed to the ability of black skin to allow an easier passage of matter that would prove dangerous if retained in the body.

[This] induces me to believe, that their bodies are constitutionally better adapted to throw off this rank and noxious matter, formed in the fluids, by the outlets of the skin, than the Europeans, and that it is for this reason, that they are less subject to those putrid diseases, which originate from its retention within the body; for it cannot be supposed, that this noxious matter should be more copiously generated in their bodies, than in those of Europeans, as they seem to be intended by Nature to inhabit that country.[122]

This explanation also supplied a cause for another 'fact' invoked casually but consistently in discussions of race from at least mid-century onwards: the claim, as Kant would put it, that 'all Negroes stink [*stinken*]'.[123] Schotte argued that the smell derived from sweat containing 'rancid and putrid particles', and that European perspiration also smelled bad in the humid months, 'though its fetor is not to be compared to that of the blacks'.[124] The latter bathed regularly, he observed, so the odour could not be due 'any nastiness harbouring on the surface of the skin'.[125] Instead, it must derive from the sweat itself, which did a better job in their bodies than in those of mulattoes or whites in removing toxic elements from their bodies.

Schotte would seem to have been flirting with polygenism with his suggestion that 'Nature' had intended blacks to live in warm climates and hence had purposefully adapted their skin to aid them there. Alexander Wilson, who had studied under Cullen at Edinburgh, was not so coy. In *Some Observations Relative to the Influence of Climate on Vegetable and Animal Bodies* (1780), he made arguments that combined phlogiston theory with claims about the cause of the blackness of skin, the capacity of such skin to keep its possessors healthier under the tropical sun, and the concomitant smell of 'phlogisticated' sweat:

[121] Ibid., 115–16.
[122] Ibid., 105.
[123] Kant, 151. The essay is reproduced, with the same pagination, in Robert Bernasconi, ed. *Concepts of Race in the Eighteenth Century. Volume 3: Kant and Forster* (Bristol: Thoemmes Press, 2001). See also Long, who listed the 'bestial or fetid smell' of negroes as one of five physical differences between them and whites. 'This rancid exhalation', he noted somewhat later, 'for which so many of the Negroes are remarkable, does not seem to proceed from uncleanliness, nor the quality of their diet'. Long, *The History of Jamaica*, I, 352, 425.
[124] Schotte, *A Treatise on the Synochus Atrabiliosa, a Contagious Fever, Which Raged at Senegal in the Year 1778, and Proved Fatal to the Greatest Part of the Europeans, and to a Number of the Natives.*, 105. Cf. Curtin, *The Image of Africa: British Ideas and Action, 1780–1850*, 85.
[125] Schotte, *A Treatise on the Synochus Atrabiliosa, a Contagious Fever, Which Raged at Senegal in the Year 1778, and Proved Fatal to the Greatest Part of the Europeans, and to a Number of the Natives.*, 104.

The perspiration of negroes is of a strong pungent alkaline odour, which seems to arise from some peculiar property or power in the reticular covering which gives colour to the skin. This extraordinary reticulated perspiration, so remarkable in blacks, we suppose, depends on the powers of secretion in the *rete mucosum*, by which the putrescent matter is more copiously discharged from the surface of the body; and undoubtedly a more free discharge of the putrescent effluvium by the skin, may not only liberate the constitution in a certain degree, but tend to produce the very blackness in the *rete mucosum* itself.[126]

We see in Wilson's text perhaps the best example of the close interlocking of polygenist and medical arguments in the later eighteenth century. 'From these very distinguishing marks', he concluded, 'negroes seem a peculiar variety of the human species, better fitted by nature than those of fair complexions to discharge by the pores of the skin the phlogiston evolved from their bodies, and consequently much better adapted to the warm climates'.[127] What is perhaps most striking about Wilson's claims, however, is that they made explicit the profound limitations of medical polygenist arguments in this period. His polygenist contentions only concerned black people, while his arguments about medicalised racial characteristics were limited to assertions about the *benefits* of black skin in warm climes. Otherwise, as the title of his book might have suggested, almost all of his arguments dealt with the role played by climate in producing (neither fixed nor racialised) differences in animal and vegetable bodies.

On the matter of skin colour, for example, Wilson argued that it was caused by the discharge of phlogiston through the skin, and that phlogiston was released when bodies putrefied. Putrefaction was greater in warmer climates, hence the darker skin of those living nearer the equator. The darker skin of those near the poles, on the other hand, was due to their great consumption of animal food, particularly fish (which putrefied easily), coupled with the fact that cold weather hindered perspiration and the carrying off of putrid matter, thus allowing it to remain and build up in the body.[128] Much less phlogiston passed through the skin in temperate climates, 'and in consequence the colour and appearances of body, and faculties of mind, of the nations of the middle regions, are as widely different from those of the torrid and frigid zones, as the climates which produce and nourish them'.[129] Brownness of skin was thus 'acquirable ... by a long continued habitual putrescency' but it could also be reversed: within even a few generations 'a better colour, form, and understanding' could be brought to Indians, for example, if they were brought to the temperate latitudes

[126] Wilson, Andrew, 270.

[127] Ibid., 270–1.

[128] . 'A putrescent tendency is the only point in which the inhabitants of the torrid and frigid zones are necessarily alike from circumstances of climate, and this cause alone', he opined, 'seems capable of regulating their external appearance, as well as mental faculties'. Ibid., 261–2.

[129] Ibid., 263.

of the globe.[130] Blackness, however, could be neither gained nor lost. Negroes, and negroes alone, were the result of a creation separate to that of the rest of humanity.

And yet, in spite of this original difference, black bodies *ceteris paribus* largely suffered from the same diseases and for the same reasons, as whites. Unusually for the time, Wilson claimed that a diet largely made up of animal food was a positive thing in warm climates. In the heat, such food was broken down more easily and provided strength to the entire bodily frame. If it was strong in health, however, it was also more prone to putrid illnesses. Thus it was that negroes – deprived of meat, for the most part – were seldom afflicted by such distempers. It was therefore diet and not race that made the difference in medical terms, as Wilson would state explicitly: 'what proves this in a still stronger manner is, that negro domestics, who live on animal food, are as subject to putrid epidemics as the white inhabitants'.[131] If whites and 'negro domestics' were thus more inclined to some diseases by their shared mode of life, they were also spared in common. Neither were often struck down by tetanus, unless (in the case of whites) they were 'reduced to a low and very relaxed state by long sickness or excessive debauchery', while the disease was common among labourers.[132] Once again, diseases were, for the most part, caused by climate, diet, and behaviour.

We have looked here at three texts, published within less than a decade of one another. The authors of each were very different. Long had no formal medical training while Schotte and Wilson were both physicians. Long was drawing on his experiences in the West Indies, Schotte from Senegal, and Wilson from unspecified 'warm climates'.[133] Yet, in terms of their claims, the similarities are abundant. All either explicitly or implicitly denied monogenist orthodoxy; all pointed to the black skin of those from Africa as a racial peculiarity; but all also seemed to suggest that the truly significant medical characteristic of black skin was not primarily its colour, but rather the protection it afforded its possessor in warm climates. And they identified that protection in the same way. Franklin had argued natural philosophically, so to speak, positing that dark skin allowed the easier passage of perspiration, which then evaporated on the outer surface of the skin. Long, Schotte, and Wilson on the other hand, argued medically, stressing not the perspiration alone, but rather what it carried with it: black skin allowed dangerous matter (bad humours for Long, rancid and putrid particles for Schotte, phlogiston for Wilson) to be expelled from the body more easily than white skin, one side effect being the racialised smell supposedly typical

---

[130] Ibid., 271, 72.
[131] Ibid., 173.
[132] Ibid., 182.
[133] Ibid., v.

of negroes. The three also held in common what they did *not* argue. Race did not make much of a difference in susceptibility to the vast majority of diseases. And where blacks might be *afflicted* disproportionately, rather than protected, the cause was never innate. Of course, we should not be misled or confused by claims that suggested black superiority on any issue, particularly not when such arguments were made by those arguing that all humans were not of the same species. The ability to function better than whites meant, fundamentally, the ability to labour better than whites. One does not find here anything like Rush's attempts to assert the suitability of Africans for their own climates, but their fundamental unsuitability to work as slaves in the new world. This was a medicine either explicitly or implicitly in defence of unfreedom.

Black Beneath the Skin

In Chapter 4 I discussed Benjamin Moseley as one of the first writers on the diseases of warm climates to turn against the putrefactive paradigm. In its place, he proffered a nervous theory of tropical diseases, relying particularly on the work of Albrecht von Haller and William Cullen. It was Haller's distinction between the 'sensible' and 'irritable' parts of animals that Moseley would draw upon in attempting to elucidate the differences between black and white bodies.[134] In Moseley's hands, the distinction between the irritable and the sensible became a racial trait. His *Treatise on Tropical Diseases* (1787) tended not to discuss the afflictions of the enslaved population in any detail, but in considering tetanus, he drew a number of observations together. The locked jaw, he asserted, was a disease 'entirely of irritability' and not of sensibility, meaning it affected only the muscles and not the nerves. Negroes, he observed (as had many medical men before him, citing various different reasons) were particularly subject to the disease. And Negroes, he continued:

whatever the cause may be, are void of sensibility to a surprising degree. They are not subject to nervous diseases. They sleep sound in every disease; nor does any mental disturbance ever keep them awake. They bear chirurgical operations much better than white people; and what would be the cause of insupportable pain to a white man, a Negro would almost disregard.[135]

---

[134] 'I call that part of the human body irritable', Haller had written, 'which becomes shorter upon being touched … I call that a sensible part of the human body, which upon being touched transmits the impression of it to the soul; and in brutes, in whom the existence of a soul is not so clear, I call those parts sensible, the irritation of which occasions evident signs of pain and disquiet in the animal'. Only those parts of the body that possessed nerves, Haller discovered, were sensible, while irritability was a property of muscle fibres. Albrecht von Haller, *A Dissertation on the Sensible and Irritable Parts of Animals [London, J. Nourse, 1755]* (Baltimore. Johns Hopkins Press, 1936), 8–9.

[135] Moseley, *A Treatise on Tropical Diseases; And on the Climate of the West-Indies*, 472 3.

It does not take a cynical reader to suspect that Moseley's interest in reporting his beliefs on black insensitivity to pain and suffering (however firmly believed) might be related to criticisms levelled by abolitionists against planters and their harsh treatment of the enslaved. That suspicion seems confirmed when one notes that, having made so much of essential differences between the two main racial groups on the island, and having suggested that there might be some connection between a given, apparently racial, characteristic and a specific disease, Moseley did little with this racial difference in his further analysis of the disease. He noted, as had many others, that black children were 'chiefly the victims of this disease in the West-Indies', that the numbers of those who perished by it annually 'are scarcely to be credited', and 'This drain of native inhabitants is far more detrimental to estates in the course of time, than all other casualties put together'.[136] But in adducing the causes, neither irritability nor sensibility was mentioned. Moseley rejected a range of previous explanations, from the intemperance or even wickedness of the mother, to irritation of the navel after birth, to the impact of damp, cold, or smoke upon the newborn. Instead, he suggested simply that the ignorance of the mother and the lack of necessities in keeping the child dry and clean were to blame.

If Moseley was somewhat vague about the precise connections between race and susceptibility to disease, Dr Collins was clearer. In 1811, under the pseudonym 'A Professional Planter', Collins published his *Practical Rules for the Management and Medical Treatment of Negro Slaves in the Sugar Colonies*. In it, he was critical of earlier authors on the diseases of the climate (Moseley included) who had not 'devoted their pens very particularly to the subject of negro disorders', effectively generalising from their treatment of whites. Yet whites, Collins noted, 'have all the advantages of good nursing, lodging, and medical attendance' that were usually denied slaves.[137] Thus far, Collins was following the dietetic and environmentalist orthodoxy I described in Section 7.1, but he proceeded to add a further, seemingly fixed and innatist distinction: 'Besides, there are many striking variations between the temperaments of the whites, and those of the negroes, sufficient almost to induce a belief of a different organization, which the knife of the anatomist, however, has never been able to detect'. The first was one with which the reader is now familiar: levels of heat that were 'intolerable' to whites were 'pleasant' and 'even necessary' to the negro.[138] The import of such a claim should be equally familiar. Collins rejected utterly the claims of abolitionists that the fields of

---

[136] Ibid., 508, 12.
[137] A Professional Planter (Dr Collins), *Practical Rules for the Management and Medical Treatment of Negro Slaves in the Sugar Colonies* (New York: Books for Libraries Press, 1971), 199–200.
[138] Ibid., 200.

the West Indies could be worked by free men, whether white or black. For all races, heat 'not only extinguishes the power, but the will, for exertion', and for Europeans who were under a 'corporeal disability', the effect was even greater.[139] Not only slavery, but specifically black slavery, was an economic and physical necessity.

The other medical differences of 'temperament' between whites and blacks were somewhat more novel. Europeans were vastly more susceptible to fevers, Collins claimed. More than nineteen out of twenty Europeans were killed by them, while barely one in a hundred negroes were. On the other hand, negroes were more subject to bowel complaints than whites, a fact that Collins put down not to any intrinsic variation, but to food, clothing, housing, and exposure to the elements. Most significantly for our purposes, Collins insisted that in terms of treatments, neither nauseous drugs nor blisters had the effects of black bodies that they did on whites. '[T]here is reason to think', Collins concluded, 'that the sensibilities, both of their minds and bodies, are much less exquisite than our own'. Travelling the same road as Moseley, he added: 'they are able to endure, with few expressions of pain, the accidents of nature, which agonize white people'. Yet where Moseley left the matter there, Collins offered an explanation. 'It is difficult to account for this otherwise than by supposing (which probably is the case) that animal sufferings derive a great part of their activity from the operations of the intellect'.[140] The power of such a set of claims should be clear. On the one hand, Collins could stand with the orthodox when discussing disease causation, relating it to dietetic, behavioural, and environmental factors. There were no diseases, he acknowledged, 'peculiar to either constitution, which may not be entertained by both'.[141] Differences were a matter of degree and not kind. On the other hand, he could still deploy racialist and essentialist arguments that denigrated the intellectual and emotional capacities of black people. Such arguments required no concrete anatomical evidence, since they were apparently undetectable by the 'knife of the anatomist', but they had palpable effects in terms of the day to day practice of medicine. 'It will be observed', he wrote, 'that in the treatment of negro disorders, I have frequently departed from the rules laid down by European practitioners; and that has been done, as well from a regard to the peculiarities of their constitutions, as to their general habits of life, which neither require, nor admit of the refinement practiced with respect to white patients'.[142] Many physicians had simply taken it for granted that black and white patients would be treated differently.[143]

---

139 Ibid., 31.
140 Ibid., 201. On race, gender, class, and assumed sensitivity to pain, see Pernick.
141 A Professional Planter, 202.
142 Ibid., 215–16.
143 For example, Chamberlaine: '[T]he very small annual sum allowed to surgeons, for the care of negroes in the country parts, will not admit of the exhibition of very expensive medicines'.

With Collins, one finds an attempt at a justification for this rooted not in the brute social and economic realities of a slave system, but in the seemingly intangible but essential physiological peculiarities of the races.

Conclusion

I will leave for the concluding chapter a more comprehensive discussion of the multiple relationships between theories of the diseases of warm climates and theories of race. Here, I want to end by pointing to the specific stakes for the history of race and 'race science' in this chapter. In general, as Chapter 5 also showed, conceptions of the causes for the distempers of the tropics were environmentalist and variable, working almost precisely against any notion that the illnesses of any given 'race' might be innate or fixed. For most of the century, that was true, too, of the majority of theories of the origins of racial differences, which were usually ascribed to climatic causes acting on a single human species. Yet, as we have seen, even those committed to monogenism were, by the 1770s, beginning to question the extent to which climate, diet, or behaviour could explain all of the characteristic features of the peoples of the world. The doctrine of special creations remained heterodoxy – although less heterodox than earlier – but race was hardening as a concept. Medicine, I would suggest, played a not insubstantial role in this hardening, but it did so in ways that were not straightforward.

Authors trying to understand the reification of racial conceptions at the end of the eighteenth century have long pointed to the abolitionist debate as one somewhat counter-intuitive locus for discussions. Black slavery required little explicit justification prior to the 1750s – no more, that is, than the other forms of slavery common to the West from at least the classical age. In response to the strident humanitarian critiques of men like Benezet, however, one finds both explicit forms of polygenism being floated – blunting humanitarianism by weakening the African's claim to humanity – and more subtle and unexpected reactions. One of these was the attempt to pay attention to the diseases of slaves, thereby rebutting the charges of neglect and lack of care made by Ramsay and others. In tracts like Grainger's, however, what emerges is a narrow focus on those afflictions that differentiated Europeans from Afro-Caribbeans – else why produce a work separate to the extant treatises on the

---

Chamberlaine, 20. Or Makittrick-Adair: 'White children generally used the warm pediluvium for some nights before the period of eruption; but the number of negro patients was so great as to render it impracticable, at least very inconvenient'. James Makittrick-Adair, 'Observations on Regimen and Preparation under Inoculation, and on the Treatment of the Natural Small-Pox, in the West Indies. To Which Are Added, Strictures on the Suttonian Practice; in a Letter to Dr Andrew Duncan' *Medical Commentaries* 8 (1784): 240.

diseases of the climate? Such works remained Hippocratic, for the most part, in the sense that they looked at 'airs, waters, and places', yet their focus was always on difference – in diet, in customs, in housing – rather than the broader similitudes that climatic arguments might suggest. This was not a reification of race, but it did contribute to a kind of boundary-making that stressed nativity or creolisation (regardless of colour) less than it did cultural differences inscribed onto differently coloured bodies.

In more heterodox accounts, which were becoming more common, one finds a blending of anatomical conceptions of race (rooted in the skin, for example) with medical paradigms, the combination working to affirm the interests of planters and those who participated in the man-trade. General assertions about the capacity of Africans and their descendants to labour in conditions deadly to Europeans were given a medical extension. Black skin not only cooled when it should have warmed, but it also encouraged the removal of the putrefactive elements that built up within the body in hot and humid conditions. As putrefactive theories waned in the last decades of the century, medical apologists argued for other innate physical differences between blacks and whites, rooting these in the nervous system, and arguing that withholding from slaves the kind of careful and sensitive treatment that would be standard for Europeans was not merely an economic decision, but one based on physiological differences.

Whether heterodox or not, medicine and racialised forms of difference were clearly, if complexly intertwined. That complexity is part of the value of the topic. I have long been struck by a sentence in Blumenbach's dissertation at the moment where he turned away from a focus on skin towards skulls: 'I intend to treat now a little more at length upon that part of the argument which has to do with skulls', he wrote, 'since things very nearly allied may be conveniently embraced and handled at the same time'.[144] The 'things' of the sentence here would seem to include not only conceptual matters, but the objects themselves. In the quiet of a study, the natural historian might handle and compare solid representations of racial variety. Precisely this was denied to the student of race-medicine. Skulls might be considered immutable mobiles: diseases most certainly were not. Moreover, for the historian trying to reconstruct the logics behind the study of diseases *in situ*, the contexts of colonialism and slavery are unavoidable. Racial difference, whether rooted in a nominally changeable set of dietetic or cultural practices, or bred in the skin, bone, and nerves increasingly shaped the interactions between medical men and their patients. In turn, forms of medical knowledge increasingly shaped the course of colonialism and abolition.

---

[144] Blumenbach, 114.

Conclusion: Place, Race, and Empire

In the introduction I noted that this work was conceived as an example of the postcolonial history of colonial science and medicine: 'postcolonial' because it takes as its subject the emergence and maintenance in colonial settings of categories that structured colonial relations and modes of life (and that continue to function as categories in a world after formal de-colonisation). In its three parts, this book has tracked changing understandings of place, race, and empire. To end, then, let me lay out both the state of such understandings at the end of the eighteenth century and the ways in which the three were conjugated with one another.[1] How, to put it simply, were ideas about locatedness, racial pathologies, and imperial power thought together in medical texts?

Locality and Expertise

It was a common refrain, in the first part of the eighteenth century, for medical men to bemoan the paucity of texts that might guide them in their practices beyond British or even European lands. In *Sea Diseases* (1706), William Cockburn evocatively spoke of the methods used by former 'Sea-Physicians', which had left no more trace than 'the Furrows a Ship makes in the Sea'.[2] Three years later, Thomas Bates similarly lamented 'the want of Books treating of Distempers incident to Seafaring People'.[3] As late as 1751, George Cleghorn

---

[1] On the 'conjugation' of forms of discourse, see Gabrielle Hecht, 'Rupture-Talk in the Nuclear Age: Conjugating Colonial Power in Africa', *Social Studies of Science* 32 (2002).

[2] Cockburn, *Sea Diseases: Or, a Treatise of Their Nature, Causes, and Cure. Also, an Essay on Bleeding in Fevers; Shewing, the Quantities of Blood to Be Let, in Any of Their Periods. The Second Edition Corrected and Much Improved*, 3. A similar sentiment is to be found in Cockburn's 1696 work: 'the paths of former Curers are as little perceptible, as the furrows made on the face of the Angry Abyss, by our lofty floating Forts', *An Account of the Nature, Causes, Symptoms, and Cure of the Distempers That Are Incident to Seafaring People with Observations on the Diet of the Sea-Men in His Majesty's Navy: Illustrated with Some Remarkable Instances of the Sickness of the Fleet During the Last Summer, Historically Related.*

[3] Thomas Bates, *An Enchiridion of Fevers Incident to Sea-Men (During the Summer) in the Mediterranean; ... The Second Edition, Corrected and Amended. With Several Medicinal Observations ...* (London: Printed for John Barns and sold by B. Bragg, 1709), ix.

confessed that he had not been long on the island of Minorca before he began to wish that those who had tried to treat distempers there and 'who must have seen' how much they differed from those in England 'had been at Pains to furnish their Successors with some Hints, some Observations, by which the fatal Consequences frequently attending those Diseases, might have been timely foreseen, or happily prevented'.[4] By the end of the century, however, many noted that the opposite was now true. William Lempriere spent some time at the beginning of his *Practical Observations on the Diseases of the Army in Jamaica* explaining why any further publications were necessary, given that the 'public are already in possession of so many valuable observations on the diseases of tropical climates, made by several authors, and at various periods'.[5] A few years earlier Thomas Reide had described what he called 'perhaps a matter of the greatest surprise to the medical world, that within these last few years more has been written on diseases between the tropics than had been before that period from the earliest discoveries in that part of the globe'.[6] Alas, for Reide, all of that production amounted to little useful, for no two authors could seem to agree on even the most basic points.

For some, the existence of works on topics related to their own concerns was a positive. Edward Ives noted in 1773 that he had once planned to write about the diseases to which Europeans were subject in the East Indies, but found no need to do so after Lind had published on similar matters.[7] But most saw the sheer number of new essays and books to be a problem: works abounded, but still left sizeable omissions and errors. Benjamin Moseley seemed to identify the root cause of the problem in the kinds of people who were writing the new studies. They were 'transient practitioners', men who 'make a few months voyage to the West Indies and bring home materials for a book, or a method of treating diseases', rather than acquiring the kind of knowledge that came only through a long residence.[8] In a twist on a debate that we have examined in several forms, Moseley was insisting that knowledge *in situ* was not itself sufficient. It was not enough to make observations on the spot, for these needed to be repeated over much time. The point might seem obvious, but he had particular targets in mind, namely those military men who used their (brief) time stationed in a country within the tropics to gather material for a publication. 'A transient practitioner', he wrote, 'more zealous to distinguish himself, than to benefit mankind, no sooner meets with a disease which he has never seen before, and perhaps does not remain long enough in a situation

---

[4] Cleghorn, vi.
[5] Lempriere, ix.
[6] Reide, xi.
[7] Ives, 447.
[8] Moseley, *A Treatise on Tropical Diseases; And on the Climate of the West-Indies*, 384.

to see again, than he transmits an account of it to his agent, who transmits it to his literary friend'.[9] Hence his specific warning, to 'inexperienced and transient practitioners; and such in the navy and army, whose residence may not be long enough to acquire a thorough and competent knowledge of the endemics of those countries'.[10] Those who had noticed a proliferation of works on the diseases of warm climates in the last decades of the century were not wrong, and the majority of the authors of such works were military men, seeing a market that they (and perhaps their 'agents' and 'literary friends') could exploit. Claiming 'twelve years extensive practice' in the West Indies, Moseley was unwilling to grant them the claimed expertise that they believed their time in the tropics had bought them.[11]

By the time of Moseley's writing, the most basic part of the debate over whether knowledge gained solely in the metropole could suffice in the colonies had been settled. Conditions were different enough in warm climates that a practitioner needed *some* local experience to have the authority to speak and be heard. One cannot imagine, in the late eighteenth century, a text like Cockburn's, which confessed openly to its author's complete lack of direct knowledge of climates far from Europe. Gilbert Blane's *Observations of the Diseases of Seamen* may stand as the polar opposite of Cockburn's, for Blane's confession in 1785 was that he *only* had experience of the diseases at sea in warm climates.[12] The question left was not *whether* local expertise was necessary, but rather, as Moseley made clear, how much was sufficient.

Moseley's text is remembered today in part because it was the first book to use the term 'tropical diseases' in its title. One must be wary of reading too much into this singular fact, but it is true that, by the beginning of the nineteenth century, there was a growing sense *both* that the diseases of the tropics were similar across widely divergent longitudes *and* that they were fundamentally different from those in more temperate latitudes, and particularly Britain. That is, it had come to be accepted (where, as we have seen, it had not been before) that there existed what might be called fundamental intra-zonal similitudes and inter-zonal differences when it came to disease environments.[13] Thus, for example, in 1788 John Hunter claimed generally, that there 'is much similarity among the diseases of warm climates', and more specifically, that the remittent fever 'described on the Coast of Africa and the banks of the Ganges would

---

[9] Ibid., 389–90.
[10] Ibid., 393.
[11] Ibid., xvii.
[12] Blane, 227.
[13] As I argued in Chapter 1, this is one of the issues on which I disagree with Harrison's similar attempts to explain how it came to be that the tropics were understood as a distinct disease zone. One cannot assume that such conceptions of difference were already extant in the West Indies in the late seventeenth century.

seem to be nearly the same as in Jamaica'.[14] Blane, similarly, was willing to admit that 'most of the diseases of one hot climate resemble those of another, so far as I know', although inflammation of the liver seemed to be an exception, being common in the East Indies and not often met with in the West.[15] Several authors explicitly paired similitude and difference. When troops were sent on an expedition into warm climates, Donald Monro advised, 'particular care should be taken to guard them against the diseases peculiar to such climates, which are different from those common to our more northern latitudes'.[16] For Moseley, there was a fundamental difference between 'the delightful climates of the earth, in temperate regions' and those, in the torrid zone, 'such as no care, nor art, can ever make agreeable'.[17] Lempriere shared Moseley's dismay, noting that 'the climate between the tropics, on so many occasions, has proved destructive to our fleets and armies' so that many now deemed extensive casualties to be unavoidable, with even the best regulations and discipline still involving the sacrifice of troops to the climate. Lempriere held out some hope, however. It was true 'that a tropical climate is unfavourable to the European constitution', but rational and judicious practices offered the possibility, at least, of alleviating its effects.[18]

Race and Place

It is not only in analyses of disease environments that this doubled move – the elision of 'smaller' differences in some areas and the expansion and elaboration of 'larger' ones – can be observed at the end of the eighteenth century. One finds it also in studies of the variation of human physical differences, or the races of humankind. Nineteenth-century racial thinking was characterised by three main tenets: first, that humankind could be divided into a comparatively small number of races, the characteristics of which were not easily modified (if at all) by cultural or physical causes; second, that races were not equal in terms of their intellectual and moral capacities; and third, that these intellectual and moral capacities bore measurable relationships to physical characteristics

[14] Hunter, *Observations on the Diseases of the Army in Jamaica; and on the Best Means of Preserving the Health of Europeans, in That Climate*, viii, ix.

[15] Blane, 91.

[16] Monro, *An Account of the Diseases Which Were Most Frequent in the British Military Hospitals in Germany, from January 1761 to the Return of the Troops to England in March 1763. To Which Is Added, an Essay on the Means of Preserving the Health of Soldiers, and Conducting Military Hospitals*, 331. The sentence is reproduced in the second edition, *Observations on the Means of Preserving the Health of Soldiers and of Conducting Military Hospitals. And on the Diseases Incident to Soldiers in the Time of Service, and on the Same Diseases as They Have Appeared in London. In Two Volumes. By Donald Monro, M.D*, 44.

[17] Moseley, *A Treatise on Tropical Diseases: And on the Climate of the West-Indies*, 1–2.

[18] Lempriere, 240–1.

of the body.[19] Unsurprisingly, most of the literature on the history of racial thinking has been concerned with uncovering the roots and fruits of the latter two ideas, reasoning (probably rightly) that the horrors of the nineteenth and twentieth centuries were more properly laid at the feet of biological determinism than the mere idea of racial division. One may note, at the very least, that of the three tenets listed, the only one that has remained continuously scientifically viable since the 1950 UNESCO Statement on Race is the first.[20]

That the first tenet feels familiar to a twenty-first century reader who still thinks (however informally) of five major races, each located on their own continent, should not blind us to its historical oddity. As Nicholas Hudson has shown in a now-classic essay, the word 'race' was originally used to designate a common bloodline or origin and was commonly used synonymously with the Latin term *gens*, often translated to mean 'peoples'.[21] Medieval and classical authors often identified as many peoples as there were cities or kingdoms. And, for the most part, such peoples were distinguished by what we would term cultural, rather than physical characteristics. Differences in language, custom, and religion thus trumped putative similarities in physical features – like skin colour or hair type – even when these could be found. It was far from natural, for example, for visitors to the New World to regard all the peoples they met as belonging to a single group. The Baron de Lahontan, travelling through Canada in the late seventeenth century, identified what he understood as eighty-five different 'nations'.[22] By contrast, for Immanuel Kant, in 1777, one needed only to speak of a single 'copper-red' American race, one of only four major divisions of humanity.[23] At some point during the eighteenth century, eyes that saw near-innumerable cultural differences among non-European peoples began only to see physical commonality.

To conclude this study of race, medicine, and empire, then, I wish to offer some reasons to explain the emergence of each pairing of inter-zonal difference and intra-zonal similarity and – however incompletely – to point to ways in which each is related to the other. Many authors have tried to explain why race should have emerged as an essentialist category at the end of the Enlightenment. Fewer have identified the same period as one in which the

---

[19] In Augstein's words, 'that mental endowments are bound up with certain physiognomical specificities which, being defined as racial characteristics, are considered to reveal the inward nature of the individual or the population in question'. Augstein, x.

[20] As Reardon has shown, the UNESCO statement actually enshrined this idea as scientific or expert orthodoxy, even as it advocated removing talk of race from popular or lay discourse. Jenny Reardon, *Race to the Finish: Identity and Governance in an Age of Genomics* (Princeton: Princeton University Press, 2005), 17–44.

[21] Hudson.

[22] Ibid., 250.

[23] Kant.

major opposition between 'tropical diseases' and those of Northern latitudes first emerged. I would contend that the two are not unconnected, for medicine was essential to the making of difference, and racial differences became integral to the theories and practices of medicine in the last decades of the eighteenth century.

I have pointed to some of these reasons already. The most obvious may be the slave trade. I noted in Chapter 2 that scholars have suggested that major demographic shifts can explain the *production* of a similar disease environment in the West Indies and the Guinea Coast where one had not existed before. The number of slaves brought from Africa to Jamaica increased dramatically across the eighteenth century. Insofar as diseases could be transmitted by the movement of people and goods, one would expect the introduction of distempers with a new population. William Hillary was in good company in claiming that many diseases had been 'imported with the African Negroes'. That said, many also disagreed with Hillary on some of his specific arguments. In 1784, for example, James Hendy wrote that he had asked 'many of the most intelligent *negroes* who have come from *Africa*' whether the yellow fever had been known in their country. They answered in the negative. Hendy claimed that it was not his intention to argue that a similar distemper did not exist in Africa, but rather that the disorder suffered in Barbados had not been brought from there. Agreeing with Hillary about the fact that the same disease could be found in two very different locations, Hendy was arguing over its aetiology. The point is worth stressing, for in explaining why actors *believed* that disease environments were similar (or had become so) in widely separated geographical regions, we must be careful not to impute modern beliefs and suppositions to them. Particularly in the case of yellow fever, we should be wary in awarding the laurel to either side of an eighteenth-century debate.[24]

The slave trade also, of course, played a role in the emergence of the concept of race, although not in the naïve way that some imagine. Race was not invented, in an instrumentalist fashion, in order to justify black slavery. Slavery had long pre-dated the use of Africans as slaves, and had long traditions of justifications within the West that did not rely on essentialist physical differences. As Hudson argued, however, the practices of slavery certainly provided the conditions of possibility for the elision of differences between

---

[24] It would not be until the twentieth century that it was generally accepted that the mosquito was the vector responsible for spreading the disease. Eighteenth-century contagionists were partly right, by our standards, for they had noted that the disease spread when large populations of the infected were located together, but they were not correct in imagining that the distemper was passed from person to person. Miasmatists may have been incorrect in imagining that the air around swamps was responsible for the illness, but of course such environments are prime breeding grounds for mosquitos.

slaves from widely different parts of the African continent: 'the process of shipping and marketing slaves literally stripped the signs of national difference from the bodies of Africans' as they were deprived of clothing, jewellery, and other cultural markers, while also being forced to learn a new and common language.[25] Evidence from slave holders also came to question the once-assumed obviousness of climatic explanations of physical difference. Black slaves seemed not to change colour over several generations; nor did white children born in the tropics. Observations made in locations in which black slaves were common seemed to point to a greater 'stickiness' of racial characteristics than had previously been imagined.

However, a more likely cause of the emergence of rigid racial conceptions, as I have argued, was not the beginning, but rather debates over the end of slavery. The practices of the trade in humans tended to produced similarities between diverse locations and similarities among diverse peoples. The abolitionist debate focused attention on differences. Proponents of slavery were more likely than others to invoke radical racial differences to justify their stance, but they too trod carefully. Even Edward Long balked, in his *History of Jamaica* (1774) at the straightforward association of human slaves with beasts of burden, managing to defend the trade and polygenism in the most odious terms without making this final step. Within medicine, particularly in the last decades of the century, one finds some examples of physicians ready to argue that racial difference was the cause of variations in physiology and pathology between whites and blacks. I have identified two foci for such arguments. First, attempts to evidence and defend the claim that black skin protected against the harsh sun, so that Negroes could labour without inconvenience in conditions potentially fatal to whites. And, second, arguments that deployed the new nervous theories of physiology and disease to provide reasons for the putative lesser sensitivity of black bodies to pain. This latter, in turn, served as a kind of license for precisely the kinds of neglect and poor medical treatment with which slave owners had been charged in anti-slavery propaganda.

More common and more orthodox medical arguments – across the century – tended not to invoke essentialist physical differences to explain diseases peculiar to given locations, following instead the broad logic of Hippocrates' *Airs, Waters, and Places*. Yet even these changed in response to abolitionist critiques, as plantation owners were forced to pay attention – or be seen to pay attention – to the tremendous losses of life among Afro-Caribbeans, both during the passage and the 'seasoning' and throughout the life cycle in the West Indies. Where climatic arguments worked well to explain why inhabitants of the Gold Coast, for example, suffered from different ailments to the English

---

[25] Hudson, 251.

(because the climate of each location was distinct), such arguments clearly seemed to do less work in explaining why black slaves and white Europeans in similar locations should be afflicted differently. In most texts that grappled with this problem, one does not find an emphasis on race, but one does find increasing attention to the medical differences that variations in culture and custom could make. For the most part, as well, differences in susceptibility to diseases were not given hard racialist explanations. Lind was only one of the first to argue that negroes should be used instead of white soldiers and sailors in tasks deemed dangerous. Yet he, like others, did not rely on differences in physical characteristics as justification, arguing instead that assigning such work to 'brave seamen' and 'gallant soldiers' did 'not seem consistent with British humanity'.[26] When Hunter offered a medical justification for a similar position, it was not on the grounds of essential difference, but rather because 'negroes afford a striking example of the power acquired by habit of resisting the causes of fevers'.[27] This emphasis on habituation should not surprise, given the discussion of the relative gendering of susceptibility offered in Chapter 5. The inhabitants of warm climates were deemed more immune to attacks of yellow fever, for example, because the climate rendered their bodily fibres more lax. Robust and masculine Englishmen would pay a price for their strength in such climates, but if they survived the seasoning they, too, would become more effeminate. Susceptibility was due to differences of degree, not kind.

New and newly focused forms of difference thus emerged over the bodies of slaves. They also emerged over the bodies of sailors and soldiers. I pointed in Chapter 3 to the effect of catastrophic losses at Cartagena in the 1740s as a particular turning point in the British public's understandings of the West Indies and the Americas as peculiarly dangerous locations for military men in service of the Empire. Cartagena cast a long shadow.[28] In 1787, Moseley observed that the debacle was unfortunately now better remembered for the 'flagrant enmity and jealousy between the commanders' than from the illnesses that 'made the crimes of individuals so expensive to the nation'.[29] A year later, Hunter made a somewhat different claim about the ways the venture were now recalled, but one that nonetheless emphasised losses due to disease: 'The unfortunate expedition against Carthagena is still remembered, more from the mortality

---

[26] See Chapter 3.
[27] Hunter, *Observations on the Diseases of the Army in Jamaica; and on the Best Means of Preserving the Health of Europeans, in That Climate*, 24.
[28] Harrison makes a related argument in Harrison, *Medicine in an Age of Commerce and Empire: Britain and its Tropical Colonies, 1660–1830*, pointing in particular to the significance of the Seven Years War for spreading the belief that the diseases of warm climates were quite radically distinct from those in colder regions. See also Charters.
[29] Moseley, *A Treatise on Tropical Diseases; And on the Climate of the West-Indies*, 75.

that attended it, than the want of success'.[30] The Seven Years War and subsequent campaigns provided further evidence for the differences between battles fought in the Old World and the New. 'The late dreadful mortality of the troops at *Lucia*, as well as at other parts of *America*', wrote Thomas Dancer, who had served in the campaign against Fort San Juan, 'serve to evince the insalubrity of these climates, and the difficulty attending all military operations in this part of the world'.[31] Lempriere, writing at the end of the century, concurred. 'Since Great Britain has been in possession of West India colonies', he wrote, 'every succeeding war in which they have been concerned, has afforded additional proofs of the dreadful mortality with which all our expeditions have been attended and which our troops ... must ever experience in a tropical climate'.[32] John Bell, in his *Inquiry into the Causes which Produce, and the Means of Preventing Diseases among British Officers, Soldiers and Others in the West Indies* (1791), was not alone in noting that many more soldiers died in the West Indies from disease than the sword, but Hunter made the point most clearly by claiming that in one period, of less than four years, 3, 500 men died in Jamaica, with half that number again discharged because of 'the climate and other causes of mortality, without a man dying by the hands of the enemy'.[33] Bell, on the other hand, made the argument explicitly comparative, emphasising not only the danger of the West Indies, but the relative mildness of Northern Europe. Fighting in Germany, British forces had outnumbered those in Jamaica by a factor of ten. Yet in comparable periods, close to the same absolute number of men were lost to disease in each location.[34]

Africa, as Philip Curtin has shown, had long been seen as 'the White Man's Grave' because of its hostile climate, but that popular image was not widely publicised until after the loss of the American War of Independence. In part due to failed attempts to replace the lost thirteen American colonies with new settlements in West Africa, in the half century after 1780 'the "deadly climate" of the African coast became gradually more common knowledge'.[35] India may have occupied a somewhat more ambiguous role within a discourse about the peculiar deadliness of hot climates. On the one hand, as we have seen, it was often included within claims about the diseases common to the tropics. And

---

[30] Hunter, *Observations on the Diseases of the Army in Jamaica; and on the Best Means of Preserving the Health of Europeans, in That Climate*, 12–13.

[31] Dancer, Note, 20.

[32] Lempriere, 1.

[33] Bell. Hunter, *Observations on the Diseases of the Army in Jamaica; and on the Best Means of Preserving the Health of Europeans, in That Climate*, 70–71.

[34] 'In the last war, British forces in Germany outnumbered those in Jamaica 10 to 1. Yet in 4.5 years, only 6500 men were lost to disease, which in four years 5250 were lost to disease in Jamaica alone'. Bell, 38–9.

[35] Curtin, '"The White Man's Grave": Image and Reality, 1780–1850', 102.

it was increasingly cast as utterly different from Britain in terms of its characteristic afflictions. In Stephen Mathews' eyes, the diseases of each Indian settlement were similar to one another and different to those found in Europe. They were, moreover more similar to one another – despite their geographical distance from each other – than one would expect in other regions. Reflecting a trope that went back to Hippocrates' *Airs, Waters, and Places*, then, Asia was cast as a realm of remarkable sameness, compared to the more vibrant changeability of Europe. '[T]he diseases peculiar to [each settlement]', Mathews wrote, 'are similar in their fundamental origin; and by a just comparison of the air, soil, and situation of the different presidencies, we do not find such an essential difference arise as is common to places describing similar parallels which are suited without the tropics'.[36] Charles Curtis in 1807 was even more emphatic about the peculiarity of medicine in the East, insisting that 'European nosology and definitions would, in India, prove but uncertain or fallacious guides', and that the newly arrived physician would need to unlearn a good deal in 'a country, where scarce a single production, whether of the animal or vegetable kingdom, is to be met with, bearing a true resemblance to its prototype in Europe'.[37] On the other hand, by the end of the eighteenth century, it could also be seen as a relative success story, compared to the perils of the West Indies and, particularly, the West African Coast. 'Forty years ago', Bell wrote in 1791, 'we could not send a ship to the East Indies, without often being deprived of one half of the crew, either by death, or by diseases which rendered the men unfit for service'.[38] But now the situation had changed and India might teach by its example. 'The West Indies has been emphatically and often too justly, stiled the grave of the British army', Bell insisted. 'To what causes is it owing, that the same mortality does not happen among our troops on the continent of Asia?'. Answering his own question, Bell implicitly played down climatic differences between eastern and western colonies. Soldiers suffered more in the West Indies not because of 'any particularly noxious power in the climate', but because of 'irregularity and inattention', as well as diet, matters that could be altered with more care and a more rational approach to victualling. The tropics would remain dangerous, but there was no reason that one part should be more deadly than another

---

[36] Mathews, 37–8.
[37] Charles Curtis, *An Account of the Diseases of India: As They Appeared in the English Fleet, and in the Naval Hospital at Madras, in 1782 and 1783, with Observations on Ulcers, and the Hospital Sores of That Country &C. &C., to Which Is Prefixed a View of the Diseases of an Expedition, and Passage of a Fleet and Armament to India in 1781* (Edinburgh: W. Laing, 1807), xvi–vii. Cf Harrison, ' "The Tender Frame of Man": Disease, Climate and Racial Difference in India and the West Indies, 1760 1860', 71.
[38] Bell, 122.

Medicine and the Making of Empire

Forms of distinctness and similarity in ideas about disease environments and race have been two major pre-occupations of this book. A third has been relationships between theories of medicine and conceptions of empire. Let me end, then, by discussing the ways in which imperial medicine helped to bring about 'tropical diseases' and distinct races of humankind. I noted, in the introduction, my unwillingness to follow those who have declared military texts to be the most valuable and important in understanding diseases outside Britain in the eighteenth century. The problem with such an assumption can be revealed quickly by noting that the five most important works on the distempers of the West Indies from the late 1670s to the late 1760s were all written by – and largely for – civilians.[39] But matters would change as an effect of the dramatic expansion of the British Empire after the end of the Seven Years' War in 1763. Lind's *Essay on Diseases Incidental to Europeans in Hot Climates* (1768) marked the beginning of a new era, one in which 'location-specific' texts diminished in importance compared to works intended for use by military men throughout the empire.

It is the characteristics of such works – as a *genre* – upon which I wish to focus, for those characteristics are quite strikingly different from those found in works devoted to the diseases of a specific place, written by practitioners living there for a sizeable period.[40] Both works, at least after the first decades of the eighteenth century, tended to emphasise personal experience *in situ*. A local practitioner-author like Towne, or Warren, however tended to invoke their experiences to position themselves as local experts, aiming to help those who laboured with them in Jamaica or Barbados. Hillary, too, cast that part of his 1759 work on diseases 'indigenous or endemial, in the West India Islands, or in the Torrid Zone' as being for the 'Good of the Inhabitants, and the Benefit of those who commonly practice in the West-India Islands'.[41] The authors of military texts, however, had broader ambitions, seeing their audience in terms of the network of medical men practicing their craft in multiple geographically distinct locations. Thus, for example, Cleghorn's treatise on the afflictions common to Minorca was not addressed solely to physicians and surgeons there.

---

[39] Trapham. Sloane. Towne. Warren. Hillary, *Observations on the Changes of the Air and the Concomitant Epidemical Diseases, in the Island of Barbados. To Which Is Added a Treatise on the Putrid Bilious Fever, Commonly Called the Yellow Fever; and Such Other Diseases as Are Indigenous or Endemial, in the West India Islands, or in the Torrid Zone.*

[40] On military texts as a genre, see Alsop.

[41] Hillary, *Observations on the Changes of the Air and the Concomitant Epidemical Diseases, in the Island of Barbados. To Which Is Added a Treatise on the Putrid Bilious Fever, Commonly Called the Yellow Fever; and Such Other Diseases as Are Indigenous or Endemial, in the West India Islands, or in the Torrid Zone*, Preface, unnumbered, 142.

Minorca, Cleghorn confessed, was only 'a small, remote Part of the *British Dominions*', albeit one in which a large number of British subjects could be found, both in times of peace and war. To make the case for the more general utility of a close study of Minorca's illnesses in other British dominions, Cleghorn needed to play down the peculiarity of the island's climate. Since 'the Qualities of the Air, and the Course of the Seasons in *Minorca* correspond nearly with those in several other Parts of the World, to which our Fleets frequently repair, it is probable the Diseases may likewise be similar'.[42] Texts written for the benefit of local readers tended to emphasise local particularity, often emphasising how far from homogenous a given location could be. Those aiming to be used in multiple sites within the empire stressed the difference between the site in which experience had been gained and the metropole – hence the need for the book for men trained within Europe – but tended to gloss differences between the author's site and those in other peripheral locations. The number of military medical texts – and their share of the global market – expanded with the number of troops stationed overseas. Thus, increasingly, emphases on the particularity of any given island or country faded compared to stress on the similarities between the countries of a given region.[43] Towne's text was essential for those working in Barbados: Lind's was carried throughout the empire.

The attempt to reach a broader market was not the only reason that military texts did not dwell on the geographical quirks or specificities of given places. In many, if not most, cases practitioners did not have time enough in the places they were to practice. Those in his Majesty's service, Cleghorn noted, 'are often obliged to take Care of Numbers of their Fellow Subjects, in Climates exposed to such Disorders; whilst at the same Time their quick Transition from one Place to another, prevents their acquiring a competent Knowledge of the various Epidemicks from their own Observation'.[44] Blane confessed of himself that 'the fleets I belonged to seldom remained more than six weeks or two months at any one place, so that any series of observation that might have been instituted was interrupted'.[45] Moseley, in other words, may have been right about the limitations of some forms of military service compared to a long residence in a given locale.

Naval service, in particular, may have led to a distorted vision of the countries men served in. Curtis acknowledged openly what few others did. In his *Account of the Diseases of India: as they appeared in the English Fleet, and*

---

[42] Cleghorn, iv.
[43] On the character of British military medicine after 1688, see Cook, 'Practical Medicine and the British Armed Forces after the "Glorious Revolution"'.
[44] Cleghorn, xii.
[45] Blane, xi.

in the Naval Hospital in Madras, he noted the limitations of his own experience: 'Let it be observed, however, that what is here stated, applies properly to *maritime* India only, and not to all the variety of inland country comprehended within that vast peninsula'. Curtis was thus honest about an aspect that strikes the reader familiar with civilian works as well as those written by military men: accounts of the diseases that strike sailors throughout the British Empire tend to treat ports as synecdoches for entire countries. Flattening, or simply ignoring, local differences of place also made it easier to connect ports at considerable geographical distance within a single discourse of tropical climates.

One might note, finally, that the bodies that inhabit military medical texts are not as varied as those found in civilian works. '[T]his was a peculiar body', J. D. Alsop has written, 'gendered male, identified as a young adult, characterized as temperamentally childlike and in need of firm guidance'.[46] To be sure, observations drawn from experience both with women and with non-Europeans are to be found in such texts, for not all practitioners were as limited as Hunter professed himself to be.[47] Lempriere served as regimental-surgeon and then superintendent of the military hospitals in Jamaica, but he also drew on a 'very extensive line of private practice in Spanish Town', which no doubt explains, for example, how he was able to observe that tetanus was much more common among the black than the white population.[48] On the other hand, those involved in extensive military practice could not have the same depth of experience as local practitioners in the West Indies, who purported to treat thousands of slaves, of all ages and both sexes, every year. And there is certainly some element of truth in the observation that, in military texts, both women and those of African descent appear more as counter-examples to the male experience than fully-fledged figures in their own right.[49] Differences of both race and sex tended to be amplified in texts that took young white males as largely uncontested exemplars of what it was to be British.

The causes were multiple, but the effect was striking. It was an outcome that was far from inevitable and produced by forces far from constant. A Briton looking back nearly a century in 1800 would not recognise a good deal that was familiar in the Britain of 1707. A Briton looking back in 1900, however, could see at least the frame of the empire shared across a century. Above all, I think, they would recognise the divisions that were as essential to empire as its unities. By 1800, the fissures that ran throughout a network of imperial control could be seen. The differences – by place and by race – that would characterise the British Empire for the next century and a half, had emerged.

[46] Alsop, 37.
[47] See Introduction, page x.
[48] Lempriere, 47–8.
[49] Alsop, 37–8.

Bibliography

Adams, Charles Kendall. *Representative British Orations*. New York: Putnam, 1884.

Adams, Vincenne and Warwick Anderson. 'Pramoedya's Chickens: Postcolonial Studies of Technoscience'. In *The Handbook of Science and Technology Studies*, edited by Edward J. Hackett, Olga Amsterdamska, Michael Lynch and Judy Wajcman, 181–207. Cambridge, MA: MIT Press, 2007.

Addison, William. *English Spas*. London: B. T. Batsford Ltd., 1951.

African Merchant, An. *A Treatise Upon the Trade from Great-Britain to Africa. Humbly Recommended to the Attention of Government*. London: R. Baldwin, 1772.

Alexander, William. *An Experimental Enquiry Concerning the Causes Which Have Generally Been Said to Produce Putrid Diseases*. London: T. Becket and P. A. de Hondt and T. Cadell, 1771.

Experimental Essays on the Following Subjects: I. On the External Application of Antiseptics in Putrid Diseases. II. On the Doses and Effects of Medicines. III. On Diuretics and Sudorifics. London: Edward and Charles Dilly, 1768.

Alpini, Prosper. *La Médicine des Egyptiens*. Translated by R. de Fenoyl. Paris: Institut français d'archéologie orientale, 1980.

Alpinus, Prosper and Jacobus Bontius. *P. Alpini, de Medicina Aegyptiorum & Jacobus Bontii, de Medicina Indorum*. Paris: Nicalaus Redelichuysen, 1645.

Prosperi Alpini, Medicina Aegyptiorum … Ut et Jacobi Bontii, Medicina Indorum. Lugduni Batavorum: Apud Gerardum Potvliet, 1745.

Alsop, J. D. 'Warfare and the Creation of British Imperial Medicine, 1600–1800'. In *British Military and Naval Medicine, 1600–1830*, edited by Geoffrey L. Hudson, 23–50. Amsterdam: Rodopi, 2007.

Altink, Henrice. 'Deviant and Dangerous: Pro-Slavery Representation of Jamaican Slave Women's Sexuality, c. 1780–1834'. *Slavery and Abolition* 26 (2005): 271–88.

Representations of Slave Women in Discourses on Slavery and Abolition, 1780–1838. New York and London: Routledge, 2007.

Anderson, Warwick. *Colonial Pathologies: American Tropical Medicine, Race, and Hygiene in the Philippines*. Durham, NC and London: Duke University Press, 2006.

The Cultivation of Whiteness: Science, Health and Racial Destiny in Australia. New York: Basic Books, 2003.

Anonymous. *Practical Remarks on West India Diseases*. London: F. Newbery; F. Blyth, 1776.

'Review of Dale Ingram, "A Historical Account of Several Plagues that Have Appeared in the World since the Year 1346" '. *The Monthly Review* (1755): 129–40.

Anson, George. *A Voyage Round the World: In the Years MDCCXL, I, II, III, IV. By George Anson ... Compiled from Papers and Other Materials Of ... George Lord Anson, and Published under His Direction, by Richard Walter ... Illustrated with Forty-Two Copper-Plates*. London: John and Paul Knapton, 1748.

Aranda, Marcelo, Katherine Arner, Lina Del Castillo, Helen Cowie, Matthew Crawford, Joseph Cullon, Marcelo Figueroa, et al. 'The History of Atlantic Science: Collective Reflections from the 2009 Harvard Seminar on Atlantic History'. *Atlantic Studies* 7 (2010): 493–509.

Arber, Edward, ed. *Capt. John Smith, of Willoughby by Alford, Lincolnshire; President of Virginia, and Admiral of New England: Works. 1608–1631*. Birmingham: The English Scholars Library, 1884.

Arbuthnot, John. *An Essay Concerning the Effects of Air on Human Bodies*. London: Printed for J. Tonson, 1733.

Arnold, David. *Colonizing the Body: State Medicine and Epidemic Disease in Nineteenth-Century India*. Berkeley: University of California Press, 1993.

'India's Place in the Tropical World, 1770–1930'. *Journal of Imperial and Commonwealth History* 26, no. 1 (1998): 1–21.

Warm Climates and Western Medicine: The Emergence of Tropical Medicine, 1500–1900. Amsterdam and Atlanta: Rodopi, 1996.

Arrizabalaga, Jon. 'Facing the Black Death: Perceptions and Reactions of University Medical Practitioners'. In *Practical Medicine from Salerno to the Black Death*, edited by Luis Garcia-Ballester, Roger French, Jon Arrizabalaga and Andrew Cunningham, 237–88. Cambridge: Cambridge University Press, 1994.

Ashcroft, M. T. 'Tercentenary of the First English Book on Tropical Medicine, by Thomas Trapham of Jamaica'. *British Medical Journal* 2 (1979): 475–7.

Atchison, Robert. 'Observations on the Dysentery, as it Appears among the Negroes on the Coast of Guinea'. *Medical Commentaries* 9 (1785): 268–71.

Atkins, John. *The Navy-Surgeon; Or, Practical System of Surgery with a Dissertation on Cold and Hot Mineral Springs; and Physical Observations on the Coast of Guiney*. London: J. Hodges, 1742.

The Navy-Surgeon: Or, a Practical System of Surgery. 1st ed. London: Caesar Ward and Richard Chandler, 1734.

The Navy-Surgeon: Or, a Practical System of Surgery. Illustrated with Observations on Such Remarkable Cases, as Have Occurred to the Author's Practice in the Service of the Royal Navy. To Which Is Added, a Treatise on the Venereal Disease, the Causes, Symptoms, and Method of Cure by Mercury: An Enquiry into the Origin of That Distemper; in Which the Dispute between Dr Dover and Dr Turner, Concerning Crude Mercury, Is Fully Consider'd; with Useful Remarks Thereon. Also an Appendix, Containing Physical Observations on the Heat, Moisture and Density of the Air on the Coast of Guiney; the Colour of the Natives; the Sicknesses Which They and the Europeans Trading Thither Are Subject to; with a Method of Cure. 2nd ed. London: W. Warner, 1737.

A Treatise on the Following Chirurgical Subjects ... London: T. Warner, 1724.

A Voyage to Guinea, Brasil, and the West-Indies; in His Majesty's Ships, the Swallow and Weymouth. London: Caesar Ward and Richard Chandler, 1735.

Aubrey, T. *The Sea-Surgeon, or the Guinea Man's Vade Mecum*. London: John Clarke, 1729.

Augstein, Hannah Franziska. *Race: The Origins of an Idea, 1760–1850*. Bristol: Thoemmes Press, 1996.

Baker, Richard. *A Chronicle of the Kings of England: From the Time of the Roman's Government Unto the Death of King James. Containing All Passages of State and Church, with All Other Observations Proper for a Chronicle. Faithfully Collected out of Authors Ancient and Modern; and Digested into a New Method*. London: Nathaniel Ranew and Jonathan Robinson, 1665.

Barker, Anthony J. *The African Link: British Attitudes to the Negro in the Era of the Atlantic Slave Trade, 1550–1807*. London: Frank Cass and Company, Ltd., 1978.

Barnard, Alan J. 'Orang Outang and the Definition of *Man*: The Legacy of Lord Monboddo'. In *Fieldwork and Footnotes: Studies in the History of European Anthropology*, edited by Han F. Vermeulen and Arturo Alvarez Roldán. London: Routledge, 1995.

Barrère, Pierre. *Dissertation sur la Cause physique de la couleur des nègres, de la qualité de leurs cheveux, et de la dégénération de l'un et de l'autre*. Paris: Pierre-Guillaume Simon, 1741.

Bates, Thomas. *An Enchiridion of Fevers Incident to Sea-Men (During the Summer) in the Mediterranean; ... The Second Edition, Corrected and Amended. With Several Medicinal Observations ...* London: Printed for John Barns and sold by B. Bragg, 1709.

Bayly, C. A. *Imperial Meridian: The British Empire and the World, 1780–1830*. London and New York: Routledge, 1989.

Beckles, Hilary McD. 'Property Rights in Pleasure: The Marketing of Slave Women's Sexuality in the West Indies'. In *West Indies Accounts: Essays on the History of the British Caribbean and the Atlantic Economy, in Honour of Richard Sheridan*, edited by Roderick A. McDonald, 169–87. Kingston, Jamaica: University of the West Indies Press, 1996.

Bell, John. *An Inquiry into the Causes Which Produce, and the Means of Preventing Diseases among British Officers, Soldiers, and Others in the West Indies*. London: J. Murray, 1791.

Benezet, Anthony. *A Short Account of That Part of Africa, Inhabited by the Negroes*. Philadelphia: William Dunlap, 1762.

Bergerus, Gottlieb Benjamin and Friedrich Hoffmann. *Dissertatio Physicomedica Inauguralis de Putredinis Doctrina Amplissimi in Medicina Usus*. Halle: 1722.

Berlin, Ira and Philip D. Morgan, eds. *Cultivation and Culture: Labor and the Shaping of Slave Life in the Americas*. Charlottesville and London: University Press of Virginia, 1993.

Bernasconi, Robert, ed. *Concepts of Race in the Eighteenth Century. Volume 3: Kant and Forster*. Bristol: Thoemmes Press, 2001.

'Who Invented the Concept of Race? Kant's Role in the Enlightenment Construction of Race'. In *Race*, edited by Robert Bernasconi, 11–36. Malden, MA and Oxford: Blackwell, 2001.

Bernier, François. 'A New Division of the Earth'. In *The Idea of Race*, edited by Robert Bernasconi and Tommy L. Lott, 1–4. Indianapolis: Hackett, 2000.

Bethencourt, Francisco. *Racisms: From the Crusades to the Twentieth Century*. Princeton: Princeton University Press, 2013.

Bethencourt, Francisco and A. J. Pearce, eds. *Racism and Ethnic Relations in the Portuguese Speaking World*. New York: Oxford University Press, 2012.

Beverley, Robert. *The History and Present State of Virginia, in Four Parts. I. The History of the First Settlement of Virginia, and the Government Thereof, to the Present Time. II. The Natural Productions and Conveniencies of the Country, Suited to Trade and Improvement. III. The Native Indians, Their Religion, Laws, and Customs, in War and Peace. IV. The Present State of the Country, as to the Polity of the Government, and the Improvements of the Land. By a Native and Inhabitant of the Place*. 1st ed. London: R. Parker, 1705.

Bewell, Alan. *Romanticism and Colonial Disease*. Baltimore: Johns Hopkins University Press, 1999.

Birch, Thomas, ed. *A Collection of the State Papers of John Thurloe, Esq; Secretary First to the Council of State and Afterwards to the Two Protectors Oliver and Richard Cromwell*. Burlington: TannerRitchie, 2005.

Bisset, Charles. *An Essay on the Medical Constitution of Great Britain, to Which Are Added Observations on the Weather, and the Diseases Which Appeared in the Period Included Betwixt the First of January 1758, and the Summer Solstice in 1760*. London: A. Millar and D. Wilson, 1762.

A Treatise on the Scurvy. Design'd Chiefly for the Use of the British Navy. London: R. and J. Dodsley, in Pall-Mall, 1755.

Blane, Gilbert. *Observations on the Diseases of Seamen*. London: Joseph Cooper, 1785.

Bleichmar, Daniela. 'Books, Bodies, and Fields: Sixteenth-Century Transatlantic Encounters with New World Materia Medica'. In *Colonial Botany: Science, Commerce, and Politics in the Early Modern World*, edited by Londa Schiebinger and Claudia Swan, 83–99. Philadelphia: University of Pennsylvania Press, 2005.

Blumenbach, Johann. 'De Generis Humani Varietate Nativa (1775)'. In *The Anthropological Treatises of Johann Friedrich Blumenbach*, edited by Thomas Bendyshe, 65–143. London: Longman, Green, Longman, Roberts, & Green, 1865.

Boerhaave, Hermann. *Boerhaave's Aphorisms: Concerning the Knowledge and Cure of Diseases. Translated from the Last Edition Printed in Latin at Leyden, 1715. With Useful Observations and Explanations, by J. Delacoste, M.D.* London: Printed for B. Cowse, and W. Innys, 1725.

'Discourse on Chemistry Purging Itself of Its Own Errors'. In *Boerhaave's Orations: Translated with Introductions and Notes by E. Kegel-Brinkgreve and A. M. Luyendijk-Elshout*, edited by E. Kegel-Brinkgreve and A. M. Luyendijk-Elshout, 180–213. Leiden: Brill, 1983.

Elements of Chemistry: Being the Annual Lectures of Herman Boerhaave, M. D. Translated by Timothy Dallowe. 2 vols. Vol. I. London: J. and J. Pemberton, 1735. Latin ed. (1731).

Elements of Chemistry: Being the Annual Lectures of Herman Boerhaave, M. D. Translated by Timothy Dallowe. 2 vols. Vol. II. London: J. and J. Pemberton, 1735. Latin ed. (1731).

Bontius, James. *An Account of the Diseases, Natural History, and Medicines of the East Indies*. London: John Donaldson, 1776.

Booth, C. C. 'William Hillary: A Pupil of Boerhaave'. *Medical History* 7, no. 4 (1963): 297–316.

Bosman, Willem. *A New and Accurate Description of the Coast of Guinea, Divided into the Gold, the Slave, and the Ivory Coasts ... Illustrated with Several Cutts. Written Originally in Dutch by William Bosman ... To Which Is Prefix'd, an Exact Map of the Whole Coast of Guinea*. London: Printed for James Knapton and Dan. Midwinter, 1705.

Boswell, John. *Christianity, Social Tolerance, and Homosexuality: Gay People in Western Europe from the Beginning of the Christian Era to the Fourteenth Century*. Chicago: Chicago University Press, 1980.

Boyle, Robert. 'General Heads for a Natural History of a Countrey, Great or Small, Imparted Likewise by Mr. Boyle'. *Philosophical Transactions* 1 (1666): 186–9.

Braude, Benjamin. 'The Sons of Noah and the Construction of Ethnic and Geographical Identities in the Medieval and Early Modern Periods'. *The William and Mary Quarterly* 54, no. 1 (1997): 103–42.

Brocklesby, Richard. *Oeconomical and Medical Observations, in Two Parts. From the Year 1758 to the Year 1763, Inclusive*. London: T. Becket and P. A. de Hondt, 1764.

Brown, Theodore M. 'Medicine in the Shadow of the Principia'. *Journal of the History of Ideas* 48, no. 4 (1987): 629–48.

Brown, Vincent. *The Reaper's Garden: Death and Power in the World of Atlantic Slavery*. Cambridge, MA: Harvard University Press, 2008.

Buffon, Georges Louis Leclerc. 'Of the Varieties in the Human Species'. In *Barr's Buffon. Buffon's Natural History Containing a Theory of the Earth, a General History of Man, of the Brute Creation, and of Vegetables, Minerals &C. &C.*, 190–352. London: H. D. Symonds, 1807.

Burnard, Trevor. '"Rioting in Goatish Embraces": Marriage and Improvement in Early British Jamaica'. *The History of the Family* 11 (2006): 185–97.

Burnard, Trevor and Richard Follett. 'Caribbean Slavery, British Anti-Slavery, and the Cultural Politics of Venereal Disease'. *The Historical Journal* 55 (2012): 427–51.

Burnard, Trevor and John Garrigus. *The Plantation Machine: Atlantic Capitalism in French Saint-Domingue and British Jamaica*. Philadelphia: University of Pennsylvania Press, 2016.

Bush, Barbara. *Slave Women in Caribbean Society*. Bloomington: Indiana University Press, 1990.

Bush-Slimani, Barbara. 'Hard Labour: Women, Childbirth, and Resistance in British Caribbean Slave Societies'. *History Workshop Journal* 36 (1993): 83–99.

Bynum, W. F. 'Cullen and the Study of Fevers in Britain, 1760–1820'. *Medical History (Supplement)* 1 (1981): 135–47.

C., T. 'Lind, James, M. D. (1736–1812)'. In *Dictionary of National Biography*, edited by Sidney Lee, 272–3. London: Smith, Elder, and Co., 1893.

Cañizares-Esguerra, Jorge. *How to Write the History of the New World: Histories, Epistemologies, and Identities in the Eighteenth-Century Atlantic World*. Stanford: Stanford University Press, 2001.

    'New Worlds, New Stars: Patriotic Astrology and the Invention of Indian and Creole Bodies in Colonial Spanish America, 1600–1650'. *American Historical Review* 104 (1999): 33–68.

Carpenter, Kenneth J. *The History of Scurvy and Vitamin C*. Cambridge: Cambridge University Press, 1986.

Carretta, Vincent. 'Who Was Francis Williams?'. *Early American Literature* 38 (2003): 213–37.

Carter, Henry Rose. *Yellow Fever: An Epidemiological and Historical Study of Its Place of Origin*. Baltimore: The Williams and Wilkins Company, 1931.

Chakrabarti, Pratik. *Materials and Medicine: Trade, Conquest and Therapeutics in the Eighteenth Century*. Manchester: Manchester University Press, 2011.

Chakrabarty, Dipesh. *Provincializing Europe: Postcolonial Thought and Historical Difference*. Princeton: Princeton University Press, 2000.

Chamberlaine, William. *A Practical Treatise on the Efficacy of Stizolobium, or Cowhage, Internally Administered, in Diseases Occasioned by Worms. To Which Are Added, Observations on Other Anthelmintic Medicines of the West Indies*. London: J. Murray, 1784.

Chaplin, Joyce E. 'Earthsickness: Circumnavigation and the Terrestrial Human Body, 1520–1800'. *Bulletin of the History of Medicine* 86, no. 4 (2012): 515–42.

  Subject Matter: Technology, the Body, and Science on the Anglo-American Frontier, 1500–1676. Cambridge, MA: Harvard University Press, 2001.

Charters, Erica. *Disease, War, and the Imperial State: The Welfare of the British Armed Forces During the Seven Years War*. Chicago and London: University of Chicago Press, 2014.

Chisholm, C. 'The History of a Singular Affection of the Liver, Which Prevailed Epidemically in Some Parts of the West Indies'. *Medical Commentaries* Second Decade, 1 (1787): 353–72.

Christie, J. *An Abstract of Some Years Observations Concerning Such General and Unperceived Occasions of Sickliness in Fleets and Ships of War*. 1709.

Churchill, Wendy D. 'Bodily Differences?: Gender, Race, and Class in Hans Sloane's Jamaican Medical Practice, 1687–1688'. *Journal of the History of Medicine and Allied Sciences* 60, no. 4 (2005): 391–444.

Clark, John. *Observations on the Diseases in Long Voyages to Hot Countries, and Particularly on Those Which Prevail in the East Indies*. London: Printed for D. Wilson and G. Nicol, 1773.

Cleghorn, George. *Observations on the Epidemical Diseases in Minorca. From the Year 1744 to 1749*. London: Printed for D. Wilson, 1751.

Cleve, George van. 'Somerset's Case Revisited: Somerset's Case and its Antecedents in Imperial Perspective'. *Law and History Review* 24, no. 3 (2006): 601–45.

Cockburn, William. *An Account of the Nature, Causes, Symptoms, and Cure of the Distempers that are Incident to Seafaring People with Observations on the Diet of the Sea-Men in His Majesty's Navy: Illustrated with Some Remarkable Instances of the Sickness of the Fleet During the Last Summer, Historically Related*. London: Hugh Newman, 1696.

  Sea Diseases: Or, a Treatise of Their Nature, Causes, and Cure. Also, an Essay on Bleeding in Fevers; Shewing, the Quantities of Blood to Be Let, in Any of Their Periods. The Second Edition Corrected and Much Improved. London: Geo. Strahan, 1706.

Cohler, Anne M., Basia C. Miller, and Harold S. Stone, eds. *Montesquieu: The Spirit of the Laws*. Cambridge: Cambridge University Press, 2010.

Colley, Linda. 'Britishness and Otherness: An Argument'. *Journal of British Studies* 31 (1992): 309–29.

Britons: Forging the Nation, 1707–1837. New Haven and London: Yale University Press, 2009.

Cook, Harold J. 'Global Economies and Local Knowledge in the East Indies: Jacobus Bontius Learns the Facts of Nature'. In *Colonial Botany: Science, Commerce, and Politics in the Early Modern World*, edited by Londa Schiebinger and Claudia Swan, 100–18. Philadelphia: University of Pennsylvania Press, 2005.

Matters of Exchange: Commerce, Medicine, and Science in the Dutch Golden Age. New Haven and London: Yale University Press, 2007.

'Practical Medicine and the British Armed Forces after the "Glorious Revolution"'. *Medical History* 34 (1990): 1–26.

Cooke, Ebenezer. *The Sot-Weed Factor, or, a Voyage to Maryland a Satyr: In Which Is Describ'd, the Laws, Government, Courts and Constitutions of the Country, and Also the Buildings, Feasts, Frolicks, Entertainments and Drunken Humours of the Inhabitants of That Part of America: In Burlesque Verse*. London: B. Bragg, 1708.

Cowley, Abraham. *The Poetical Works of Abraham Cowley in Four Volumes*. Edinburgh: Apollo Press, 1784.

Crawford, Matthew. *The Andean Wonder Drug: Cinchona Bark and Imperial Science in the Spanish Atlantic, 1630–1800*. Pittsburgh: University of Pittsburgh Press, 2016.

Creighton, Charles. *A History of Epidemics in Britain. Vol. II. From the Extinction of Plague to the Present Time*. Cambridge: Cambridge University Press, 1894.

Crosby, David L., ed. *The Complete Antislavery Writings of Anthony Benezet, 1754–1783*. Baton Rouge: Louisiana State University Press, 2013.

Cullen, William. 'First Lines of the Practice of Physic (1784)'. In *The Works of William Cullen*, edited by John Thomson, 465–676. Edinburgh and London: William Blackwood; T. & G. Underwood, 1827.

First Lines of the Practice of Physic. For the Use of Students in the University of Edinburgh. Vol. 1, London and Edinburgh: J. Murray; William Creech, 1777.

Cunningham, Andrew. 'Sydenham Versus Newton: The Edinburgh Fever Dispute of the 1690s between Andrew Brown and Archibald Pitcairne'. *Medical History, Supplement* 1 (1981): 71–98.

'Thomas Sydenham: Epidemics, Experiment, and the "Good Old Cause"'. In *The Medical Revolution of the Seventeenth Century*, edited by Roger French and Andrew Wear, 164–91. Cambridge: Cambridge University Press, 1989.

Curran, Andrew S. *The Anatomy of Blackness: Science & Slavery in an Age of Enlightenment*. Baltimore: Johns Hopkins University Press, 2011.

Curtin, Philip D. 'Epidemiology and the Slave Trade'. *Political Science Quarterly* 83, no. 2 (1968): 190–216.

The Image of Africa: British Ideas and Action, 1780–1850. Madison: University of Wisconsin Press, 1964.

'"The White Man's Grave": Image and Reality, 1780–1850'. *Journal of British Studies* 1 (1961): 94–110.

Curtis, Charles. *An Account of the Diseases of India: As They Appeared in the English Fleet, and in the Naval Hospital at Madras, in 1782 and 1783, with Observations on Ulcers, and the Hospital Sores of That Country &C. &C., to Which Is Prefixed a View of the Diseases of an Expedition, and Passage of a Fleet and Armament to India in 1781*. Edinburgh: W. Laing, 1807.

Dampier, William. *A New Voyage Round the World: Describing Particularly the Isthmus of America, Several Coasts and Islands in the West Indies, the Isles of Cape Verd, the Passage by Terra Del Fuego, the South Sea Coasts of Chili, Peru and Mexico, the Isle of Guam One of the Ladrones, Mindanao, and Other Philippine and East-India Islands near Cambodia, China, Formosa, Luconia, Celebes, &C., New Holland, Sumatra, Nicobar Isles, the Cape of Good Hope, and Santa Hellena: Their Soil, Rivers, Harbours, Plants, Fruits, Animals, and Inhabitants: Their Customs, Religion, Government, Trade, &C.* London: James Knapton, 1697–1703.

Dancer, Thomas. *A Brief History of the Late Expedition against Fort San Juan, So Far as it Relates to the Diseases of the Troops; Together with Some Observations on Climate, Infection, and Contagion.* Kingston: D. Douglass & W. Aikman, 1781.

Davidson, Arnold I. *The Emergence of Sexuality: Historical Epistemology and the Formation of Concepts.* Cambridge, MA: Harvard University Press, 2001.

Davis, David Brion. *The Problem of Slavery in the Age of Revolution, 1770–1823.* Ithaca: Cornell University Press, 1975.

The Problem of Slavery in Western Culture. Ithaca: Cornell University Press, 1966.

Debus, Allen G. *The Chemical Philosophy.* Mineola: Dover, 2002.

Defoe, Daniel. *A Tour Thro' the Whole Island of Great Britain: Divided into Circuits or Journeys. Giving a Particular and Entertaining Account of Whatever Is Curious, and Worth Observation; ... By a Gentleman.* 4 vols. vol. I. London: J. Osborn, S. Birt, D. Browne, J. Hodges, A. Millar, J. Whiston, and J. Robinson, 1742.

DeLacy, Margaret. 'The Conceptualization of Influenza in Eighteenth-Century Britain: Specificity and Contagion'. *Bulletin of the History of Medicine* 67 (1993): 74–118.

'Nosology, Mortality, and Disease Theory in the Eighteenth Century'. *Journal of the History of Medicine* 54 (1999): 261–84.

Delbourgo, James. *Collecting the World: Hans Sloane and the Origins of the British Museum.* Cambridge, MA: Belknap Press, 2017.

A Most Amazing Scene of Wonders: Electricity and Enlightenment in Early America. Cambridge, MA: Harvard University Press, 2006.

'The Newtonian Slave Body: Racial Enlightenment in the Atlantic World'. *Atlantic Studies* 9 (2012): 185–207.

'Slavery in the Cabinet of Curiosities: Hans Sloane's Atlantic World'. www. britishmuseum.org/research/news/hans_sloanes_atlantic_world.aspx (2007).

Dellon, Gabriel. *A Voyage to the East-Indies: Giving an Account of the Isles of Madagascar, and Mascareigne, of Suratte, the Coast of Malabar, of Goa, Gameron, Ormus: As Also a Treatise of the Distempers Peculiar to the Eastern Countries: to Which is Annexed an Abstract of Monsieur de Rennefort's History of the East-Indies, with His Propositions for the Improvement of the East-India Company.* London: D. Browne, A. Roper, D. Leigh, 1698.

Denton, Daniel. *A Brief Description of New-York, Formerly Called New-Netherlands: With the Places Thereunto Adjoyning: Together with the Manner of Its Situation, Fertility of the Soyle, Healthfulness of the Climate, and the Commodities Thence Produced: Also Some Directions and Advice to Such as Shall Go Thither ... Likewise a Brief Relation of the Customs of the Indians There.* London: John Hancock and William Bradley, 1670.

Doig, A., J. P. S. Ferguson, I. A. Milne, and R. Passmore, eds. *William Cullen and the Eighteenth Century Medical World: A Bicentenary Exhibition and Symposium Arranged by the Royal College of Physicians of Edinburgh in 1990.* Edinburgh: Edinburgh University Press, 1993.

Drescher, Seymour. *Capitalism and Antislavery: British Mobilization in Comparative Perspective.* Oxford: Oxford University Press, 1987.

'The Ending of the Slave Trade and the Evolution of European Scientific Racism'. *Social Science History* 14 (1990): 415–50.

The Mighty Experiment: Free Labor Versus Slavery in British Emancipation. Oxford: Oxford University Press, 2002.

Duden, Barbara. *The Woman beneath the Skin: A Doctor's Patients in Eighteenth-Century Germany.* Cambridge, MA: Harvard University Press, 1991.

Dunn, Richard S. *Sugar and Slaves: The Rise of the Planter Class in the English West Indies, 1624–1713.* Chapel Hill and London: University of North Carolina Press, 2000.

'Sugar Production and Slave Women in Jamaica'. In *Cultivation and Culture: Labor and the Shaping of Slave Life in the Americas*, edited by Ira Berlin and Philip D. Morgan, 49–72. Charlottesville and London: University Press of Virginia, 1993.

Eliav-Feldon, Miriam, Benjamin H. Isaac, and Joseph Ziegler, eds. *The Origin of Racism in the West.* Cambridge: Cambridge University Press, 2009.

Estwick, Samuel. *Considerations on the Negroe Cause, Commonly So Called, Addressed to the Right Honourable Lord Mansfield, Lord Chief Justice of King's Bench, &C. By a West Indian.* London: J. Dodsley, 1772.

Considerations on the Negroe Cause, Commonly So Called, Addressed to the Right Honourable Lord Mansfield, Lord Chief Justice of the Court of King's Bench, &C. 2nd ed. London: J. Dodsley, 1773.

Fabian, Johannes. *Time and the Other: How Anthropology Makes Its Object.* New York: Columbia University Press, 1983.

Fett, Sharla M. *Working Cures: Healing, Health, and Power on Southern Slave Plantations.* Chapel Hill and London: The University of North Carolina Press, 2002.

Findlay, G. M. 'John Williams and the Early History of Yellow Fever'. *The British Medical Journal* 2, no. 4574 (1948): 474–6.

Foa, Anna. 'The New and the Old: The Spread of Syphilis (1494–1530)'. Translated by Carole C. Gallucci. In *Sex and Gender in Historical Perspective*, edited by Edward Muir and Guido Ruggiero, 26–45. Baltimore: Johns Hopkins University Press, 1990.

Foot, Jesse. *A Defence of the Planters in the West Indies; Comprised in Four Arguments.* London: J. Debrett, 1792.

Forster, Georg. 'Noch etwas über die Menschenraßen. An Herrn Dr. Biester'. *Teutsche Merkur* October and November (1786): 57–86, 150–66.

Fortescue, J. W. *A History of the British Army.* 2nd ed. Vol. II. London: Macmillan, 1910.

Fothergill, John. *An Account of the Sore Throat Attended with Ulcers; a Disease Which Hath of Late Years Appeared in This City, and the Parts Adjacent.* London: C. Davis, 1747.

Foucault, Michel. *The History of Sexuality*. 3 vols. Vol. I. London: Allen Lane, 1978.
'Of Other Spaces: Utopias and Heterotopias'. *Architecture/Mouvement/Continuité*, no. October (1984).
Frängsmyr, Tore, J L. Heilbron, and Robin E. Rider. *The Quantifying Spirit in the Eighteenth Century*. Berkeley: University of California Press, 1990.
Franklin, Benjamin. *Experiments and Observations on Electricity*. London: Printed for David Henry, 1769.
Gibbes, Philip. *Instruction for the Treatment of Negroes &C. &C. &C.* 2nd ed. London: Shepperson and Reynolds, 1797. 1786.
Golinski, Jan. 'American Climate and the Civilization of Nature'. In *Science and Empire in the Atlantic World*, edited by James Delbourgo and Nicholas Dew, 153–74. New York and London: Routledge, 2008.
British Weather and the Climate of Enlightenment. Chicago: University of Chicago Press, 2007.
Gómez, Pablo F. 'The Circulation of Bodily Knowledge in the Seventeenth-Century Black Spanish Caribbean'. *Social History of Medicine* 26 (2013): 383–402.
The Experiential Caribbean: Creating Knowledge and Healing in the Early Modern Atlantic. Chapel Hill: University of North Carolina Press, 2017.
'Incommensurable Epistemologies?: The Atlantic Geography of Healing in the Early Modern Caribbean'. *Small Axe* 18 (2014): 95–107.
Goodeve, H. H. 'Sketch of Medical Progress in the East'. *The Quarterly Journal of the Calcutta Medical and Physical Society* (1837): 124–56.
Gossett, Thomas. *Race: The History of an Idea in America*. Oxford: Oxford University Press, 1997.
Gould, Stephen Jay. *The Mismeasure of Man*. New York: Norton, 1981.
Goveia, Elsa V. *Slave Society in the British Leeward Islands at the End of the Eighteenth Century*. New Haven and London: Yale University Press, 1965.
'The West Indian Slave Laws of the Eighteenth Century'. *Chapters in Caribbean History* 2 (1970): 7–53.
Govier, Mark. 'The Royal Society, Slavery, and the Island of Jamaica, 1660–1700'. *Notes and Records of the Royal Society of London* 53 (1999): 203–17.
Graham, Richard, ed. *The Idea of Race in Latin America, 1870–1940*. Austin: University of Texas Press, 1990.
Grainger, James. 'An Essay on the More Common West-India Diseases, James Grainger, MD (1764), with Additional Notes by William Wright, MD, FRS (1802)'. In *On the Treatment and Management of the More Common West-India Diseases (1750–1802)*, edited by J. Edward Hutson, 1–56. Kingston, Jamaica: University of the West Indies Press, 2005.
'The Sugar-Cane (1764). Book IV'. In *On the Treatment and Management of the More Common West-India Diseases (1750–1802)*, edited by J. Edward Hutson, 57–84. Kingston, Jamaica: University of the West Indies Press, 2005.
Grosse, Pascal. *Kolonialismus, Eugenik und Bürgerliche Gesellschaft in Deutschland 1850–1918*. Frankfurt and New York: Campus, 2000.
'Turning Native? Anthropology, German Colonialism, and the Paradoxes of the "Acclimatization Question", 1885–1914'. In *Worldly Provincialism: German Anthropology in the Age of Empire*, edited by H. Glenn Penny and Matti Bunzl, 179–96. Ann Arbor: University of Michigan Press, 2003.

Guerrini, Anita. 'Archibald Pitcairne and Newtonian Medicine'. *Medical History* 31 (1987): 70–83.

'Isaac Newton, George Cheyne, and the "Principia Medicinae"'. In *The Medical Revolution of the Seventeenth Century*, edited by Roger French and Andrew Wear, 222–45. Cambridge: Cambridge University Press, 1989.

'James Keill, George Cheyne, and Newtonian Physiology, 1690–1740'. *Journal of the History of Biology* 8 (1985): 247–66.

Obesity and Depression in the Enlightenment: The Life and Times of George Cheyne. Norman: University of Oklahoma Press, 2000.

'The Tory Newtonians: Gregory, Pitcairne, and Their Circle'. *Journal of British Studies* 25 (1986): 288–311.

Hales, Stephen. *A Description of Ventilators: Whereby Great Quantities of Fresh Air May with Ease Be Conveyed into Mines, Goals, Hospitals, Work-Houses and Ships, in Exchange for Their Noxious Air. An Account Also of Their Great Usefulness in Many Other Respects: As in Preserving All Sorts of Grain Dry, Sweet, and Free from Being Destroyed by Weevels, Both in Grainaries and Ships: And in Preserving Many Other Sorts of Goods. As Also in Drying Corn, Malt, Hops, Gun-Powder, &C. And for Many Other Useful Purposes*. London: W. Innys and R. Manby; T. Woodward, 1743.

Philosophical Experiments Containing Useful, and Necessary Instructions for Such as Undertake Long Voyages at Sea. Shewing How Sea-Water May Be Made Fresh and Wholsome: And How Fresh-Water May Be Preserv'd Sweet. London: W. Innys and R. Manby; T Woodward, 1739.

Hall, Catherine. *Civilising Subjects: Colony and Metropole in the English Imagination, 1830–1867*. Chicago: Chicago University Press, 2002.

Haller, Albrecht von. *A Dissertation on the Sensible and Irritable Parts of Animals [London, J. Nourse, 1755]*. Baltimore: Johns Hopkins Press, 1936.

Haller, John S. 'The Negro and the Southern Physician: A Study of Medical and Racial Attitudes, 1800–1860'. *Medical History* 16 (1972): 238–53.

Hamlin, Christopher. 'Chemistry, Medicine, and the Legitimization of English Spas, 1740–1840'. *Medical History. Supplement* 10 (1990): 67–81.

More Than Hot: A Short History of Fever. Baltimore: Johns Hopkins University Press, 2014.

'Predisposing Causes and Public Health in Early Nineteenth-Century Medical Thought'. *Social History of Medicine* 5 (1992): 43–70.

'What Is Putrid About Putrid Fever?' In *History of Science Society Annual Meeting*, Chicago, 2014.

Handler, Jerome S. 'Diseases and Medical Disabilities of Enslaved Barbadians, from the Seventeenth Century to around 1838 (Part I)'. *The Journal of Caribbean History* 40 (2006): 1–38.

'Diseases and Medical Disabilities of Enslaved Barbadians, from the Seventeenth Century to around 1838 (Part II)'. *The Journal of Caribbean History* 40 (2006): 177–214.

Hargrave, Francis. *An Argument in the Case of James Sommersett, a Negro, Lately Determined by the Court of King's Bench: Wherein It Is Attempted to Demonstrate the Present Unlawfulness of Domestic Slavery in England. To Which Is Prefixed a State of the Case*. London: W. Ostridge, 1772.

Harrison, Mark. *Climates & Constitutions: Health, Race, Environment and British Imperialism in India, 1600–1850.* New Delhi and New York: Oxford University Press, 1999.

Medicine in an Age of Commerce and Empire: Britain and Its Tropical Colonies, 1660–1830. Oxford: Oxford University Press, 2010.

'"The Tender Frame of Man": Disease, Climate and Racial Difference in India and the West Indies, 1760–1860'. *Bulletin of the History of Medicine* 70, no. 1 (1996): 68–93.

Harvey, Gideon. *A Treatise of the Small-Pox and Measles: Describing Their Nature, Causes, and Signs, Diagnostick and Prognostick, in a Different Way to What Hath Hitherto Been Known: Together, with the Method of Curing the Said Distempers, and All, or Most, of the Best Remedies: Also, a Particular Discourse of Opium, Diacodium, and Other Sleeping Medicines: With a Reference to a Very Great Case.* London: W. Freeman, 1696.

Headley, John M. 'The Sixteenth-Century Venetian Celebration of the Earth's Total Habitability: The Issue of the Fully Habitable World for Renaissance Europe'. *Journal of World History* 8, no. 1 (1997): 1–27.

Hecht, Gabrielle. 'Rupture-Talk in the Nuclear Age: Conjugating Colonial Power in Africa'. *Social Studies of Science* 32 (2002): 691–727.

Hendy, James. *A Treatise on the Glandular Disease of Barbadoes: Proving It to Be Seated in the Lymphatic System.* London: C. Dilly, 1784.

Hickeringill, Edmund. *Jamaica Viewed with All the Ports, Harbours, and Their Several Soundings, Towns, and Settlements Thereunto Belonging.* 3rd ed. London: Printed and sold by B. Bragg, 1705.

Hillary, William. 'An Account of the Principal Variations of the Weather, and the Concomitant Epidemic Diseases, as They Appeared in Rippon, and the Circumjacent Parts of Yorkshire, from the Year 1726 to the End of 1734'. In *A Practical Essay on the Small-Pox.* London: C. Hitch and J. Leake, 1740.

An Inquiry into the Contents and Medicinal Virtues of Lincomb Spaw Water, near Bath. By William Hillary, M.D [in English]. London: Printed for J. Leake, in Bath; and sold by C. Hitch [London], 1742.

Observations on the Changes of the Air and the Concomitant Epidemical Diseases, in the Island of Barbados. To Which Is Added a Treatise on the Putrid Bilious Fever, Commonly Called the Yellow Fever; and Such Other Diseases as Are Indigenous or Endemial, in the West India Islands, or in the Torrid Zone. London: C. Hitch and L. Hawes, 1759.

A Practical Essay on the Small-Pox: Wherein a Method of Preparing the Body before the Disease Comes on, and of Deriving the Variolous Matter from the Vital to the Remote Parts of the Body after the Accession ...; to Which is Added, an Account of the Principal Variations of the Weather, and the Concomitant Epidemic Diseases, as They Appeared at Rippon ... From the Year 1726, to the End of 1734. 2nd ed. London: C. Hitch and J. Leake, 1740.

A Rational and Mechanical Essay on the Small-Pox: Wherein the Cause, Nature, and Diathesis of That Disease, Its Symptoms, Their Causes, and Manner of Production, Are Explained ... With the Diagnostic and Prognostic Symptoms ... To Which Is Prefixed, a Short History of the First Rise and Progress of That Disease; and an

Essay on a New Method of Curing It, as We Do Other Inflammatory Diseases. London: G. Strahan, 1735.

Hippocrates. 'On Airs, Waters, and Places', *The Genuine Works of Hippocrates*, Translated from the Greek by Francis Adams, with a preliminary discourse and annotations. In two volumes, vol. 1, 190–222. London: Sydenham Society, 1849.

'Epidemics I', *The Genuine Works of Hippocrates*, Translated from the Greek by Francis Adams, with a preliminary discourse and annotations. In two volumes, vol. 1, 352–382. London: Sydenham Society, 1849.

'Epidemics III', *The Genuine Works of Hippocrates*, Translated from the Greek by Francis Adams, with a preliminary discourse and annotations. In two volumes, vol. 1, 388–420. London: Sydenham Society, 1849.

Hoffmann, Friedrich and Bernardino Ramazzini. *A Dissertation on Endemial Diseases or, Those Disorders Which Arise from Particular Climates, Situations, and Methods of Living; Together with a Treatise on the Diseases of Tradesmen ... The First by the Celebrated Frederick Hoffman ... The Second by Bern. Ramazini ... Newly Translated with a Preface and an Appendix by Dr. James*. London: Printed for Thomas Osborne, and J. Hildyard at York, 1746.

Hogarth, Rana Asali. 'Comparing Anatomies, Constructing Races: Medicine and Slavery in the Atlantic World, 1787–1838'. PhD Thesis. New Haven: Yale University, 2012.

Holwell, J. Z. *An Account of the Manner of Inoculating for the Small Pox in the East Indies*. London: T. Becket and P. A. De Hondt, 1767.

Houstoun, James. *Some New and Accurate Observations Geographical, Natural and Historical. Containing a True and Impartial Account of the Situation, Product, and Natural History of the Coast of Guinea*. London: J. Peele, 1725.

Hudson, Nicholas. 'From "Nation" to "Race": The Origin of Racial Classification in Eighteenth-Century Thought'. *Eighteenth-Century Studies* 29, no. 3 (1996): 246–64.

Hughes, Griffith. 'The Natural History of the Island of Barbados, Book II (1750)'. In *On the Treatment and Management of the More Common West-India Diseases (1750–1802)*, edited by J. Edward Hutson, 85–99. Kingston, Jamaica: University of the West Indies Press, 2005.

Hume, David. 'Of National Characters'. In *Hume: Essays, Moral, Political, and Literary*, edited by E. F. Miller. Indianapolis: Online Library of Liberty, 1987.

Hume, John. 'An Account of the True Bilious, or Yellow Fever; and of the Remitting Fevers of the West Indies'. In *Letters and Essays on the Small-Pox and Inoculation, the Measles, the Dry Belly-Ache, the Yellow, and Remitting, and Intermitting Fevers of the West Indies*, 195–248. London: J. Murray, 1778.

Hunter, John. *Disputatio Inauguralis, Quaedam de Hominum Varietatibus, et Harum Causis, Exponens*. Edinburgh: Balfour and Smellie, 1775.

Observations on the Diseases of the Army in Jamaica; and on the Best Means of Preserving the Health of Europeans, in That Climate. London: G. Nicol, 1788.

Huxham, John. *A Dissertation on the Malignant, Ulcerous Sore-Throat*. London: J. Hinton, 1757.

An Essay on Fevers, and Their Various Kinds, as Depending on Different Constitutions of the Blood: With Dissertations on Slow Nervous Fevers; on Putrid, Pestilential,

Spotted Fevers; on the Small-Pox; and on Pleurisies and Peripneumonies. London: S. Austen, 1750.

Observationes de Aëre et Morbis Epidemicis: Ab Anno MDCCXXVIII ad Finem Anni MDCCXXXVII, Plymuthi Fact. His Accedit Opusculum de Morbo Colico Damnoniensi. London: S. Austen, 1739.

Observations on the Air and Epidemical Diseases, Made at Plymouth from the Year MDCCXXVIII [1728] to the End of the Year MDCCXXXVII [1737], to Which Is Added a Short Treatise on the Devonshire Colic. 2 vols. Vol. I, London: J. Coote; J. Staples, 1758.

The Works of John Huxham, M. D. F. R. S. In Two Volumes. II vols. Vol. I, London: W. Bent, 1788.

Ince, Joseph. 'Prosper Alpinus, de Medicina Aegyptiorum Libri Quatuor. A. D. 1591'. *Pharmaceutical Journal and Transactions* II (1860): 367–72.

Ingram, Dale. *Essay on the Nature, Cause, and Seat of Dysentery's, in a Letter to Dr. Henry Warren of Barbados.* Barbados: William Beeby, 1744.

An Historical Account of the Several Plagues That Have Appeared in the World since the Year 1346. With an Enquiry into the Present Prevailing Opinion, That the Plague Is a Contagious Distemper ... In Which the Absurdity of Such Notions Is Exposed ... To Which Are Added a Particular Account of the Yellow Fever ... Also Observations on Dr Mackenzie's Letters; ... And an Abstract of Capt. Isaac Clemens's Voyage in the Sloop Fawey. London: R. Baldwin and J. Clark, 1755.

Isaac, Benjamin H. *The Invention of Racism in Classical Antiquity.* Princeton: Princeton University Press, 2004.

Ives, Edward. *A Voyage from England to India, in the Year MDCCLIV: And an Historical Narrative of the Operations of the Squadron and Army in India, Under ... Watson And ... Clive ... Also, a Journey from Persia to England, by an Unusual Route. With an Appendix, Containing an Account of the Diseases Prevalent in Admiral Watson's Squadron: A Description of Most of the Trees, Shrubs, and Plants, of India ... Illustrated with a Chart, Maps, and Other Copper-Plates.* London: Edward and Charles Dilly, 1773.

Jackson, Maurice. *Let This Voice Be Heard: Anthony Benezet, Father of Atlantic Abolitionism.* Philadelphia: University of Pennsylvania Press, 2009.

Jamaica, Assembly. *Two Reports (One Presented the 16th of October, the Other on the 12th of November, 1788) from the Committee of the Honourable House of Assembly of Jamaica, Appointed to Examine into ... The Slave-Trade ... Published, by Order of the House of Assembly, by Stephen Fuller ... Agent for Jamaica.* London: B. White and Son; J. Sewell; R. Faulder; and J. Debrett, and J. Stockdale, 1789.

Jamaica Planter, A. *Notes on the Two Reports from the Committee of the Honourable House of Assembly of Jamaica.* London: James Phillips, 1789.

Jennings, Eric T. *Curing the Colonizers: Hydrotherapy, Climatology, and French Colonialism.* Durham, NC: Duke University Press, 2006.

Johnson, Howard. 'Introduction'. In *The History of Jamaica.* Montreal: McGill-Queens University Press, 2002.

Johnston, Katherine. 'The Constitution of Empire: Place and Bodily Health in the Eighteenth-Century Atlantic'. *Atlantic Studies* 10 (2013): 443–66.

Johnstone, James. *An Historical Dissertation Concerning the Malignant Epidemical Fever of 1756.* London: W. Johnstone, 1758.

Jordan, Winthrop D. *White over Black: American Attitudes toward the Negro, 1550–1812*. Chapel Hill: University of North Carolina Press, 1968.

Jordanova, L. J. 'Earth Science and Environmental Medicine: The Synthesis of the Late Enlightenment'. In *Images of the Earth: Essays in the History of the Environmental Sciences*, edited by L. J. Jordanova and Roy S. Porter, 119–46. London: The British Society for the History of Science, 1979.

Kant, Immanuel. 'Of the Different Human Races'. In *The Idea of Race*, edited by Robert Bernasconi and Tommy L. Lott, 8–22. Indianapolis: Hackett, 2000.

'Von den Verschiedenen Racen der Menschen'. In *Der Philosoph Für Die Welt*, edited by J. J. Engel, 125–64, Liepzig: Dr Stintzings Bibl.,1777

Kidd, Colin. 'Ethnicity in the British Atlantic World, 1688–1830'. In *A New Imperial History: Culture, Identity, and Modernity in Britain and the Empire, 1660–1840*, edited by Kathleen Wilson, 260–77. Cambridge: Cambridge University Press, 2004.

The Forging of Races: Race and Scripture in the Protestant Atlantic World, 1600–2000. Cambridge: Cambridge University Press, 2006.

King, Lester S. *The Medical World of the Eighteenth Century*. Chicago: University of Chicago Press, 1958.

The Philosophy of Medicine: The Early Eighteenth Century. Cambridge, MA: Harvard University Press, 1978.

Kiple, Kenneth F. *The Caribbean Slave: A Biological History*. Cambridge: Cambridge University Press, 1984.

Kiple, Kenneth F. and Kriemhild Coneé Ornelas. 'Race, War, and Tropical Medicine in the Eighteenth-Century Caribbean'. In *Warm Climates and Western Medicine: The Emergence of Tropical Medicine, 1500–1900*, edited by David Arnold, 65–79. Amsterdam and Atlanta: Rodopi, 1996.

Kirkwood, James. *The History of the Twenty Seven Gods of Linlithgow Being an Exact and True Account of a Famous Plea Betwixt the Town-Council of the Said Burgh, and Mr. Kirkwood*. Edinburgh: 1711.

Knox, Robert. *The Races of Men: A Fragment*. London: H. Renshaw, 1850.

Kuefler, Mathew, ed. *The Boswell Thesis: Essays on Christianity, Social Tolerance, and Homosexuality*. Chicago: University of Chicago Press, 2006.

Kuhn, Thomas S. *'The Structure of Scientific Revolutions'*. Chicago: University of Chicago Press, 1962.

Kupperman, Karen. "Fear of Hot Climates in the Anglo-American Experience". *William and Mary Quarterly* 41 (1984): 213–40.

'The Puzzle of the American Climate in the Early Colonial Period'. *The American Historical Review* 87 (1982): 1262–89.

Lancisi, Giovanni Maria. 'Of Marshes and Their Effluvia'. Translated by Samuel Latham Mitchill. In *The Medical Repository*, edited by Samuel Latham Mitchill and Edward Miller, 9–18, 126–35, 237–45, 326–30. New York: Collins & Perkins, 1810.

Laqueur, Thomas. *Making Sex: Body and Gender from the Greeks to Freud*. Cambridge, MA: Harvard University Press, 1990.

Lassone, M. de. 'Histoire de divers Accidens graves, occasionnés par les miasmes d'animaux en putrefaction, et de la nouvelle methode de traitment qui a été employé avec succés dans cette circonstance'. *Medical Commentaries* 9 (1785): 57–63.

Lawrence, Christopher. 'Priestley in Tahiti: The Medical Interests of a Dissenting Chemist'. In *Science, Medicine, and Dissent: Joseph Priestley*, edited by C. J. Lawrence and R. Anderson. London: Wellcome Trust/Science Museum, 1987.

Le Cat, Mons. 'An Account of Those Malignant Fevers, That Raged at Rouen, at the End of the Year 1753, and the Beginning of 1754'. *Philosophical Transactions* 49 (1755–6): 49–61.

Lecaan, John Polus. *Advice to the Gentlemen of the Army of Her Majesty's Forces in Spain and Portugal: With a Short Method How to Preserve Their Health; and Some Observations Upon Several Distempers Incident to Those Countries, and All Other Hot Climates, as Our Plantations in the West-Indies, &C. To Which Are Added the Medicinal Virtues of Many Peculiar Plants Growing Naturally in Those Parts, and Not Wild in England*. London: P. Varenne, 1708.

Lempriere, William. *Practical Observations on the Diseases of the Army in Jamaica, as They Occurred between the Years 1792 and 1797*. 2 vols. London: T. N. Longham and O. Rees, 1799.

Leslie, Charles. *A New History of Jamaica: From the Earliest Accounts, to the Taking of Porto Bello by Vice-Admiral Vernon. In Thirteen Letters from a Gentleman to His Friend*. London: Printed for J. Hodges, 1740.

Ligon, Richard. *A True and Exact History of the Island of Barbados*. London: Humphrey Moseley, 1657.

Lind, James. *An Essay on Diseases Incidental to Europeans in Hot Climates: With the Method of Preventing Their Fatal Consequences. To Which Is Added, an Appendix Concerning Intermittent Fevers*. London: T. Becket and P. A. de Hondt, 1768.

An Essay of the Most Effectual Means of Preserving the Health of Seamen in the Royal Navy. 2nd ed. London: D. Wilson, 1762.

A Treatise of the Scurvy. In Three Parts. Containing an Inquiry into the Nature, Causes, and Cure of That Disease. Together with a Critical and Chronological View of What Has Been Published on the Subject. London: A. Millar, 1753.

A Treatise on the Scurvy. In Three Parts. Containing an Inquiry into the Nature, Causes, and Cure, of That Disease. Together with a Critical and Chronological View of What Has Been Published on the Subject. 3rd ed. London: S. Crowder, D. Wilson and G. Nicholls, T. Cadell, T. Becket and Co. G. Pearch, and W. Woodfall, 1772.

Lind, James. *A Treatise on the Putrid and Remitting Marsh Fever, Which Raged at Bengal in the Year 1762*. Edinburgh: C. Elliot, 1776.

Lindeboom, G. A. *Herman Boerhaave: The Man and His Work*. London: Methuen, 1968.

Lining, John. *A Description of the American Yellow Fever*. Edinburgh: G. Hamilton and J. Balfour, 1756.

A Description of the American Yellow Fever, Which Prevailed at Charleston, in South Carolina, in the Year 1748. Philadelphia: Thomas Dobson, 1799.

Livingstone, David N. *Adam's Ancestors: Race, Religion, and the Politics of Human Origins*. Baltimore: Johns Hopkins University Press, 2008.

'Human Acclimatization: Perspectives on a Contested Field of Inquiry in Science, Medicine, and Geography'. *History of Science* 25 (1987): 359–94.

'Tropical Climate and Moral Hygiene: The Anatomy of a Victorian Debate'. *British Journal for the History of Science* 32, no. 1 (1999): 93–110.

Lockyer, Charles. *An Account of the Trade in India Containing Rules for Good Government in Trade … With Descriptions of Fort St. George … Calicut … To Which Is Added, an Account of the Management of the Dutch in Their Affairs in India.* London: Samuel Crouch, 1711.

Long, Edward. *Candid Reflections Upon the Judgement Lately Awarded by the Court of King's Bench in Westminster Hall, on What Is Commonly Called the Negroe-Cause, by a Planter.* London: T. Lowndes, 1772.

The History of Jamaica, or, General Survey of the Antient and Modern State of the Island: With Reflections on Its Situation Settlements, Inhabitants, Climate, Products, Commerce, Laws, and Government: Illustrated with Copper Plates. 3 vols. London: T. Lowndes, 1774.

Lovejoy, Arthur O. *The Great Chain of Being: A Study of the History of an Idea.* Cambridge, MA: Harvard University Press, 1936.

M., N. 'Atkins, John (1685–1757)'. *Dictionary of National Biography* 2 (1885): 220.

Major, Andrea. *Slavery, Abolitionism, and Empire in India, 1772–1843.* Liverpool: Liverpool University Press, 2012.

Makittrick-Adair, James. 'Observations on Regimen and Preparation under Inoculation, and on the Treatment of the Natural Small-Pox, in the West Indies. To Which Are Added, Strictures on the Suttonian Practice; in a Letter to Dr Andrew Duncan'. *Medical Commentaries* 8 (1784): 211–47.

Malcolmson, Cristina. *Studies of Skin Color in the Early Royal Society: Boyle, Cavendish, Swift.* Farnham: Ashgate, 2013.

Marshall, Woodville K. 'Provision Ground and Plantation Labor in Four Windward Islands: Competition for Resources During Slavery'. In *Cultivation and Culture: Labor and the Shaping of Slave Life in the Americas*, edited by Ira Berlin and Philip D. Morgan, 203–20. Charlottesville and London: University Press of Virginia, 1993.

Mathews, Stephen. *Observations on Hepatic Diseases Incidental to Europeans in the East-Indies.* London: T. Cadell, 1783.

Mazzolini, Renato G. 'Skin Color and the Origin of Physical Anthropology (1640–1850)'. In *Reproduction, Race, and Gender in Philosophy and the Early Life Sciences*, edited by Susanne Lettow, 131–61: New York: SUNY Press, 2014.

McClellan III, James 'Science & Empire Studies and Postcolonial Studies: A Report from the Contact Zone'. In *Entangled Knowledge: Scientific Discourses and Cultural Difference*, edited by Klaus Hock and Gesa Mackenthun, 51–74. Münster: Waxmann, 2012.

McConaghey, R. M. 'John Huxham'. *Medical History* 13, no. 3 (1969): 280–7.

McCoskey, Denise Eileen. 'On Black Athena, Hippocratic Medicine, and Roman Imperial Edicts: Egyptians and the Problem of Race in Classical Antiquity'. In Race and Ethnicity: Across Time, Space, and Discipline, edited by Rodney D. Coates, 297–330. Leiden: Brill, 2004.

McDaniel, W. Caleb. 'Philadelphia Abolitionists and Antislavery Cosmopolitanism'. In *Antislavery and Abolition in Philadelphia: Emancipation and the Long Struggle for Racial Justice in the City of Brotherly Love*, edited by Richard Newman and James Mueller, 149–73. Baton Rouge: Louisiana State University Press, 2011.

McNeill, John Robert. *Mosquito Empires: Ecology and War in the Greater Caribbean, 1620–1914.* New York: Cambridge University Press, 2010.

Mead, Richard. 'Discourse on the Scurvy'. In *An Historical Account of a New Method for Extracting the Foul Air out of Ships, &C with the Description and Draught of the Machines, by Which It Is Performed: In Two Letters to a Friend, by Samuel Sutton, the Inventor*, edited by Samuel Sutton, 93–120. London: J. Brindley, 1749.

    A Mechanical Account of Poisons: In Several Essays. London: Printed by J.R. for Ralph South, 1702.

    'A Mechanical Account of Poisons: In Several Essays (4th Ed.)'. In *The Medical Works of Richard Mead*, iii-111. Dublin: Thomas Ewing, 1767.

    A Short Discourse Concerning Pestilential Contagion and the Methods to Be Used to Prevent It. London: Printed [by William Bowyer] for Sam. Buckley, and Ralph Smith, 1720.

    A Short Discourse Concerning Pestilential Contagion and the Methods to Be Used to Prevent It. Eighth, with large Additions ed. London: Sam. Buckley, 1722.

Meli, Domenico Bertoloni, ed. *Marcello Malpighi: Anatomist and Physician*. Firenze: Leo. S. Olschki, 1997.

Merret, Christopher. 'An Account of Several Observables in Lincolnshire, Not Taken Notice of in Camden, or Any Other Author'. *Philosophical Transactions* 19 (1695–7): 343–53.

Miller, G. '"Airs, Waters, and Places" in History'. *Journal of the History of Medicine* 17 (1962): 129–40.

Milman, Francis. 'An Account of Two Instances of the True Scurvy, Seemingly Occasioned by the Want of Due Nourishment; Being an Extract of a Letter Addressed to Dr. Baker, by Francis Milman'. *Medical Transactions, Published by the College of Physicians in London* 2 (1772): 471–85.

    An Enquiry into the Source from Whence the Symptoms of the Scurvy and of Putrid Fevers Arise. London: J. Dodsley, 1782.

Mitchell, John. 'An Essay Upon the Causes of the Different Colours of People in Different Climates'. *Philosophical Transaction* 43 (1744–5): 102–50.

Moll, Herman. *Atlas Geographus: Or, a Compleat System of Geography, Ancient and Modern*. Vol. V, London: J. Nutt, 1717.

Monchy, Solomon de. *An Essay on the Causes and Cure of the Usual Diseases in Voyages to the West Indies*. London: T. Becket and P. A. De Hondt, 1762.

Monro, Donald. *An Account of the Diseases Which Were Most Frequent in the British Military Hospitals in Germany, from January 1761 to the Return of the Troops to England in March 1763. To Which Is Added, an Essay on the Means of Preserving the Health of Soldiers, and Conducting Military Hospitals*. London: A. Millar, D. Wilson, and T. Durham, 1764.

    Observations on the Means of Preserving the Health of Soldiers and of Conducting Military Hospitals. And on the Diseases Incident to Soldiers in the Time of Service, and on the Same Diseases as They Have Appeared in London. In Two Volumes. By Donald Monro, M.D. 2nd ed. London: J. Murray; and G. Robinson, 1780.

    John Quier, Thomas Fraser, John Hume, George Monro, and Ambrose Dawson. *Letters and Essays on the Small-Pox and Inoculation, the Measles, the Dry Belly-Ache, the Yellow, and Remitting, an Intermitting Fevers of the West Indies*. London: J. Murray, 1778.

Montagu, Ashley. *Man's Most Dangerous Myth: The Fallacy of Race*. 2nd ed. New York: Columbia University Press, 1945.

Morgan, Jennifer L. *Laboring Women: Reproduction and Gender in New World Slavery*. Philadelphia: University of Pennsylvania Press, 2004.

'"Some Could Suckle over Their Shoulder": Male Travelers, Female Bodies, and the Gendering of Racial Ideology, 1500–1770'. *The William and Mary Quarterly* 54 (1997): 167–92.

Morgan, Philip D. 'The Black Experience and the British Empire, 1680–1810'. In *Black Experience and the Empire*, edited by Philip D. Morgan and Sean Hawkins, 86–110. Oxford: Oxford University Press, 2006.

Moseley, Benjamin. *A Treatise on Sugar*. London: Printed for G.G. and J. Robinson, 1799.

A Treatise on Tropical Diseases; And on the Climate of the West-Indies. London: T. Cadell, 1787.

Mosse, George L. *Toward the Final Solution: A History of European Racism*. New York: H. Fertig, 1978.

Nash, D. W. 'The Welsh Indians: To the Editor of the Cambrian Journal'. *The Cambrian Journal* (1860): 142.

Nisbet, Richard. *Slavery Not Forbidden by Scripture. Or a Defence of the West-India Planters*. Philadelphia: 1773.

Norris, John. *Profitable Advice for Rich and Poor: In a Dialogue, or Discourse between James Freeman, a Carolina Planter, and Simon Question, a West Country Farmer. Containing a Description ... Of South Carolina*. London: J. How, 1712.

Northrup, David. *Africa's Discovery of Europe, 1450–1850*. Oxford: Oxford University Press, 2002.

Numbers, Ronald and Todd L. Savitt, eds. *Science and Medicine in the Old South*. Baton Rouge: Louisiana State University Press, 1999.

Nutton, Vivian. 'Hippocrates in the Renaissance'. *Sudhoffs Archiv* 27 (1989): 420–39.

Ogborn, Miles. 'Talking Plants: Botany and Speech in Eighteenth-Century Jamaica'. *History of Science* 51 (2013): 251–82.

Oglethorpe, J. Edward. *A New and Accurate Account of the Provinces of South-Carolina and Georgia: With Many Curious and Useful Observations on the Trade, Navigation and Plantations of Great-Britain*. London: J. Worrall, 1732.

Orland, Barbara. 'The Fluid Mechanics of Nutrition: Herman Boerhaave's Synthesis of Seventeenth-Century Circulation Physiology'. *Studies in History and Philosophy of Biological and Biomedical Sciences* 43 (2012): 357–69.

Orta, Garcia de, Francisco Manuel de Melo Ficalho, and Clements R. Markham. *Colloquies on the Simples and Drugs of India*. London: H. Sotheran, 1913.

Osborne, Michael A. 'Acclimatizing the World: A History of the Paradigmatic Colonial Science'. *Osiris* 15 (2000): 135–51.

Nature, the Exotic and the Science of French Colonialism. Bloomington: Indiana University Press, 1994.

O'Shaugnessy, Andrew Jackson. *An Empire Divided: The American Revolution and the British Caribbean*. Philadelphia: University of Pennsylvania Press, 2000.

Ovington, John. 'A Voyage to Suratt in the Year 1689'. In *India in the Seventeenth Century: Being an Account of the Two Voyages to India by Ovington and Thevenot. To Which Is Added the Indian Travels of Careri*, edited by J. P. Guha. New Delhi: Associated Publishing House, 1976.

P., L. *Two Essays Sent in a Letter from Oxford to a Nobleman in London*. London: R. Baldwin, 1695.

Pagel, Walter. 'Van Helmont's Concept of Disease – to Be or Not to Be? The Influence of Paracelsus'. *Bulletin of the History of Medicine* XLVI, no. 5 (1972): 419–54.

'Van Helmont's Ideas on Gastric Digestion and the Gastric Acid'. *Bulletin of the History of Medicine* 30 (1956): 524–36.

Parliament., Great Britain. *A Collection of the Parliamentary Debates in England, from the Year MDCLXVIII. To the Present Time*. Vol. 17, London: John Torbuck, 1739–42.

Parrish, Susan Scott. *American Curiosity: Cultures of Natural History in the Colonial British Atlantic World*. Chapel Hill: University of North Carolina Press, 2006.

Paugh, Katherine. 'The Curious Case of Mary Hylas: Wives, Slaves, and the Limits of British Abolitionism'. *Slavery and Abolition* 35 (2014): 629–51.

'The Politics of Childbearing in the British Caribbean and the Atlantic World During the Age of Abolition, 1776–1838'. *Past and Present*, no. 221 (2013): 119–60.

The Politics of Reproduction: Race, Medicine, and Fertility in the Age of Abolition. Oxford: Oxford University Press, 2017.

Pernick, Martin S. *A Calculus of Suffering: Pain, Professionalism, and Anesthesia in Nineteenth-Century America*. New York: Columbia University Press, 1985.

Petley, Christer. 'Gluttony, Excess, and the Fall of the Planter Class in the British Caribbean'. *Atlantic Studies* 9 (2012): 85–106.

Philips, John. *An Authentic Account of Commodore Anson's Expedition: Containing All That Was Remarkable, Curious and Entertaining, During That Long and Dangerous Voyage: ... Taken from a Private Journal*. London: J. Robinson, 1744.

Phillips, Edward. *The New World of Words: Or, Universal English Dictionary*. 6th ed. London: J. Phillips, 1706.

Pinckard, George and Andrew Dickson White, *Notes On the West Indies, Including Observations Relative to the Creoles and Slaves of the Western Colonies, and the Indians of South America: Interspersed with Remarks Upon the Seasoning Or Yellow Fever of Hot Climates*. 2d ed. London: Baldwin, Cradock and Joy [etc.], 1816.

Popkin, Richard H. *Isaac La Peyrère (1596–1676): His Life, Work, and Influence*. Leiden: E. J. Brill, 1987.

Pormann, Peter E. and Emilie Savage-Smith. *Medieval Islamic Medicine*. Washington, DC: Georgetown University Press, 2007.

Porter, Roy. 'Cleaning up the Great Wen: Public Health in Eighteenth-Century London'. *Medical History. Supplement* 11 (1991): 61–75.

ed. *The Medical History of Waters and Spas, Medical History Supplement 10*. London: Wellcome Institute for the History of Medicine, 1990.

Powers, John C. *Inventing Chemistry: Herman Boerhaave and the Reform of the Chemical Arts*. Chicago: University of Chicago Press, 2012.

Prakash, Gyan. *Another Reason: Science and the Imagination of Modern India*. Princeton: Princeton University Press, 1999.

Pratt, Mary Louise. *Imperial Eyes: Travel Writing and Transculturation*. 2nd ed. London and New York: Routledge, 2008.

Price, Richard. *Observations on Reversionary Payments; on Schemes for Providing Annuities for Widows, and for Persons in Old Age; on the Method of Calculating the Values of Assurances on Lives; and on the National Debt*. London: T. Cadell, 1771.

Priestley, J. 'On the Noxious Quality of the Effluvia of Putrid Marshes. A Letter from the Rev. Dr. Priestley to Sir John Pringle'. *Philosophical Transactions* 64 (1774): 90–5.

Pringle, John. *A Discourse on the Different Kinds of Air, Delivered at the Anniversary Meeting of the Royal Society, November 30, 1773*. London: Royal Society, 1774.

Observations on the Diseases of the Army. 7th ed. London: W. Strahan, J. and F. Rivington, W. Johnston, T. Payne, T. Longman, Wilson and Nicoll, T. Durham, and T. Cadell, 1775.

Observations on the Diseases of the Army: In Camp and Garrison. In Three Parts. With an Appendix. London: A. Millar, and D. Wilson; and T. Payne, 1752.

Observations on the Nature and Cure of Hospital and Jayl-Fevers, in a Letter to Doctor Mead, Physician to His Majesty, &C. London: A. Millar and D. Wilson, 1750.

Professional Planter, A (Dr Collins). *Practical Rules for the Management and Medical Treatment of Negro Slaves in the Sugar Colonies*. New York: Books for Libraries Press, 1971. 1811.

Quinlan, Sean. 'Colonial Bodies, Hygiene, and Abolitionist Politics in Eighteenth-Century France'. *History Workshop Journal* 42 (1996): 106–25.

Rabin, Dana. '"In a Country of Liberty?": Slavery, Villeinage, and the Making of Whiteness in the Somerset Case (1772)'. *History Workshop Journal* 72 (2011): 5–29.

Raj, Kapil. 'Beyond Postcolonialism ... And Postpositivism: Circulation and the Global History of Science'. *Isis* 104 (2013): 337–47.

Relocating Modern Science: Circulation and the Construction of Knowledge in South Asia and Europe, 1650–1900. Basingstoke: Palgrave Macmillan, 2007.

Ramsay, James. *An Essay on the Treatment and Conversion of African Slaves in the British Sugar Colonies*. Dublin: T. Walker, C. Jenkin, R. Marchbank, L. White, R. Burton, P. Byrne, 1784.

Ray, John. *The Correspondence of John Ray: Consisting of Selections from the Philosophical Letters Published by Dr. Derham: And Original Letters of John Ray in the Collection of the British Museum / Edited by Edwin Lankester*. London: Printed for the Ray Society, 1848.

Reardon, Jenny. *Race to the Finish: Identity and Governance in an Age of Genomics*. Princeton: Princeton University Press, 2005.

Reide, Thomas Dickson. *A View of the Diseases of the Army in Great Britain, America, the West Indies, and on Board of King's Ships and Transports, from the Beginning of the Late War to the Present Time*. London: J. Johnson, 1793.

Reviewer. 'Essay on the Medical Constitution of Great Britain'. *The Critical Review, or Annals of Literature* (1763): 186–9.

Richardson, David. 'Through a Looking Glass: Olaudah Equiano and African Experiences of the British Atlantic Slave Trade'. In *Black Experience and the Empire*, edited by Philip D. Morgan and Sean Hawkins, 58–85. Oxford: Oxford University Press, 2006.

Robertson, Robert. *A Physical Journal Kept on Board His Majesty's Ship Rainbow, During Three Voyages to the Coast of Africa, and West Indies, in the Years 1772, 1773, and 1774*. London: E. & C. Dilly, J. Robson, T. Cadell, and T. Evans, 1777.

Roddis, Louis H. *James Lind: Founder of Nautical Medicine*. New York: Henry Schuman, 1950.

Rouppe, Lewis. *Observations on Diseases Incidental to Seamen*. Translated from the Latin Edition [1764], Printed at Leyden ed. London: T. Carnan and F. Newbery, 1772.

Rush, Benjamin. *An Address to the Inhabitants of the British Settlements in America Upon Slave-Keeping (the Second Edition). To Which Are Added, Observations on a Pamphlet, Entitled, 'Slavery Not Forbidden by Scripture; or, a Defence of the West-India Planters'. By a Pennsylvanian*. Philadelphia: John Dunlap, 1773.

Rusnock, Andrea A. 'Hippocrates, Bacon, and Medical Meteorology at the Royal Society, 1700–1750'. In *Reinventing Hippocrates*, edited by David Cantor. Burlington: Ashgate, 2001.

   Vital Accounts: Quantifying Health and Population in Eighteenth-Century England and France. Cambridge: Cambridge University Press, 2002.

Rutman, Darrett B. and Anita H. Rutman. 'Of Agues and Fevers: Malaria in the Early Chesapeake'. *The William and Mary Quarterly* 33, no. 1 (1976): 31–60.

Saakwa-Mante, Norris. 'Western Medicine and Racial Constitutions: Surgeon John Atkins Theory of Polygenism and Sleepy Distemper in the 1730s'. In *Race, Science, and Medicine, 1700–1960*, edited by Waltraud Ernst and Bernard Harris, 28–57. London and New York: Routledge, 1999.

Said, Edward W. *Orientalism*. New York: Vintage, 2003.

Sargent, Frederick. *Hippocratic Heritage: A History of Ideas About Weather and Human Health*. New York: Pergamon Press, 1982.

Savitt, Todd L. *Medicine and Slavery: The Diseases and Health Care of Blacks in Antebellum Virginia*. Champaign: University of Illinois Press, 1978.

   'Slave Health and Southern Distinctiveness'. In *Disease and Distinctiveness in the American South*, edited by Todd L. Savitt and James Harvey Young, 120–53. Knoxville: University of Tennessee Press, 1988.

   'The Use of Blacks for Medical Experimentation and Demonstration in the Old South'. *The Journal of Southern History* 48 (1982): 331–48.

Schaffer, Simon, Lissa Roberts, Kapil Raj, and James Delbourgo, eds. *The Brokered World: Go-Betweens and Global Intelligence, 1770–1820*. Sagamore Beach: Science History Publications, 2009.

Schiebinger, Londa. 'Human Experimentation in the Eighteenth Century: Natural Boundaries and Valid Testing'. In *The Moral Authority of Nature*, edited by Lorraine Daston and Fernando Vidal, 384–408. Chicago: University of Chicago Press, 2004.

   'Scientific Exchange in the Eighteenth-Century Atlantic World'. In *Soundings in Atlantic History: Latent Structures and Intellectual Currents, 1500–1830*, edited by Bernard Bailyn and Patricia L. Denault, 294–328. Cambridge, MA: Harvard University Press, 2009.

   Secret Cures of Slaves: People, Plants, and Medicine in the Eighteenth-Century Atlantic World. Stanford: Stanford University Press, 2017.

Schotte, J. P. 'A Description of a Species of Sarcocele of a Most Astonishing Size in a Black Man in the Island of Senegal: With Some Account of Its Being an Endemial Disease in the Country of Galam'. *Philosophical Transactions* 73 (1783): 85–93.

   'Journal of the Weather at Senegambia, During the Prevalence of a Very Fatal Putrid Disorder, with Remarks on That Country'. *Philosophical Transactions* 70 (1780): 478–506.

A Treatise on the Synochus Atrabiliosa, a Contagious Fever, Which Raged at Senegal in the Year 1778, and Proved Fatal to the Greatest Part of the Europeans, and to a Number of the Natives. London: M. Scott, 1782.

Seth, Suman. 'Colonial History and Postcolonial Science Studies'. *Radical History Review* 127 (2017): 63–85.

'Crisis and the Construction of Modern Theoretical Physics'. *British Journal for the History of Science* 40, no. 144 (2007): 25–51.

ed. 'Focus: Re-Locating Race'. *Isis* 105, no 4 (2014): 759–814.

'The History of Physics after the Cultural Turn'. *Historical Studies in the Natural Sciences* 41 (2011): 112–22.

Sharp, Granville. *A Representation of the Injustice and Dangerous Tendency of Tolerating Slavery; or of Admitting the Least Claim of Private Property in the Persons of Men, in England.* London: Printed for Benjamin White, (no. 63) in Fleet-Street, and Robert Horsfield, (no. 22) in Ludgate Street, 1769.

Sheridan, Richard B. 'Africa and the Caribbean in the Atlantic Slave Trade'. *The American Historical Review* 77, no. 1 (1972): 15–35.

'The Doctor and the Buccaneer: Sir Hans Sloane's Case History of Sir Henry Morgan, Jamaica, 1688'. *Journal of the History of Medicine and Allied Sciences* 41 (1986): 76–87.

Doctors and Slaves; A Medical and Demographic History of Slavery in the British West Indies, 1680–1834. Cambridge: Cambridge University Press, 1985.

'The Guinea Surgeons on the Middle Passage: The Provision of Medical Services in the British Slave Trade'. *The International Journal of African Historical Studies* 14, no. 4 (1981): 601–25.

Short, Thomas. *A Comparative History of the Increase and Decrease of Mankind in England, and Several Countries Abroad ... To Which Is Added, a Syllabus of the General States of Health, Air, Seasons, and Food for the Last Three Hundred Years: And Also a Meteorological Discourse.* London: W. Nicoll, 1767.

Sims, James. *Observations on Epidemic Disorders, with Remarks on Nervous and Malignant Fevers.* London: J. Johnson; G. Robinson, 1773.

Singer, Dorothea. 'Sir John Pringle and His Circle. Part I. Life'. *Annals of Science* 6, no. 2 (1949): 127–80.

'Sir John Pringle and His Circle, II'. *Annals of Science* 6, no. 3 (1950): 229–47.

Siraisi, Nancy. *History, Medicine, and the Traditions of Renaissance Learning.* Ann Arbor: University of Michigan Press, 2007.

Sivasundaram, Sujit. 'Sciences and the Global: On Methods, Questions, and Theory'. *Isis* 101 (2010): 146–58.

Skidmore, Thomas E. *Black into White: Race and Nationality in Brazilian Thought.* New York: Oxford University Press, 1974.

Sloan, Phillip R. 'Buffon, German Biology, and the Historical Interpretation of Biological Species'. *The British Journal for the History of Science* 12, no. 2 (1979): 109.

'The Idea of Racial Degeneracy in Buffon's *Histoire Naturelle*'. *Studies in Eighteenth-Century Culture* 3 (1973): 293–321.

Sloane, Hans. *A Voyage to the Islands Madera, Barbados, Nieves, S. Christophers and Jamaica, with the Natural History of the Herbs and Trees, Four-Footed Beasts, Fishes, Birds, Insects, Reptiles, &C. Of the Last of Those Islands; to Which Is*

Prefix'd an Introduction, Wherein is an Account of the Inhabitants, Air, Waters, Diseases, Trade, &C. of That Place, with Some Relations Concerning the Neighbouring Continent, and Islands of America. 2 vols. London: printed by B. M. for the author, 1707 & 1725.

Sloane, Hans and Christoph L. Becker. *Johann Sloane … Von den Krankheiten, Welche er in Jamaika Beobachtet und Behandelt hat: aus dem Englischen Übersetzt und mit Einigen Zusätzen Begleitet.* Augsburg: Klett, 1784.

Smith, Dale C. 'Medical Science, Medical Practice, and the Emerging Concept of Typhus in Mid-Eighteenth-Century Britain'. *Medical History (Supplement)* 1 (1981): 121–34.

Smith, Justin E. H. *Nature, Human Nature, and Human Difference: Race in Early Modern Philosophy.* Princeton: Princeton University Press, 2015.

Smith, Sean Morey. 'Seasoning and Abolition: Humoural Medicine in the Eighteenth-Century British Atlantic'. *Slavery and Abolition* 36 (2015): 684–703.

Snelders, Stephen. 'Leprosy and Slavery in Suriname: Godfried Schilling and the Framing of a Racial Pathology in the Eighteenth Century'. *Social History of Medicine* 26 (2013): 432–50.

Stannard, Jerry. 'Alpini, Prospero'. In *Complete Dictionary of Scientific Biography*, 124–5. Detroit: Charles Scribner's Sons, 2008.

Stepan, Nancy. *The Idea of Race in Science: Great Britain, 1800–1960.* Hamden: Archon, 1982.

Stewart, Larry. 'The Edge of Utility: Slaves and Smallpox in the Early Eighteenth Century'. *Medical History* 29 (1985): 54–70.

Stubbes, Henry. 'An Enlargement of the Observations, Formerly Publisht Numb. 27, Made and Generously Imparted by That Learn'd and Inquisitive Physician, Dr. Stubbes'. *Philosophical Transactions* 3 (1668): 699–709.

'Observations Made by a Curious and Learned Person, Sailing from England, to the Caribe-Islands'. *Philosophical Transactions* 2 (1666): 493–502.

Stuurman, Siep. 'François Bernier and the Invention of Racial Classification'. *History Workshop Journal* 50 (2000): 1–21.

Sweet, James H. *Domingo Álvares, African Healing, and the Intellectual History of the Atlantic World.* Chapel Hill: University of North Carolina Press, 2011.

Sweet, John Wood. *Bodies Politic: Negotiating Race in the American North, 1730–1830.* Baltimore: Johns Hopkins University Press, 2003.

Sydenham, Thomas. *The Whole Works of That Excellent Practical Physician, Dr. Thomas Sydenham Wherein Not Only the History and Cures of Acute Diseases Are Treated Of … But Also the Shortest and Fastest Way of Curing Most Chronical Diseases.* 9th ed. London: Printed for J. Darby, A. Bettesworth, and F. Clay, in trust for Richard, James, and Bethel Wellington, 1729.

Sydenham, Thomas and Benjamin Rush. *The Works of Thomas Sydenham, M.D., on Acute and Chronic Diseases with Their Histories and Modes of Cure: With Notes, Intended to Accommodate Them to the Present State of Medicine, and to the Climate and Diseases of the United States.* Philadelphia: B. & T. Kite, 1815.

Tadman, Michael. 'The Demographic Cost of Sugar: Debates on Slave Societies and Natural Increase in the Americas'. *The American Historical Review* 105 (2000): 1534–75.

Tennent, John. *A Reprieve from Death: In Two Physical Chapters ... With an Appendix. Dedicated to the Right Honourable Sir Robert Walpole.* London: Printed for John Clarke, 1741.

 Physical Enquiries Discovering the Mode of Translation in the Constitutions of Northern Inhabitants, on Going to, and for Some Time after Arriving in Southern Climates ... An Error ... In Recommending Vinegar to His Majesty's Fleet in the West Indies, to Prevent the Epidemic Fever ... And the Barren State of Useful Physical Knowledge, as Well as the Mercenary Practice of Physicians, by an Impartial State of Dr. Ward's Qualifications for the Practice of Physic ... Illustrated with Remarks Upon a Printed Letter to a Member of Parliament, Signed Philanthropos. London: T. Gardner, 1742.

Thevenot, Jean de. 'The Third Part of the Travels of Mr. De Thevenot, Containing the Relation of Indostan, the New Moguls and of Other People and Countries of the Indies'. In *India in the Seventeenth Century: Being an Account of the Two Voyages to India by Ovington and Thevenot. To Which Is Added the Indian Travels of Careri*, edited by J. P. Guha, 1–186. New Delhi: Associated Publishing House, 1976 [1687].

Thomas, Robert. *Medical Advice to the Inhabitants of Warm Climates, on the Domestic Treatment of All the Diseases Incidental Therein: With a Few Useful Hints to New Settlers, for the Preservation of Health, and the Prevention of Sickness.* London: J. Strahan and W. Richardson, 1790.

Tilley, Helen. 'Global Histories, Vernacular Science, and African Genealogies: Or, Is the History of Science Ready for the World?'. *Isis* 101 (2010): 110–19.

Timberland, Ebenezer. *The History and Proceedings of the House of Lords from the Restoration in 1660 to the Present Time: Containing the Most Remarkable Motions, Speeches, Debates, Orders and Resolutions.* London: Printed for Ebenezer Timberland in Ship-Yard, Temple Bar, 1742.

Tise, Larry E. *Proslavery: A History of the Defense of Slavery in America, 1701–1840.* Athens and London: University of Georgia Press, 1987.

Towne, Richard. *A Treatise of the Diseases Most Frequent in the West-Indies, and Herein More Particularly of Those Which Occur in Barbadoes.* London: J. Clarke, 1726.

Trapham, Thomas. *A Discourse of the State of Health in the Island of Jamaica with a Provision Therefore Calculated from the Air, the Place, and the Water, the Customs and Manner of Living &C.* London: Printed for R. Boulter, 1679.

Tubbs, F. 'John Atkins: An Eighteenth-Century Naval Surgeon'. *British Medical Bulletin* 5 (1947–8): 83–4.

Turner, Daniel. *Syphilis. A Practical Dissertation on the Venereal Disease ... In Two Parts.* London: Printed for R. Bonwicke, Tim. Goodwin, J. Walthoe, M. Wotton, S. Manship, Richard Wilkin, Benj. Tooke, R. Smith and Tho. Ward, 1717.

Turner, Sasha. 'Home-Grown Slaves: Women, Reproduction, and the Abolition of the Slave Trade, Jamaica 1788–1807'. *Journal of Women's History* 23 (2011): 39–62.

Van Dantzig, Albert. 'English Bosman and Dutch Bosman: A Comparison of Texts'. *History in Africa* 2 (1975): 185–216.

 'Willem Bosman's "New and Accurate Description of the Coast of Guinea": How Accurate Is It?'. *History in Africa* 1 (1974): 101–8.

Van der Star, Peter, ed. *Fahrenheit's Letters to Leibniz and Boerhaave.* Leiden: Rodopi, 1983.

Vaughan, Megan. *Curing Their Ills: Colonial Power and African Illness*. Stanford: Stanford University Press, 1991.

Voltaire. *The Philosophy of History*. London: I. Allcock, 1766.

W., G. 'The Cures of the Diseased in Forraine Attempts of the English Nation, London, 1598. Reproduced in Facsimile', edited by Charles Joseph Singer. Oxford: Clarendon Press, 1915.

Walker, Timothy. 'Acquisition and Circulation of Medical Knowledge within the Early Modern Portuguese Colonial Empire'. In *Science in the Spanish and Portuguese Empires, 1500–1800*, edited by Daniela Bleichmar, Paula De Vos and Kristin Huffine, 247–70. Stanford: Stanford University Press, 2008.

Waller, Edmund. *The Works of Edmund Waller, Esq., in Verse and Prose: Published by Mr. Fenton*. London: J. and R. Tonton and S. Draper, 1744.

Wallis, Faith. 'Medicine, Theoretical'. In *Medieval Science, Technology, and Medicine: An Encyclopedia*, edited by Thomas F. Glick, Stephen Livesy and Faith Wallis, 336–40. New York: Routledge, 2005.

Wallis, P. J. and R. V. Wallis. *Eighteenth Century Medics (Subscriptions, Licences, Apprenticeships)*. 2nd ed. Newcastle Upon Tyne: Project for Historical Bibliography, 1988.

Ward, Estelle Frances. *Christopher Monck, Duke of Albemarle*. London: J. Murray, 1915.

Warren, Henry. *A Treatise Concerning the Malignant Fever in Barbados and the Neighbouring Islands: With an Account of the Seasons There, from the Year 1734 to 1738. In a Letter to Dr. Mead*. London: Printed for Fletcher Gyles against Grays-Inn in Holborn, 1740.

Watt, James. 'Surgeon James Ramsay, 1733–1789: The Navy and the Slave Trade'. *Journal of the Royal Society of Medicine* 87 (1994): 773–6.

Wear, Andrew. 'Health and the Environment in Early Modern England'. In *Medicine in Society: Historical Essays*, edited by Andrew Wear. Cambridge: Cambridge University Press, 1992.

   Knowledge and Practice in English Medicine, 1550–1680. Cambridge: Cambridge University Press, 2000.

   'Place, Health, and Disease: The Airs, Waters, Places Tradition in Early Modern England and North America'. *Journal of Medieval and Early Modern Studies* 38, no. 3 (2008): 443–65.

Weaver, Karol. *Medical Revolutionaries: The Enslaved Healers of Eighteenth-Century Saint Domingue*. Urbana and Chicago: University of Illinois Press, 2006.

Wey Gómez, Nicolás. *The Tropics of Empire: Why Columbus Sailed South to the Indies*. Cambridge, MA: MIT Press, 2008.

Wheeler, Roxann. *The Complexion of Race: Categories of Difference in Eighteenth-Century British Culture*. Philadelphia: University of Pennsylvania Press, 2000.

Wiecek, William M. 'Somerset: Lord Mansfield and the Legitimacy of Slavery in the Anglo-American World'. *The University of Chicago Law Review* 42, no. 1 (1974): 86–146.

Williams, John. *[an] Essay on the Bilious, or Yellow Fever of Jamaica*. Kingston, Jamaica: William Daniell, 1750.

Williams, John and Parker Bennet. *Essays on the Bilious Fever: Containing the Different Opinions of Those Eminent Physicians John Williams and Parker Bennet, of Jamaica: Which Was the Cause of a Duel, and Terminated in the Death of Both*. Jamaica and London: T. Waller, 1752.

Wilson, Alexander. *Some Observations Relative to the Influence of Climate on Vegetable and Animal Bodies*. London: T. Cadell, 1780.

Wilson, Andrew. *Rational Advice to the Military, When Exposed to the Inclemency of Hot Climates and Seasons*. London: W. Richardson, 1780.

Wilson, Kathleen. 'Empire, Trade and Popular Politics in Mid-Hanoverian Britain: The Case of Admiral Vernon'. *Past and Present* 121 (1988): 74–109.

'Introduction: Histories, Empires, Modernities'. In *A New Imperial History: Culture, Identity, and Modernity in Britain and the Empire, 1660–1840*, edited by Kathleen Wilson, 1–26. Cambridge: Cambridge University Press, 2004.

The Island Race: Englishness, Empire and Gender in the Eighteenth Century. London: Routledge, 2003.

ed. *A New Imperial History: Culture, Identity, and Modernity in Britain and the Empire, 1660–1840*. Cambridge: Cambridge University Press, 2004.

Wisecup, Kelly. *Medical Encounters: Knowledge and Identity in Early American Literatures*. Amherst: University of Massachusetts Press, 2013.

Zuckerman, Arnold. 'Dr. Richard Mead (1673–1754): A Biographical Study'. PhD Thesis. Urbana-Champaign: University of Illinois, 1965.

'Plague and Contagionism in Eighteenth-Century England'. *Bulletin of the History of Medicine* 78, no. 2 (2004): 273–308.

Index